Methods in Bioengineering

Stem Cell Bioengineering

The Artech House Methods in Bioengineering Series

Series Editors-in-Chief
Martin L. Yarmush, M.D., Ph.D.,
Robert S. Langer, Sc.D.

Methods in Bioengineering: Stem Cell Bioengineering,
Biju Parekkadan and Martin L. Yarmush, Editors

Methods in Bioengineering: Microdevices in Biology and Medicine,
Yaakov Nahmias and Sangeeta Bhatia, Editors

Methods in Bioengineering: Systems Analysis of Biological Networks,
Arul Jayaraman and Juergen Hahn, Editors

Methods in Bioengineering: Nanoscale Bioengineering and Nanomedicine,
Kaushal Rege and Igor Medintz, Editors

Methods in Bioengineering: Biomicrofabrication and Biomicrofluidics,
Jeffrey D. Zahn and Luke P. Lee, Editors

Methods in Bioengineering

Stem Cell Bioengineering

Biju Parekkadan
Massachusetts General Hospital/Harvard Medical School

Martin L. Yarmush
Massachusetts General Hospital/Harvard Medical School

Editors

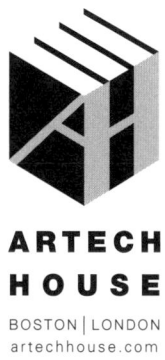

ARTECH HOUSE
BOSTON | LONDON
artechhouse.com

Library of Congress Cataloging-in-Publication Data
A catalog record for this book is available from the U. S. Library of Congress.

British Library Cataloguing in Publication Data
A catalogue record for this book is available from the British Library.

ISBN-13: 978-1-59693-402-3

Text design by Darrell Judd

Cover design by Igor Valdman

© 2009 Artech House. All rights reserved.

Printed and bound in the United States of America. No part of this book may be reproduced or utilized in any form or by any means, electronic or mechanical, including photocopying, recording, or by any information storage and retrieval system, without permission in writing from the publisher.

All terms mentioned in this book that are known to be trademarks or service marks have been appropriately capitalized. Artech House cannot attest to the accuracy of this information. Use of a term in this book should not be regarded as affecting the validity of any trademark or service mark.

10 9 8 7 6 5 4 3 2 1

Contents

Preface — xiii

CHAPTER 1
Somatic Cell Nuclear Transfer and Derivation of Embryonic Stem Cells — 1

- 1.1 Introduction — 2
- 1.2 Materials for Nuclear Transfer — 2
    - 1.2.1 Equipment for mouse nuclear transfer — 2
    - 1.2.2 Reagents for mouse nuclear transfer — 2
- 1.3 Methods for Nuclear Transfer — 4
    - 1.3.1 Preparation of enucleation and nuclear transfer pipettes — 4
    - 1.3.2 Medium preparation — 4
    - 1.3.3 Animal preparation — 5
    - 1.3.4 Nuclear transfer — 5
    - 1.3.5 Enucleation — 5
    - 1.3.6 Preparation of donor cells — 6
    - 1.3.7 Nuclear transfer — 7
    - 1.3.8 Activation — 11
    - 1.3.9 Embryo culture and embryo transfer — 12
- 1.4 Derivation of Mouse ntES Cells — 13
- 1.5 Materials for ES Cell Derivation — 13
- 1.6 Methods for ES Cell Derivation — 14
    - 1.6.1 Derivation of ntES cells — 14
    - 1.6.2 In vitro characterization of ntES cells — 15
    - 1.6.3 In vivo characterization of ntES cells — 16
- 1.7 Discussion and Commentary — 19
    - Troubleshooting Table — 19
- 1.8 Summary Points — 21
- Acknowledgments — 21
- References — 21

CHAPTER 2
Derivation of Mouse Parthenogenetic Embryonic Stem Cells — 23

- 2.1 Introduction — 24
- 2.2 Materials — 24
  - 2.2.1 Reagents — 24
  - 2.2.2 Equipment — 26
  - 2.2.3 Media recipe — 27
- 2.3 Methods — 29
  - 2.3.1 Generation of p(MI) embryos — 30
  - 2.3.2 Generation of p(MII) embryos — 30
  - 2.3.3 Generation of p(hap) embryos — 31
  - 2.3.4 Derivation of p(MI), p(MII), and p(hap) ES cells — 32
  - 2.3.5 ES cell characterization — 34
  - 2.3.6 Teratoma induction — 34
- 2.4 Data Acquisition, Anticipated Results, and Interpretation — 35
- 2.5 Discussion and Commentary — 35
  - Troubleshooting Table — 36
- 2.6 Summary Points — 36
- Acknowledgments — 37
- References — 37

CHAPTER 3
Generation of Mice from Embryonic Stem Cells Using Tetraploid Embryos as Hosts — 39

- 3.1 Introduction — 40
- 3.2 Experimental Design — 40
- 3.3 Materials — 41
  - 3.3.1 Preparation of 4n embryos: Mice and reagents — 41
  - 3.3.2 Preparation of 4n embryos: Equipment — 41
  - 3.3.3 ES cells and culture conditions — 41
  - 3.3.4 Micromanipulation system — 42
- 3.4 Methods — 42
  - 3.4.1 Preparation of host embryos — 42
  - 3.4.2 Electrofusion of two-cell stage embryos — 43
  - 3.4.3 Removal of the zona pellucida — 43
  - 3.4.4 Generation of ES ↔ multiple 4n embryos by aggregation — 43
  - 3.4.5 Generation of ES ↔ 4n embryos by blastocyst injection — 44
  - 3.4.6 Data acquisition — 45
- 3.5 Anticipated Results — 45
- 3.6 Discussion and Commentary — 45
  - Troubleshooting Table — 46
- 3.7 Application Notes — 47
- 3.8 Summary Points — 47
- Acknowledgments — 48
- References — 48

CHAPTER 4

Bioreactor Design and Implementation   49

    4.1   Introduction   50
    4.2   Experimental Methods and Materials   51
        4.2.1   General system description   51
        4.2.2   Closed system   52
        4.2.3   Hollow-fiber bioreactor   53
        4.2.4   CES fluid circuit   54
        4.2.5   Oxygenator design   55
        4.2.6   Monitoring   56
        4.2.7   User interface   56
    4.3   Anticipated Results   56
        4.3.1   MSC source 1: Loading whole BM marrow into the CES   58
        4.3.2   MSC source 2 or 3: Loading preselected MSC into the CES   59
    4.4   Discussion and Commentary   60
        Troubleshooting Table   61
    4.5   Application Notes   61
        4.5.1   Therapeutic dose of MSC grown from a whole BM sample   61
        4.5.2   Nonadherent cell culture: Kg1a cells grown in suspension   61
    4.6   Summary Points   62

CHAPTER 5

Extracellular Matrix Microarrays and Stem Cell Fate   63

    5.1   Introduction   64
    5.2   Experimental Design   65
    5.3   Materials   65
    5.4   Methods   66
        5.4.1   Preparation of substrates for arrays   66
        5.4.2   Fabrication of ECM arrays   67
        5.4.3   Cell culture on ECM arrays   68
        5.4.4   Staining, imaging, and data acquisition   68
        5.4.5   Data analysis   69
    5.5   Anticipated Results   69
    5.6   Discussion and Commentary   70
        Troubleshooting Table   71
    5.7   Application Notes   72
    5.8   Summary Points   72
    Acknowledgments   73
    References   73

CHAPTER 6

Microfluidic Culture Platform for Investigating the Proliferation and Differentiation of Stem Cells   75

    6.1   Introduction   76
    6.2   Experimental Design   76

	6.2.1	Microfluidic platform for differentiation of human neural progenitor cells	76
	6.2.2	A hybrid microfluidic platform for stem cell biology	77
	6.2.3	ESC response under dynamically controlled gradient condition	79
6.3	Materials and Methods		80
	6.3.1	Fabrication of the microfluidic device	80
	6.3.2	Fabrication of a hybrid microfluidic platform	81
	6.3.3	Human neural stem cells	81
	6.3.4	Mouse neural stem cells	82
	6.3.5	Culturing cells inside the microfluidic chamber and time-lapse microscopy	82
	6.3.6	Immunocytochemistry	83
6.4	Data Acquisition, Anticipated Results, and Interpretation		83
	6.4.1	hNSC proliferation in the gradient chamber	83
	6.4.2	Differentiation of hNSCs into astrocytes in the gradient chamber	84
	6.4.3	ESC response to BMP signaling	85
6.5	Discussion and Commentary		86
	Troubleshooting Table		86
6.6	Application Notes		87
6.7	Summary Points		87
Acknowledgments			87
References			87

CHAPTER 7

Analysis of Mouse Hematopoietic Stem and Progenitor Cells   89

7.1	Introduction		90
7.2	Experimental Design of Lineage Depletion of Whole Bone Marrow Cells		90
7.3	Materials for Lineage Depletion of Whole Bone Marrow Cells		91
	7.3.1	Tools and plasticware	91
	7.3.2	Reagents	91
	7.3.3	Additional equipment and reagents required for method 1 (MACS beads method)	91
	7.3.4	Additional equipment and reagents required for method 2 (Dynabeads method)	91
	7.3.5	Common protocols for both methods	91
	7.3.6	Discussion and commentary	93
	Troubleshooting Table for Lineage Depletion Method		94
7.4	Methylcellulose-Based in Vitro Colony-Forming Assay		95
	7.4.1	Materials	95
	7.4.2	Methods	95
	7.4.3	Data acquisition, anticipated results, and interpretation	96
	7.4.4	Discussion and commentary	96
	Troubleshooting Table for CFU Assay		97
7.5	Radiation of Mice for In Vivo Assays		97

		Troubleshooting Table for Bone Marrow Transplantation	97
7.6	Colony-Forming Unit-Spleen Assay		98
	7.6.1	Materials	98
	7.6.2	Methods	99
	7.6.3	Data acquisition, anticipated results, and interpretation	99
	7.6.4	Discussion and commentary	100
		Troubleshooting Table for CFU-S Assay	100
7.7	Quantification of HSCs Using the Limiting Dilution Assay		100
	7.7.1	Buffers and materials	101
	7.7.2	Methods	101
	7.7.3	Data acquisition, anticipated results, and interpretation	102
	7.7.4	Discussion and commentary	103
		Troubleshooting Table for Limited Dilution Assay	104
7.8	Summary Points		104
	References		105

CHAPTER 8
Skeletal Stem Cells and the Hematopoietic Microenvironment: Biology and Assays   107

8.1	Introduction		108
8.2	Experimental Design		108
8.3	Materials		109
	8.3.1	Stromal cell isolation and culture	109
	8.3.2	Isolation of CD45-CD146+ cells	109
	8.3.3	In vivo transplantation	109
8.4	Method		109
	8.4.1	Bone marrow single-cell suspensions	109
	8.4.2	Isolation of MCAM/CD146-expressing bone marrow osteoprogenitors	110
	8.4.3	In vivo transplantation	111
	8.4.4	Analysis of heterotopic ossicles	112
8.5	Anticipated Results		112
8.6	Discussion and Commentary		113
	Troubleshooting Table		114
8.7	Application Notes		114
8.8	Summary Points		115
Acknowledgments			116
References			116

CHAPTER 9
Targeting the Stem Cell Niche In Vivo   117

9.1	Introduction		118
9.2	Experimental Design		119
9.3	Materials		120
	9.3.1	PTH treatment	120

	9.3.2	Obtaining bone marrow mononuclear cells	120
	9.3.3	Immunophenotypic enumeration of HSC number	120
	9.3.4	Functional enumeration of HSC number	120
9.4	Methods		120
	9.4.1	Treatment of mice with PTH	120
	9.4.2	Immunophenotypic enumeration of HSC number	121
	9.4.3	Functional enumeration of HSC number	121
9.5	Anticipated Results		121
9.6	Discussion and Commentary		122
	Troubleshooting Table		122
9.7	Application Notes		123
9.8	Summary Points		123
References			123

CHAPTER 10
Parabiosis in Aging Research and Regenerative Medicine — 125

10.1	Introduction		126
	10.1.1	What is parabiosis?	126
	10.1.2	Animal species	126
	10.1.3	Physiology of joining	126
	10.1.4	History of parabiosis and the range of its biomedical applications	127
	10.1.5	Parabiosis in aging studies	128
10.2	Experimental Design for Aging Studies		130
10.3	Materials		131
10.4	Methods		131
	10.4.1	Parabiosis protocol	131
	10.4.2	Experimental method	132
	10.4.3	Postoperative care	135
	10.4.4	Removing the staples	135
	10.4.5	Separating a pair	135
10.5	Troubleshooting Parabiotic Disease		136
	10.5.1	"Parabiotic intoxication"	136
	10.5.2	Suggestions for the side effects associated with parabiotic disease	137
10.6	Discussion and Commentary		137
Acknowledgments			139
References			140

CHAPTER 11
Utilization of the Mixed Lymphocyte Reaction Assay to Determine Stem Cell Immunogenicity and Suppression — 143

11.1	Introduction	144
11.2	Experimental Design	146

		11.2.1	Immunogenicity assay	146
		11.2.2	Suppression assay	148
		11.2.3	T-cell priming assay	149
	11.3	Materials		152
	11.4	Methods		152
		11.4.1	General considerations	152
		11.4.2	Safety	153
		11.4.3	Media preparation	153
		11.4.4	Prepare responder cell populations	153
		11.4.5	Prepare stimulator cell populations	154
		11.4.6	Performance of immunogenicity assays	154
		11.4.7	Performance of suppression assays	154
		11.4.8	Performance of T-cell priming assays	155
		11.4.9	MLR plate culture, pulsing with ^{3}H-thymidine, cell harvest, and scintillation counting: applicable to all three MLR assays	155
	11.5	Data Acquisition, Anticipated Results, Interpretation, and Statistical Guidelines		155
		11.5.1	Immunogenicity assay	155
		11.5.2	Suppression assay	157
		11.5.3	T-cell priming assay	158
	11.6	Discussion and Commentary		160
		11.6.1	General considerations	160
		11.6.2	Immunogenicity assay	161
		11.6.3	Suppression assay	162
		11.6.4	T-cell priming assay	162
		Troubleshooting Table		163
	11.7	Application Notes		163
	11.8	Summary Points		164
	Acknowledgments			164
	References			164

CHAPTER 12

A Novel Method for the Preservation of Embryonic Stem Cells Using a Quartz Capillary Freezing System — 167

	12.1	Introduction		168
		12.1.1	Slow-freezing protocols	168
		12.1.2	Vitrification protocols	168
		12.1.3	Increasing cooling rates for vitrification	169
		12.1.4	Quartz capillary system	169
		12.1.5	Apparent vitrification of CPA-laden solutions	169
		12.1.6	Slush nitrogen	171
	12.2	Experimental Design		172
	12.3	Materials		172
		12.3.1	Required equipment	172
		12.3.2	Supplies	172

		12.3.3	Cells and reagents	172
	12.4	Methods		173
		12.4.1	Murine ES cell culture	173
		12.4.2	Preparing slush nitrogen	173
		12.4.3	Cryopreservation of murine ES cells by vitrification	173
	12.5	Anticipated Results		174
		12.5.1	Cell attachment and proliferation after vitrification	174
		12.5.2	Pluripotent properties of ES cells after vitrification	174
	12.6	Discussion and Commentary		176
		Troubleshooting Table		176
	12.7	Application Notes		176
	12.8	Summary Points		177
	Acknowledgments			177
	References			177

CHAPTER 13

In Vivo MR Tracking of hESC-Derived Oligodendrocyte Precursors in Mouse Brain 179

	13.1	Introduction		180
	13.2	Experimental Design		180
	13.3	Materials		181
	13.4	Methods		182
		13.4.1	Maintenance and differentiation of hES cells	182
		13.4.2	Preparation of magnetically labeled cells	182
		13.4.3	Confirmation of magnetically labeled cells: Histochemical staining	182
		13.4.4	Transplantation procedure	184
		13.4.5	MRI procedure	184
		13.4.6	Data analysis	186
	13.5	Anticipated Results		186
	13.6	Discussion and Commentary		187
		Troubleshooting Table		188
	13.7	Application Notes		188
	13.8	Summary Points		189
	Acknowledgments			189
	References			

About the Editors	193
List of Contributors	195
Index	201

Preface

The identification of stem cells within the human body that are capable of maintaining the homeostatic cell mass within a tissue has had a significant impact on clinical care. Perhaps one of the best demonstrations of stem cell therapy is hematopoietic stem cell transplantation, where bone marrow-derived stem cells, infused into a compromised patient, are able to reconstitute all hematopoietic lineages, ultimately saving a patient's life. However, even with the success of this therapy, several technical hurdles remain that impact the effectiveness of future strategies and treatments. How do we harvest and grow enough stem cells to treat a patient? How do we maintain their stem cell phenotype during ex vivo processing? How do we enhance the viability and engraftment of a stem cell transplant? How do we monitor the progress and side effects of a stem cell therapy? How can we direct the differentiation of stem cells towards a particular lineage? And finally, how can we develop predictive tools to perform these tasks with high efficiency, practicality, and scale? These problems are complex, systems-oriented, multidisciplinary, and demand the development of new methods and technologies. These problems, by nature, beckon the input from biomedical scientists and engineers that are well-versed in stem cell biology.

Methods are the lifeblood of scientists and engineers in any field. In stem cell research, there are several key methods that are critical for new investigators to appreciate. Once mastered these methods can be extremely powerful—they can enable one to rigorously test hypotheses and compare their results to the "gold standards." A clear-cut knowledge of existing methods can spur investigators to improve the existing protocols, or even new methods that go beyond the current scope.

This book describes many methods to derive, manipulate, target, and/or prepare stem cells for clinical use. Chapters 1 through 3 describe the derivation and testing of human embryonic stem cells. Chapters 4 through 6 outline micro- and macroscale techniques to expand stem cell populations and guide their differentiation programs. Assays to demonstrate stem cell phenotype and function are highlighted in Chapters 7 and 8. In Chapters 9 and 10, we focus on methodologies to boost endogenous stem cell populations in the adult. Graft preparation, including the immunobiology and preservation of stem cell populations, are the focus of Chapters 11 and 12. And Chapter 13 shows non-invasive methods to image stem cell transplants and monitor graft function.

The contributors of each chapter are among the best scientists and engineers in their respective fields, and have come together with one unified goal—to arm biomedical scientists and engineers with the tools they need to usher in the next generation of stem cell therapeutics to the clinic.

Martin L. Yarmush
Biju Parekkadan
Mass General Hospital/
Harvard Medical School
July 2009

CHAPTER 1

Somatic Cell Nuclear Transfer and Derivation of Embryonic Stem Cells

Li-Ying Sung,[1] Sadie L. Marjani,[2] Tomokazu Amano,[3] X. Yang,* and Cindy Tian[3]

[1]Institute of Biotechnology
National Taiwan University
Taipei 106
Taiwan ROC

[2]Department of Molecular, Cellular, and
Developmental Biology
Yale University
New Haven, CT 06520

[3]Center for Regenerative Biology and Department
of Animal Science
University of Connecticut
Storrs, CT 06269

*Xiangzhong "Jerry" died of adenocarcinoma at the age of 49 on February 5, 2009 (Nature 458, 161: 2009). He was a renowned embryo biotechnologist, stem cell biologist, and activist.

Abstract

Nuclear transfer (otherwise known as *cloning*) and embryonic stem cells have tremendous biomedical applications. The potential of therapeutic cloning, the generation of cloned embryos for the purpose of embryonic stem cell derivation, has received a boost with the recent reports of the generation of cloned human blastocysts. Nuclear transfer in mice has benefited from a decade of research and well-characterized protocols. Thus, it serves as an excellent model for establishing the sophisticated technique for those who hope to do human work in the future. This chapter describes the protocol for mouse somatic cell nuclear transfer, and provides guidance for both direct injection and electrofusion methods. It also describes the derivation and characterization of embryonic stem cells from the nuclear transfer embryos generated.

| Key Terms | Somatic cell nuclear transfer
cloning
embryonic stem cells
pluripotency |

1.1 Introduction

Nuclear transfer is a powerful technology with multiple biomedical applications. Therapeutic cloning involves using a single donor cell from a diseased patient (they can be genetically modified if needed) for nuclear transfer in order to make patient-specific embryonic stem (nuclear transfer embryonic stem [ntES]) cells. These ntES cells could then be differentiated into the desired cell type or tissue. This would offer tailored treatment without the need for life-long immunosuppression. Recently, nuclear transfer in primates, including humans, has been successful [1, 2]. Even though ntES cell lines were not produced from the cloned human blastocysts, the mere ability to produce human nuclear transfer blastocysts was a huge step forward and indicates that human ntES cells will soon be derived. The mouse was among the first mammalian species to be cloned [3], and extensive research has been carried out with the embryos and subsequent ntES cell lines. Research has shown that ntES cells have the same level of pluripotency as ES cells from fertilized embryos and indistinguishable gene expression profiles [4–6]. In addition, the therapeutic cloning proof-of-principle in mice has been established [7]. This chapter provides detailed protocols for (1) mouse nuclear transfer by both direct injection and electrofusion methods, and (2) ntES cell line derivation and characterization. These techniques require skill with a micromanipulator and, with enough practice and the aid of our thorough troubleshooting guidelines, should be successfully established in other laboratories wishing to pursue cloning and stem cell research.

1.2 Materials for Nuclear Transfer

1.2.1 Equipment for mouse nuclear transfer

- NuAire Class II Type A2 Biological Safety Cabinet (NU 440-400, LABREPCO)
- Vibration Isolation Workstations (Newport)
- Nikon TE300 microscope with inflourescence and image analysis (MVI)
- 3D Hanging Joystick Oil Hydraulic Micromanipulator (MMO-202ND, Narishige)
- Piezo Impact Drive (PMM-150FU, Sutter Instruments)
- Microwarm Plate (MPF-10-SMZ, Kitazato Supply)
- Microinjector for injection (IM-9B, Narishige)
- Microinjector for holding (IM-6, Narishige)
- Nikon Dissection Microscope (SMZ-645/600, MVI)
- BTX Electroporator (VWR)
- Micropipette Puller Instrument (P-97, Sutter Instruments)
- Microforge (MF-900, Narishige)
- Borosilicate glass (outside diameter [OD], 1 mm, inside diameter [ID], 0.75 mm; B1000-75-15, Sutter Instruments)
- Mouth control Pasteur pipette (13-678-20B, Fisher Scientific)
- 10-cm dish (35-1029, Falcon)

1.2.2 Reagents for mouse nuclear transfer

- Mercury (M-140, Fisher Scientific)
- D-mannitol (M-4125, Sigma)
- Bovine serum albumin (BSA; A-3311, Sigma)

- Pregnant mare serum gonadotropin (PMSG; G-4877, Sigma)
- Human chorionic gonadotropin (hCG; C-1063, Sigma)
- M2 medium (M-7167, Sigma)
- Hyaluronidase (H-3506, Sigma)
- Cytochalasin B (CB; C-6762, Sigma)
- Mineral oil (M-8410, Sigma)
- KSOM + Amino Acids (KSOM+AA) (MR-121-D, Chemicon Specialty Media)
- Dulbecco's modified Eagle's medium (DMEM; SLM-220-M, Chemicon Specialty Media)
- Fetal bovine serum (FBS; SH30071.03, Hyclone)
- Ultrapure water (TMS-006-B, Chemicon Specialty Media)
- Polyvinylpyrolidine (PVP; PVP360, Sigma)
- Trichostatin A (TSA; T-8552, Sigma)

Media recipes [8] (all from Sigma unless otherwise noted).

Table 1.1 Composition of the CZB Stock

Chemicals	Catalog No.	Weight (mg)	
		1,000 mL	500 mL
MiliQ water	Fresh	990 mL	495 mL
NaCl	S-5886	4,760	2,368
KCl	P-5405	360	180
$MgSO_4 \cdot 7H_2O$	M-1880	290	145
$EDTA \cdot 2Na$	E-6635	40	20
Na-Lactate	L-7900	5.3 mL	2.65 mL
D-Glucose	G-6152	1,000	500 (0.5g)
KH_2PO_4	P-5655	160	80 (0.08g)

Table 1.2 Composition of the CZB-G Medium

Chemicals	Catalog No.	Weight (mg)	
		100 mL	200 mL
CZB stock		99 mL	198 mL
$NaHCO_3$	S-5761	211	422
$CaCl_2 \cdot 2H_2O$ 100× stock	C-7902	1 mL	2 mL
Pyruvate	P-4562	3	6
Glutamine	Gibco, 21051-024	15	30
BSA	A-3311	500	1,000

Table 1.3 Composition of the HEPS-CZB-G Medium

Chemicals	Catalog No.	Weight (mg)	
		100 mL	200 mL
CZB stock		99 mL	198 mL
HEPS	8651	520	1,040
$NaHCO_3$	S-5761	42	84
$CaCl_2 \cdot 2H_2O$ 100× stock	C-7902	1 mL	2 mL
Pyruvate	P-4562	3	6
Glutamine	Gibco, 21051-024	15	30
Polyvinyl alchol (PVA)	P-8136	10	15–16

Adjust pH by 1N HCl (H-9892, Sigma) 0.9 to 1 mL = pH 7.4.

Somatic Cell Nuclear Transfer and Derivation of Embryonic Stem Cells

Table 1.4 Composition of the Ca^{2+} Free CZB-G Medium

Chemicals	Catalog No.	Weight (mg)/100 mL
CZB stock		100 mL
NaHCO$_3$	S-5761	211
Pyruvate	P-4562	3
Glutamine	Gibco, 21051-024	15
BSA	A-3311	500

Table 1.5 Composition of the Ca^{2+} Free HEPS-CZB-G Medium

Chemicals	Catalog No.	Weight (mg)	
		100 mL	200 mL
CZB stock		99 mL	198 mL
HEPS	8651	520	1,040
NaHCO$_3$	S-5761	42	84
Pyruvate	P-4562	3	6
Glutamine	Gibco, 21051-024	15	30
PVA	P-8136	10	15–16

1.3 Methods for Nuclear Transfer

1.3.1 Preparation of enucleation and nuclear transfer pipettes

1. Purchase borosilicate glass and make all pipettes using a micropipette puller and microforge before the experiment. Slightly bend (approximately 15–20 degrees) all pipettes around 0.3 cm from the end.
2. *Holding pipettes:* Pull pipettes to an outside diameter of around 80 to 100 µm and polish with microforge to an inside diameter of approximately 15 to 20 µm.
3. *Enucleation pipettes:* Pull to diameter of approximately 10 µm.
4. *Injection pipettes:* The size of the injection pipettes are dependent on donor cell type used for nuclear transfer. For direct nuclear injection, pull to approximately 5 to 7 µm; for the fusion method, pull to approximately 18 to 20 µm.
5. Load 0.2 to 0.3 cm mercury into micropipettes with long needle carefully (*Toxic! Handle with gloves in the hood.*) before starting the micromanipulation.

1.3.2 Medium preparation

1. Make CZB medium (Table 1.1) for micromanipulation and short-term culture. Prepare CZB medium biweekly using high-quality MiliQ water or purchase ultrapure water. Use a disposable container to make the solutions and aliquot 10 mL per tube; store at 4°C. CZB-G medium (Table 1.2) is for short-term culture in the 37°C incubator during micromanipulation. HEPS-CZB-G (Table 1.3) is the base medium for micromanipulation at room temperature. Ca^{2+}-free HEPS-CZB-G (Table 1.4) is the washing medium for electrofusion method, and Ca^{2+}-free CZB-G (Table 1.5) is the base medium for activation. Add glutamine (100× stock, aliquoted and stored at –20°C) to each buffer before use.
2. Electrofusion medium: 0.3M mannitol containing 0.1 mM $MgSO_4$ and 5 mg/mL BSA.

1.3.3 Animal preparation

1. *Oocyte donors:* Use female B6D2F1 (C57BL/6J × DBA/2) 8- to 12-week-old mice as oocyte donors. Superovulate mice by sequential injections of 5 IU PMSG and hCG. Collect oocytes 13 to 14 hours after the administration of hCG. Normally, approximately 30 to 40 oocytes can be harvested per female.
2. *Recipient mothers:* Use 10- to 14-week-old female CD-1 mice as the recipients of the cloned embryos. Transfer day 5 cloned blastocysts into the uterine horns (around 7–10 embryos per horn) of 2.5 days postconception (dpc) pseudopregnant recipients (mated with mature vasectomized CD-1 males). Sacrifice recipient mothers at day 19.5 and obtain live pups by cesarean section.
3. *Foster mothers:* Lactating foster mothers raise the cloned pups. To generate the foster mothers, mate 10- to 14-week-old female CD-1 mice with normal mature CD-1 males so that the due dates are the same (or 1 day earlier) as the recipient mothers.

1.3.4 Nuclear transfer

1. Prepare dishes of CZB-G droplets (approximately 50 µL per drop) and cover with mineral oil. Equilibrate in a humidified atmosphere of 5% CO_2/95% air at 37°C (Jacked CO_2 incubator, Thermo Forma) for at least 30 minutes before use.
2. *Oocyte collection:* Collect oocytes in M2 medium 13 to 14 hours after hCG injection. Treat cumulus–oocyte complexes with 0.1 mg/mL hyaluronidase and pipette up and down repeatedly with a mouth control Pasteur pipette to remove the cumulus cells. After complete removal of cumulus cells from the oocytes, transfer them to an equilibrated CZB-G dish for incubation until enucleation.

1.3.5 Enucleation

1. Make micromanipulation drops of HEPS-CZB-G medium containing 5 µg/mL CB in a 10-cm dish and cover with mineral oil as shown in Figure 1.1. Each droplet should only be used once.

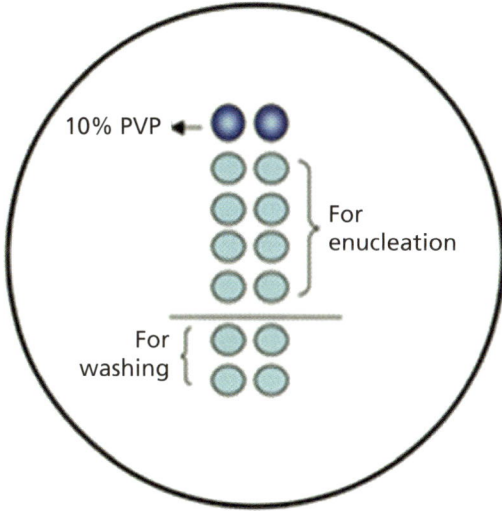

Figure 1.1 Layout of droplets for oocyte enucleation.

2. After culture in CZB-G medium, transfer groups of 20 to 30 oocytes to the droplets of HEPS-CZB-G medium with CB. The spindle is very sensitive to temperature; therefore, using a warming plate (Microwarm Plate, 37°C) will help reveal the spindle chromosome complex (Figure 1.2).
3. Perform enucleation in the HEPS-CZB-G medium with CB under an inverted microscope using a piezo-driven micromanipulator. The size of the blunt-ended enucleation pipette is approximately 10 µm. Load approximately 0.2 to 0.3 mm mercury into each pipette to generate smooth piezo pulses.
    i. Before moving the pipette into the drop with the oocytes, wash the pipette in a 10% PVP drop with a couple of piezo pulses several times.
    ii. Rotate the oocyte with the enucleation pipette to focus on the spindle chromosome complex (relatively bright area in cytoplasm).
    iii. When the oocyte is properly positioned, multiple piezo pulses will allow you to penetrate the zona pellucida. To avoid damaging the oocyte, rotate the spindle near the polar body; use the enucleation pipette and proper holding pipette pressure. This provides more space in the perivitelline space during the piezo pulses. Never give a pulse when the pipette is touching the oocyte membrane.
    iv. After penetration into the zona pellucida, move the pipette forward and focus exactly on the spindle. Carefully create a small negative suction when the pipette is touching the spindle (the whole spindle chromosome complex can be felt to move with the pipette), and aspirate the spindle with only a minimal volume of cytoplasm. If there is suction without exact focus on the spindle, too much cytoplasm will be removed. Figure 1.3 demonstrates the steps of the enucleation process.

1.3.6 Preparation of donor cells

Handle different donor cell types in the following manner:
1. *Fresh cumulus cells:* Isolate fresh cumulus cells from BDF1 oocytes by 0.1 mg/mL hyaluronidase treatment. Suspend the cumulus cells in a small volume of 3% PVP in HEPS-CZB-G and keep on ice.

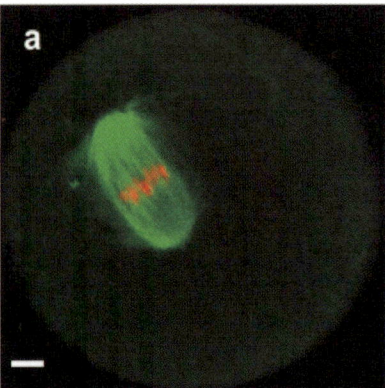 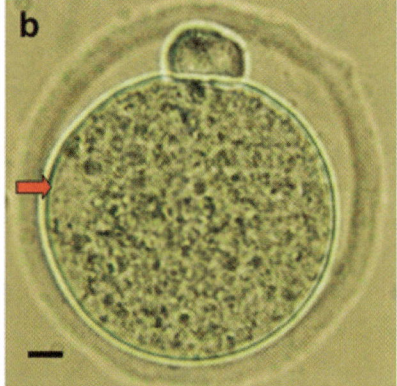

Figure 1.2 Mouse metaphase II (MLL) stage oocytes. (a) Laser scanning confocal image of a mouse oocyte. Red indicates the metaphase II chromosomes; green indicates the spindle chromosome complex. Bar = 10 µm. (b) Phase contrast image of mouse oocyte: the arrow indicates the spindle chromosome complex.

1.3 Methods for Nuclear Transfer

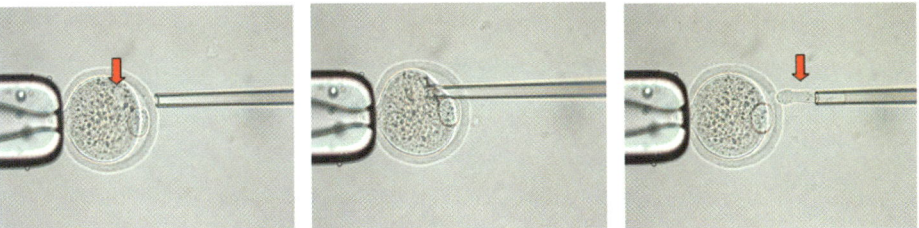

Figure 1.3 Enucleation of a mouse oocyte (a–c). Arrow indicates the spindle chromosome complex.

2. *Frozen hematopoietic cells:* In instances of great distance between collaborating laboratories, frozen cells can be alternative resource for nuclear transfer. Isolate high-purity hematopoietic cells by multiparameter fluorescence-activated cell sorting. Cryopreserve the sorted cells in liquid nitrogen. Before nuclear transfer experiments, thaw the frozen cells in a water bath at 37°C for about 30 seconds. Wash the cells carefully using HEPS-CZB-G medium and centrifuge for 5 minutes at 1,000 rpm in a 15-mL tube. Remove the supernatant, resuspend the cell pellet, and transfer to a 1.5-mL tube for another round of centrifugation. Mix the cell pellet well with a small volume of 10% PVP in HEPS-CZB-G and keep it on ice before nuclear transfer. Use a small fraction of the cells for the cell viability test (0.4% trypan blue staining).
3. *Fibroblast cells:* Culture fibroblast cells in DMEM containing 10% FBS until confluence. Further culture cells in starvation medium (0.5% FBS in DMEM) for 3 to 5 days to arrest the cell cycle in the G0/G1 phase. Before nuclear transfer, remove culture medium from the dish and wash the cells with Dulbecco's Phosphate Buffered Saline (DPBS). Add 0.05% trypsin–ethylenediaminetetraacetic acid and incubate 5 minutes at 37°C in 5% CO_2 incubator. Suspend the fibroblast cells in starvation medium and keep on ice.

1.3.7 Nuclear transfer

There are two methods of nuclear transfer, depending on the donor cell type used: direct injection of donor nuclei with a piezo drill micromanipulator or electrofusion. Typically, we prefer to use direct injection with small donor cells (e.g., cumulus, hematopoietic cells) and electrofusion with larger donor cells (e.g., fibroblast cells). Electrofusion is routinely used for nuclear transfer in domestic species. It is technically less challenging than direct injection [9]. Compared with the electrofusion method, direct nuclear injection using the piezo drill micromanipulator results in less donor cell cytoplasm introduced into enucleated oocytes [8]. Figure 1.4 illustrates the entire mouse nuclear transfer procedure.

1.3.7.1 Direct injection

1. Make micromanipulation droplets of HEPS-CZB-G medium in 10-cm dish and cover with mineral oil as shown in Figure 1.5. The droplets of 10% and 3% PVP are used for pipette washing to prevent the pipette from getting "sticky" after several injections. The droplets are not reused.

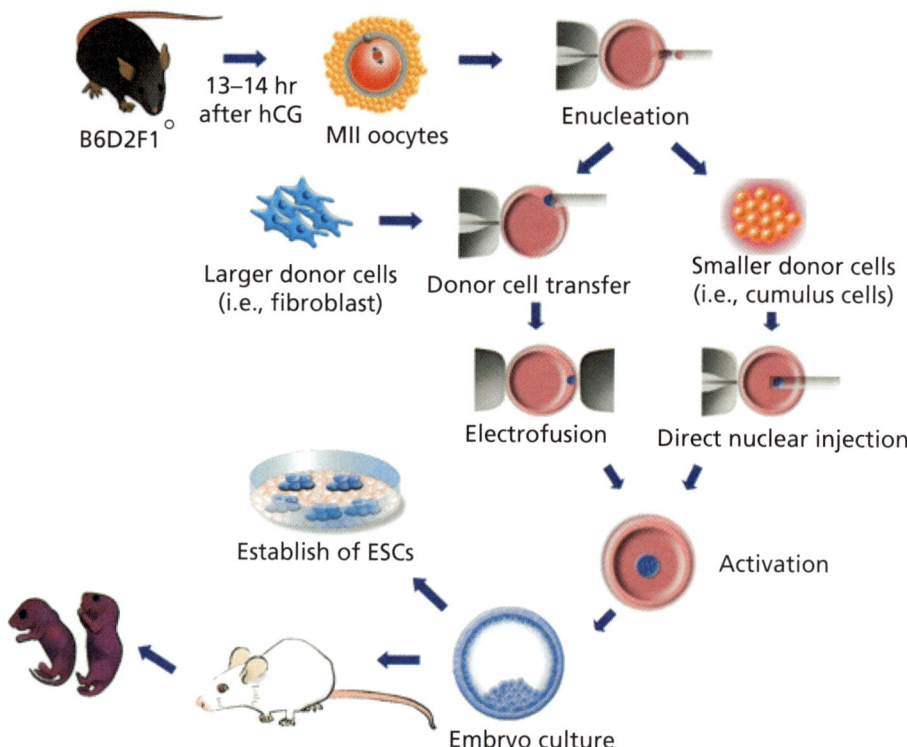

Figure 1.4 The procedure of mouse nuclear transfer.

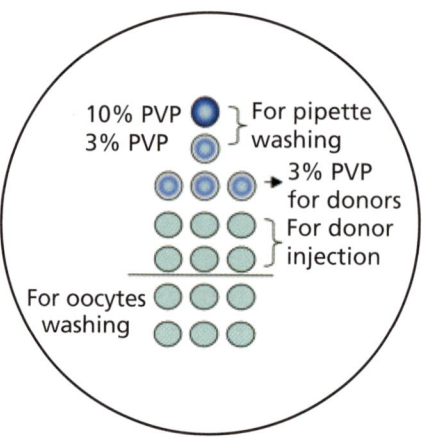

Figure 1.5 Layout of HEPS-CZB-G droplets for injection of nuclear donor cells.

2. Place a group of 10 to 15 oocytes into each HEPS-CZB-G droplet. Inject the oocytes within 15 to 20 minutes of placing them in the droplets.
3. When using cumulus cells or hematopoietic cells (5–6 μm) as nuclear donor cells, take an individual small-size cell (<10 μm) and draw in and out of the injection pipette until its plasma membrane is broken. Load four to five nuclei into the injection pipette.

4. Position one enucleated oocyte with the holding pipette; use the higher piezo pulse (approximate speed, 3–4; intensity, 2–4) to penetrate the zona pellucida.
5. After the zona pellucida is penetrated, move the injection pipette to the opposite side and give a single pulse (speed, 1; intensity, 1) to the oocyte membrane. At the same time, inject nuclei into the cytoplasm. Inject as little medium as possible and pull out the pipette quickly (Figure 1.6).
6. Keep all the oocytes in the droplet for 10 to 15 minutes at room temperature after injection. Higher lyses rates result when the reconstructed oocytes are moved back to the incubator immediately after injection. Culture the reconstructed oocytes in CZB-G medium for 1 to 3 hours before activation.

Important Points About Injection

- Very often, the donor cell membrane or oocyte membrane does not break because of poor control of piezo pulses during injection. However, a strong piezo pulse will increase oocyte lyses right after injection (as shown in Figure 1.7). In addition, the donor cell nuclear membrane can break as a result of the high piezo pulses, and this will cause the injection pipette to become sticky.

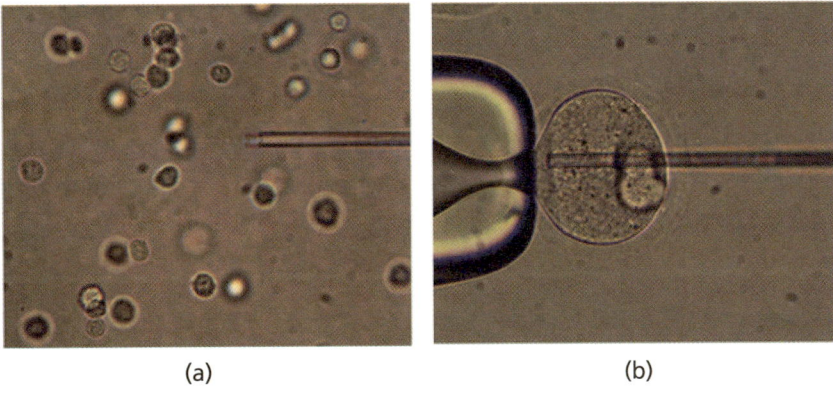

Figure 1.6 (a, b) Direct injection of donor cell by piezo drill micromanipulator.

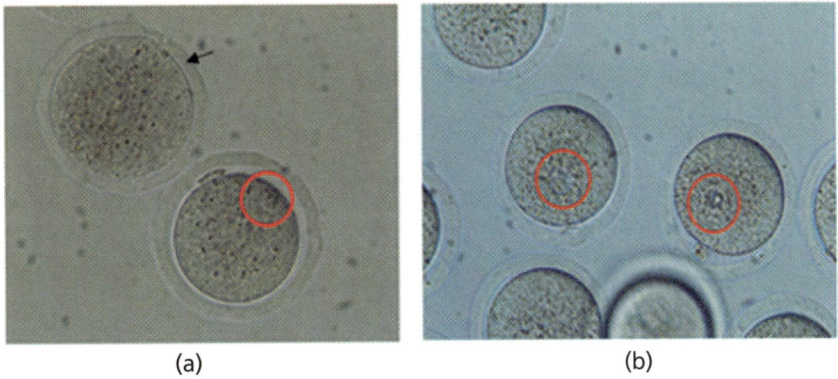

Figure 1.7 Failed injection of donor cell into enucleated oocytes. (a) Arrow indicates a lysed oocyte resulting from a piezo pulse that was too strong. The red circle indicates that the donor cell membrane did not break. (b) The red circle shows that oocyte cytoplasm was not pierced and that the injected medium formed a loop inside the cytoplasm. These reconstructed oocytes will not form pseudo-pronuclei and will become fragmented after culture.

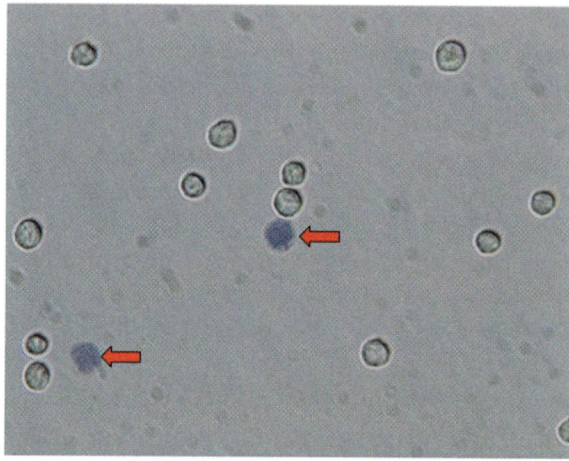

Figure 1.8 Viability of frozen hematopoietic cells after thawing. Arrows indicate dead cells after 0.4% trypan blue staining.

- When working with frozen cells, only select cells with healthy, smooth, and intact membranes (Figure 1.8). Otherwise, the lysed nuclei will clog the injection pipette and prevent injection.

1.3.7.2 Fusion method

1. Remove the polar body and its debris before donor cell transfer. This prevents confusion when it is time to hand align the oocyte–donor pair during electrofusion. If the electropulse is administered without proper alignment of the oocyte–donor pair, the fusion rate will be significantly decreased.
2. For larger donor cells like fibroblast cells, inject the intact donor cell into the perivitelline space using an 18- to 20-μm pipette as shown in Figure 1.9.
3. Wash reconstructed oocytes in Ca^{2+}-free HEPS-CZB-G medium droplets before placing into 0.3M mannitol (Figure 1.10).
4. Move a group of three to four reconstructed oocytes into fusion medium and align by hand before giving the electropulse (Figure 1.11).

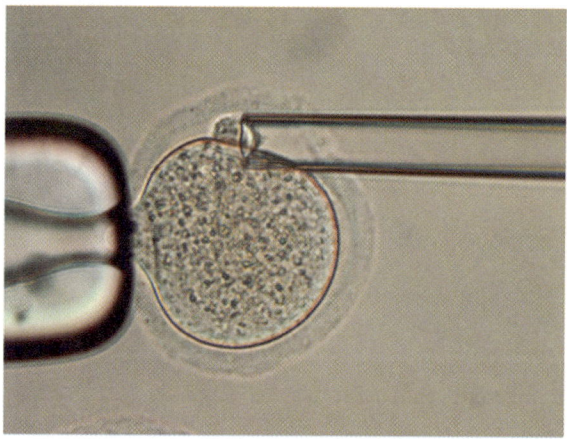

Figure 1.9 The transfer of a fibroblast donor cell into an enucleated egg.

1.3 Methods for Nuclear Transfer

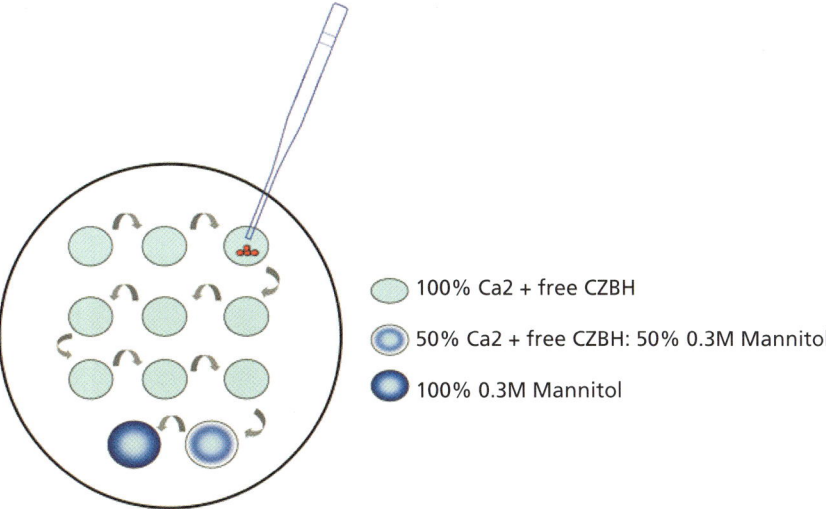

Figure 1.10 Droplet layout for washing the reconstructed oocytes before electrofusion.

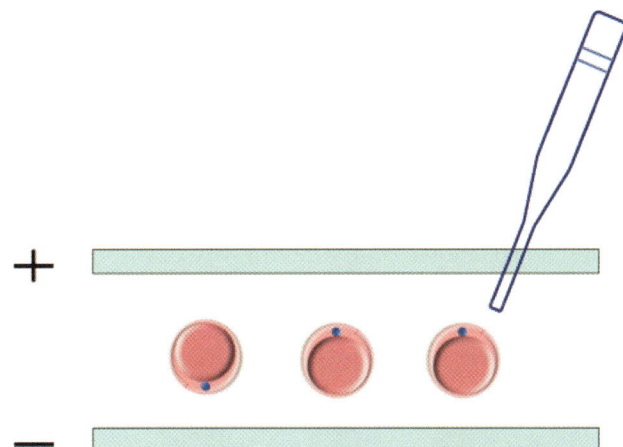

Figure 1.11 Hand alignment of reconstructed oocytes before administering electrofusion pulses.

5. Fuse the donor cell and oocyte membranes with two direct current pulses of 150V/mm for 10 μsec with a BTX ECM 2001 in 0.3M mannitol containing 0.1 mM $MgSO_4$ and 5 mg/mL BSA.
6. Transfer reconstructed oocytes to Ca^{2+}-free HEPS-CZB-G medium at 37°C on a warming plate and check the fusion rate 15 minutes later.
7. Culture in CZB-G medium for 1 to 3 hours before activation.

1.3.8 Activation

Activate the reconstructed oocytes in Ca^{2+}-free CZB-G medium containing 10 mM strontium and 5 μg/mL CB with or without 10 nM TSA (discussed later) for 6 hours. Figure 1.12 demonstrates the dynamic reorganization of the chromosomes and microtubules after nuclear transfer and activation (Sung, unpublished data).

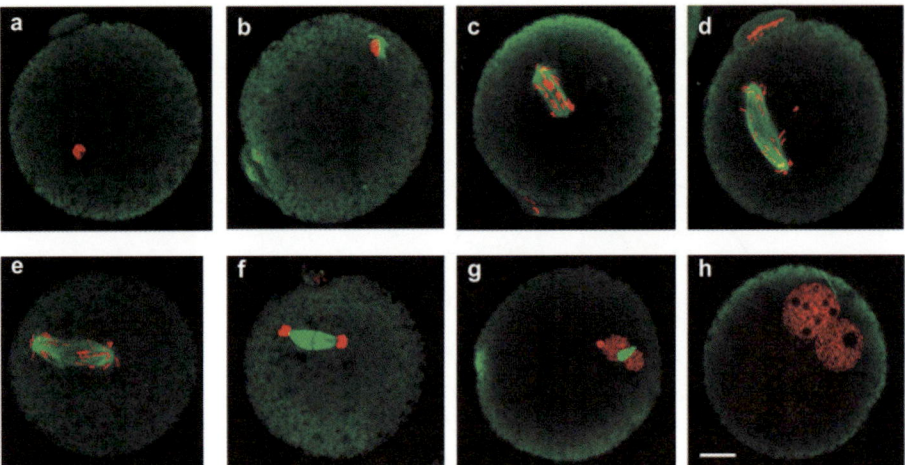

Figure 1.12 Chromatin remodeling dynamics and spindle organization in reconstructed oocytes following nuclear transfer and activation. Ten minutes (a), 30 minutes (b), 1 hour (c), and 3 hours (d) after nuclear transfer. The nuclear envelope breakdown, chromosome condensation, and spindle organization 30 minutes (e), 1 hour (f), 3 hours (g) and 6 hours (h) after activation. Chromosome decondensation and pseudo-pronuclei formation. Bar = 20 μm.

Important point: TSA treatment (10 nM for 10 hours total) significantly increases cloned embryo development [10]. Figure 1.13 shows the large number of high-quality cloned embryos generated after TSA treatment (Sung and Amano, unpublished data).

1.3.9 Embryo culture and embryo transfer

1. Culture cloned embryos in KSOM+AA with or without 10 nM TSA for 4 hours, then transfer to fresh KSOM+AA medium and culture for 4 days at 37°C in a humidified atmosphere of 5% CO_2, 5% O_2, and 90% N_2.

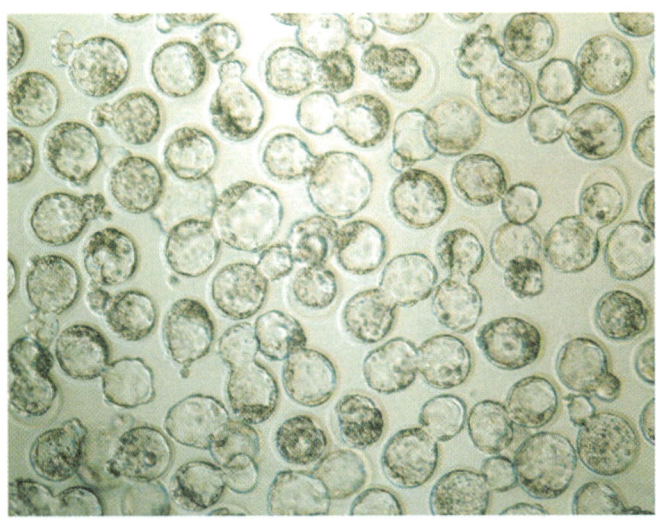

Figure 1.13 Trichostatin A (TSA) treatment significantly increases cloned embryo development. The cloned blastocysts shown were derived from tail-tip fibroblast donor cells and were treated with TSA after activation for 10 hours.

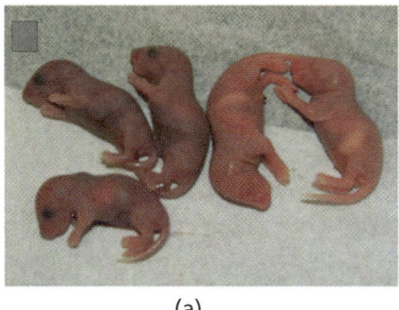
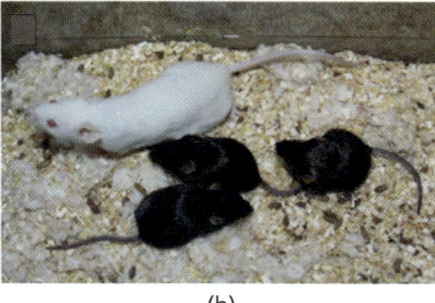

(a)   (b)

Figure 1.14 Cloned pups harvested by cesarean section. (a) The three cloned pups on the left were generated with cumulus donor cells and the two on the right were from fertilized control embryos. (b) Three cloned mice with foster mother.

2. Transfer the embryos that developed to the morula/blastocyst stage into the uteri of day 2.5 pseudopregnant CD-1 females.
3. Sacrifice recipient mothers at day 19.5 and obtain live pups by cesarean section. Place the pups with lactating foster mothers (Figure 1.14).

1.4 Derivation of Mouse ntES Cells

The following method of deriving mouse ntES cells from embryos was adapted from [6].

1.5 Materials for Embryonic Stem Cell Derivation

Embryonic Stem Cell Derivation Medium	100 mL
Knockout DMEM (Gibco, #10829)	80 mL
Knockout serum replacement (KSR, Gibco, #10828)	15 mL
Pen/Strep (100×, Specialty Media, TMS-AB-2C)	1 mL
L-glutamine (100×, Specialty Media, TMS-002-C)	1 mL
Nonessential amino acids (100×, Specialty Media, TMS-001-C)	1 mL
Nucleosides for ES cells (100×, Specialty Media, ES-008-D)	1 mL
2-Mercaptoethanol (100×, Specialty Media, ES-007-E)	1 mL
LIF (ESGROW, Gibco 13275-029)	10 μl
Embryonic Stem Cell Culture Medium	100 mL
DMEM (Specialty Media, SLM-220-M)	80 mL
FBS (Hyclone, SH30071.03)	15 mL
Pen/Strep (100×, Specialty Media, TMS-AB-2C)	1 mL
L-glutamine (100×, Specialty Media, TMS-002-C)	1 mL
Nonessential amino acids (100×, Specialty Media, TMS-001-C)	1 mL
Nucleosides for ES cells (100×, Specialty Media, ES-008-D)	1 mL
2-Mercaptoethanol (100×, Specialty Media, ES-007-E)	1 mL
LIF (ESGROW, Gibco 13275-029)	10 μL

1.6 Methods for Embryonic Stem Cell Derivation

1.6.1 Derivation of ntES cells

1. Carefully remove the zona pellucida of blastocyst stage embryos by treatment with 0.1% protease (freshly made) for 3 to 5 minutes under dissection microscope. Place a zona-free blastocyst into the well of 96-well plate containing primary mouse embryonic fibroblast (PMEF) feeder cells. Prepare the PMEF feeders 1 day earlier by treating with 10 μg/mL mitomycin C (M-4287, Sigma) and culturing in DMEM and 10% FBS medium ($0.75 \cdot 10^5$ cells/mL, 2.5 mL per well of a six-well plate).
2. Culture for 7 days at 37°C in a humidified atmosphere of 5% CO_2, 5% O_2, and 90% N_2 in ES cell derivation medium, and then pick up the small colony (outgrowth) and put it into a new well with fresh feeder cells for 3 additional days.
3. When the colony is large enough [Figure 1.15(b)], detach by trypsinization and transfer into a 48-well plate with fresh feeder cells: and culture in ES cell culture medium for another 2 to 3 days.

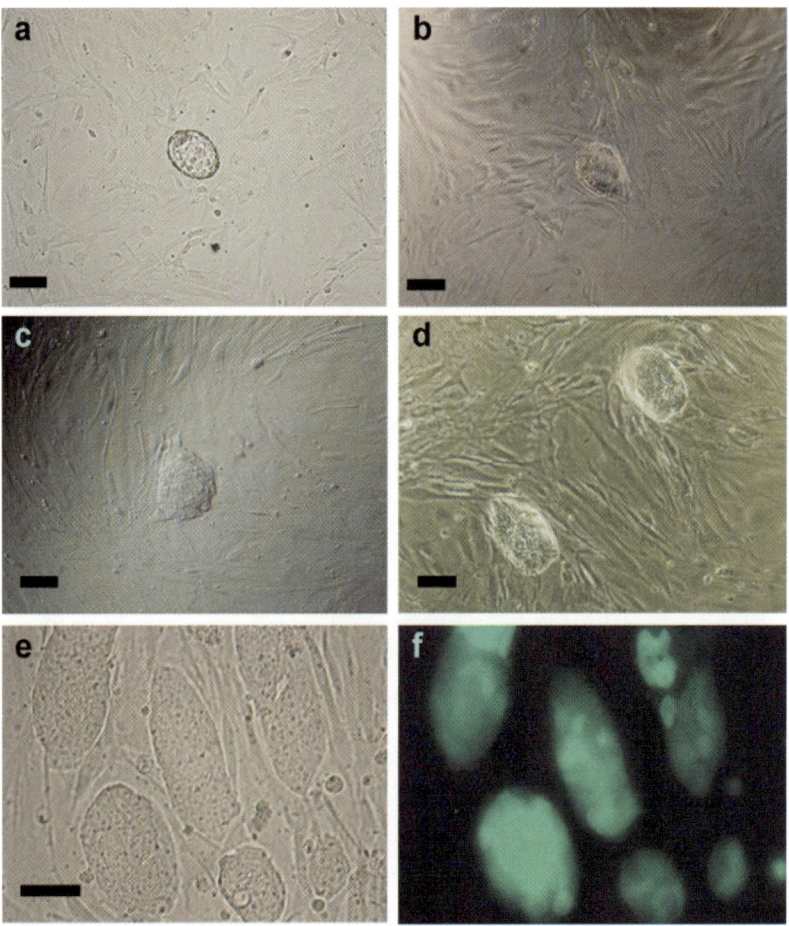

Figure 1.15 Establishment of an ntES cell line. (a) Cloned blastocyst derived from green fluorescent protein (GFP) donor is placed into mouse embryonic fibroblast (MEF) feeder cells (zona pellucida was removed by 0.1% protease). (b, c) The colony was formed after 7 and 10 days culture with primary MEF feeder cells. (d, e) Morphology of colonies at p2 and p4. (f) GFP expression in all colonies indicate that the ES cells were derived from a GFP-cloned blastocyst.

4. Clonally expand the undifferentiated colonies by mild trypsinization and sequential transfer to 24- and six-well plates, and then finally into a T-25 flask at intervals of 2 to 3 days (Figure 1.15).

1.6.2 In vitro characterization of ntES cells

Karyotyping, reverse transcription–polymerase chain reaction (RT-PCR), and immunohistochemistry determine the pluripotency of established ntES cell lines.

1.6.2.1 Karyotyping

1. Replate ntES cells onto gelatin-coated dishes without PMEF before analysis.
2. Mitotically arrest log-phase ES cells with treatment of 0.1 μg/mL demecolcine for 1 hour.
3. Scrape the ES cells from the bottom of the dish and suspend them in 0.56% KCl.
4. Fix cells with 3 methanol:1 acetic acid and then spread onto the slides with Giemsa stain.

1.6.2.2 Immunostaining

1. Add 4% paraformaldehyde to the cells for 15 minutes and then wash with PBS several times.
2. Wash fixed ntES cells in blocking solution consisting of 5% donkey or goat serum (Chemicon) with 5% BSA in PBS for 1 hour at room temperature.
3. Incubate primary antibodies: rabbit polyclonal anti-Oct4 (Santa Cruz Biotechnology), rabbit polyclonal anti-Nanog (Chemicon), rabbit polyclonal Sox2 (Abcam), and mouse monoclonal anti-SSEA-1 (Chemicon) with the cells at room temperature for 1 hour.
4. Incubate secondary antibodies (Invitrogen, Alexa Fluor 594) at room temperature for 1 hour.
5. Visualize nuclei with 4′-6-Diamidino-2-pheylindole (DAPI) (Figure 1.16).

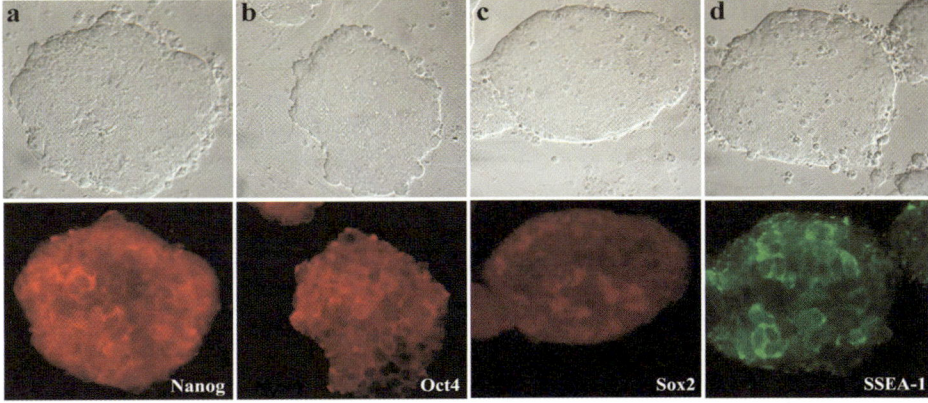

Figure 1.16 Immunostaining of ntES cell colonies for Nanog (a), Oct4 (b), Sox2 (c), and SSEA-1 (d).

1.6.2.3 RT-PCR

1. Isolate total RNA from each ntES cell line using the RNeasy kit (Qiagen).
2. Treat the RNA with DNase to remove any containing DNA (Ambion, Turbo DNA-free kit).
3. Carry out complementary DNA synthesis with cells-to-cDNA kit (Ambion).
4. Perform PCR with specific primers (final concentration, 0.3 µM) for *Oct4*, *Nanog*, and *Sox2*, and *Actb* as a control. Program 35 cycles of 94°C, 30 seconds; 60°C, 30 seconds; and 72°C, 45 seconds.
5. Visualize bands on a 2% agarose gel.

Table 1.6 Primers for RT-PCR

Gene	Primers	Size of Product (bp)
Sox2	(F):TAGAGCTAGACTCCGGGCGAT (R):TTGCCTTAAACAAGACCACGA	300
Nanog	(F):CTTAGAAGCGTGGGTCTTGG (R):GACTCCAAGGACAAGCAAGC	265
Oct4	(F):GAGGATCACCTTGGGGTACA (R):CTCATTGTTGTCGGCTTCCT	189
Actb	(F):GATGGTGGGAATGGGTCAGA (R):CGTCCCAGTTGGTAACAATGC	167

1.6.3 In vivo characterization of ntES cells

The pluripotency of ntES cell lines is confirmed by producing chimeras.

1.6.3.1 Chimera generation: Recovery of two-cell stage embryos

1. Sacrifice the superovulated, pseudo-pregnant females by cervical dislocation on day 1.5 (day 0.5 is the day of the plug).
2. Dissect the oviducts with the upper part of the uterus attached and place a drop of M2 medium in a dish.
3. Transfer one of the oviducts into small drop of M2 medium.
4. Flush the embryos with M2 medium from the end of the oviduct (infundibulum).
5. Repeat steps 3 and 4 with the remaining oviducts.
6. Collect embryos with a mouth pipette attached to a drawn-out Pasteur pipette.
7. Wash the embryos using M2 medium, transfer to KSOM drops, put into the incubator (at 37°C, 5% CO_2 in air), and culture to the blastocyst stage.

1.6.3.2 Injection of ntES cells into diploid blastocyst

1. Trypsinize ntES cells for 5 minutes to give a single cell suspension. After spinning down, remove the supernatant and resuspend the cells in ES medium and put cells into the drop on the microinjection plate.
2. Wash the injection pipette with a 10% PVP drop and set up the holding and injection pipettes at the proper position (i.e., the middle of the view).
3. Pick up 10 to 15 ntES cells and inject them into the blastocoele of a diploid blastocyst.
4. Repeat step 3 until all blastocysts are injected.
5. Transfer injected blastocysts into KSOM medium and culture them for 1 hour until embryo transfer.

1.6.3.3 Embryo transfer and germline transmission test

1. Prepare the recipient mothers by mating with vasectomized males.
2. Transfer the injected blastocysts into uteri of 2.5 dpc recipient female mice.
3. Sacrifice the recipient females at 18.5 dpc and collect the pups.

Chimeric mice are generally test bred to ascertain contribution of the ntES cells to the germline.

1. Mate sexually mature chimeric males with CD1 females. This will allow for a distinction between ntES cell-derived and host blastocyst-derived gametes.
2. Check the eyes of the offspring at birth. If ntES cells contributed to germ cells of chimera mice, the offspring will have black eyes.

Table 1.7 Time Schedule for Mouse Nuclear Transfer and ntES Cell Derivation

Time Schedule	Nuclear Transfer	ntES Cell Derivation
Pre-day 1	PM: PMSG injection of BDF-1 females for oocyte donation	
Pre-day 2	PM: Prepare CD-1 foster mothers by selecting those in estrus and mate with same strain of males	
Pre-day 3	AM: Check plug to ensure foster mothers are available on the due date of the cloned pups	
	Prepare CZB medium and pipettes for manipulation PM: hCG injection of BDF-1 females for oocyte donation	
Day 1	Nuclear transfer schedule 8:00 AM: MII oocyte collection 8:30–10:00 AM: enucleation 9:30–10:00 AM: donor cell preparation 10:00 AM–1:00 PM: donor nucleus injection (direction injection method) (10:00 AM–1:00 PM: donor cell transfer and electrofusion [fusion method]) 1:00–2:00 PM: culture 1 hour to allow premature chromosome condensation (PCC) formation 3:00–8:00 PM: activation (in $SrCl_2$ + CB + TSA medium) 8:00 PM–12:00 midnight: culture in KSOM+AA + TSA medium 12:00 midnight–day 4: culture in KSOM+AA medium	
Day 2	Check and record embryo cleavage	
	PM: Prepare surrogate mothers (select CD-1 females in estrus and mate with vasectomized males)	
Day 3	AM: Check plug to ensure surrogate mothers are ready for embryo transfer	
Day 4		Plate mitomycin C (10 μg/mL in sDMEM)-treated PMEF feeder cells (in sDMEM) into a 96-well plate
Day 5	Check and record embryo development	
	Transfer cloned embryos to day 2.5 synchronized CD-1 surrogate mothers Observe surrogate mothers' recovery every day after surgery	AM: Change feeder medium to embryonic stem cell (ESC) derivation medium PM: Place embryos into 96-well plate with feeders and culture for 6 to 7 days
Day 11		Plate mitomycin C-treated PMEF feeder cells into 48-well dish
Day 12		AM: Change feeder medium to ESC derivation medium PM: Mechanically pick up "outgrowth" and put into 48-well plate; culture for another 2 to 3 days
Day 14		Prepare mitomycin C-treated PMEF feeder cells and put into 24-well plate

(continues)

Table 1.7 (Continued)

Time Schedule	Nuclear Transfer	ntES Cell Derivation
Day 15		AM: Change feeder medium to ESC culture medium PM: Mild trypsinization of newly formed "ntES-like cell colony" Transfer to 24-well plate with feeder cells (count as passage 1), and culture another 3 to 5 days until new colonies form
Day 18		Prepare mitomycin C-treated PMEF feeder cells and put into six-well plate
Day 19		Passage ntES-like cells and move to six-well dish with feeder cells (passage 2) and culture for 2 to 3 days
Day 20		Change ESC culture medium
Day 21	Ensure that lactating foster mothers are ready for cloned pups	Change ESC culture medium
Day 22	Obtain cloned pups by cesarean section, examine/record pup health and let them be raised by lactating foster mothers	Depending on the experimental design, passage and freeze cell lines for further in vitro and in vivo characterization to confirm their pluripotency

Table 1.8 In Vitro Development of Nuclear Transfer Embryos from Different Hematopoietic Cell Types

Cell Type	No. Oocytes Injected (reps)	No. (%) Activated	No. (%) Cleaved/Activated	No. (%) M+B/Activated
LT-HSC (CD34− LKS)	573 (6)	459 (80.1)[a]	379 (82.6)[a]	19 (4.1)[a]
ST-HSC (CD34+ LKS)	681 (6)	521 (76.5)[a]	446 (85.6)[a]	41 (7.9)[a]
HPC (LKS−)	574 (6)	463 (80.7)[a]	412 (89.0)[a]	49 (10.6)[a]
Granulocyte	474 (6)	278 (58.7)[b]	196 (70.5)[b]	96 (34.5)[b]

Superscripts within a column indicate a significant difference between donor cell types in the efficiency of activation ($P < 0.05$) or the proportion of embryos that cleaved and developed to morulae/blastocysts. *Cleaved* refers to two- and four-cell stage embryos, and *M+B* means morula plus blastocyst stage embryos.

HPC, hematopoietic progenitor cells, enriched with LKS− immunophenotype; LT-HSC, long-term repopulating hematopoietic stem cells, isolated with the CD34− LKS immunophenotype; ST-HSC, short-term repopulating hematopoietic stem cells, isolated with the CD34+ LKS immunophenotype.

Data from [11]. Nuclear transfer by direct injection method.

Table 1.9 Developmental Comparison of Nuclear Transfer Embryos Reconstructed with Different Donor Cell Types

Cell Type	No. Oocytes Injected (reps)	No. (%) Activated	No. (%) Cleaved/Activated	No. (%) M+B/Activated	No. M+B Transferred (reps)	No. (%) Pups/Transferred
Granulocyte	894 (8)	555 (62.1)[a]	394 (71.0)[a]	216 (38.9)[a]	182 (11)	2 (1.1)
Cumulus cell	1022 (9)	974 (95.3)[b]	939 (96.4)[b]	519 (53.3)[b]	505 (35)	15 (3.0)
ES cells	420	412 (98.1)	349 (84.7)	202 (49.0)	197 (12)	18 (9.1)

Superscripts within a column indicate a significant difference between donor cell types in the efficiency of activation ($P < 0.05$) or the proportion of embryos that cleaved and developed to morulae/blastocysts. *Cleaved* refers to two- and four-cell stage embryos, and *M+B* means morula plus blastocyst stage embryos. *ES cells* means HM-1 ES cells. The body weight of both cloned pups derived from granulocyte was 1.837g and 1.670g; the placenta weight was 0.309g and 0.287g, respectively. Both cloned pups were alive after cesarean section, but died within 2 hours after cesarean section. Data from Sung et al. [n].

The cleavage and development to morulae/blastocysts of different cell types was statistically analyzed to compare their efficiency using the Generalized Linear Model procedures (PROC GENMOD in SAS). The point estimates of the successful proportions at each stage and their 95% confidence intervals are marked by different superscripts for significant differences for each cell type (Tables 1.8 and 1.9).

Table 1.10 Nuclear Transfer by Fusion Method

Groups	Oocyte Source	No. Enucleated Oocytes (% of survived oocytes)	No. Electrofused Oocytes (% of fused oocytes)	No. Activated Oocytes (no. of replicates)	No. Cleaved (% activated embryos)	No. M+B Embryos (%activated embryos)	No. Blastocysts (% activated embryos)
Partheno-genesis	Fresh	—	—	186 (3)	186 (100)	184 (98.9)[a]	181 (97.3)[a]
	Frozen/thawed	—	—	149 (3)	146 (98.0)	136 (91.3)[ab]	117 (78.5)[b]
fibroblast fusion	Fresh	478/480 (99.6)	376/425 (88.5)	376 (4)	357 (94.9)	322 (85.6)[b]	301 (80.1)[b]
	Frozen/thawed	394/430 (91.6)	221/310 (71.3)	192 (4)	185 (96.4)	160 (83.3)[b]	108 (56.3)[c]

From [12].

Table 1.11 ntES Cell Derivation

Embryo Source	No. Blastocysts Used	No. (%) Outgrowth ICM	No. (%) Embryonic Stem Cell Lines
Fibroblast nuclear transfer	101	50 (49.5)	25 (24.8)

From [12]. Inner cell mass (ICM).

a, b, c values within the same column with different superscripts differ significantly (P<.05).

1.7 Discussion and Commentary

Mouse nuclear transfer by direct injection using the piezo drill micromanipulator is more technically difficult than the fusion method. For the new user, the most difficult aspects are 1) handling the piezo pulse precisely to penetrate the zona pellucida; 2) recognizing the spindle chromosome complex quickly with removal of a minimal amount of cytoplasm; 3) successfully piercing the cytoplasmic membrane without damaging the enucleated oocyte. The creation of good pipettes (proper diameter and angle) and the use of mercury are very helpful during these processes. Unsatisfactory control of piezo pulses will cause the pipette to become "sticky" and will result in a high lyses rate after injection. Moreover, controlled timing of micromanipulation is also very important for embryo development. To prevent a high lyses rate of reconstructed oocytes, consider using the fusion method for the larger donor cells instead of direct injection. For the fusion method, it is critical to align the donor–oocyte pair precisely when administering the electropulses. For both nuclear transfer methods, properly synchronizing the donor cells' cell cycle in G0/G1 phase when using an MII oocyte egg is critical.

Troubleshooting Table

Problem	Explanation	Potential Solutions
Out of control of enucleation or injection pipette pressure	Oxidation of mercury, precipitate will clog pipette When working with a small pipette (approximately 4–5 μm), sucking in and out too fast during manipulation will plug the pressure	Store mercury properly to prevent oxidation. Handle pressure smoothly; do not be impatient.

(continues)

Somatic Cell Nuclear Transfer and Derivation of Embryonic Stem Cells

Problem	Explanation	Potential Solutions
Difficulty controlling piezo pulses	Not handling pipettes and micromanipulators properly	Determine whether all micromanipulator connections and screws are tight. Hold pipette with slight angle (15–20 deg). Apply proper amount of mercury (0.2–0.3 cm) inside injection pipette (not essential, can be replaced with Fluorinert, Sigma, FC-70). Mercury is toxic; handle carefully inside hood.
Cannot see spindle clearly	Check instruments (e.g., microscope or working plate/dish)	Use glass dish with differential interference contrast (DIC) microscope and plastic dish with Hoffman Modulation Contrast system.
	Room temperature too low	Spindle is sensitive to temperature, applying a warming plate (37°C, Microwarm Plate) can help.
	Not enough experience	Get more practice.
Oocyte lysed after enucleation	Enucleated oocyte without incubating long enough with CB	Incubate oocytes in CB (2.5–5 µg/mL) for approximately 10 minutes to allow it to work.
	Touched the cytoplasm membrane when giving piezo pulses for penetration of the zona	Rotate the oocyte to a proper position (near the polar body) with more space in perivitelline space then give piezo pulses.
Sticky pipette	Piezo pulses are too strong, causes nuclear membrane to break	Reduce piezo pulse power. Wash pipette in 10% PVP drop with mercury.
	Not handling the donor cells properly or keeping them at RT for too long	Suspend donor cells in 3% to 5% PVP (depends on donor cell types), keep donor cells on ice before injection and use fresh donor cells for every injection batch.
	May have picked a lysed cell; lysed nuclei clog the injection pipette	Only select cells with healthy, smooth, intact membranes; if pipette clogs, change to a new one immediately.
High lyses rate after donor cell injection	Highly dependent on personal skill	Get more practice.
	Pipettes are too big and give too strong a pulse, especially a problem for work with larger cells (i.e., fibroblast cells)	For larger cells, consider using the fusion method. Reduce piezo pulses.
	Moved reconstructed oocytes to incubator right after injection	Keep reconstructed oocytes in injection drop for approximately 15 minutes after injection.
	The pipette is sticky because of a dirty working droplet	Do not reuse working droplet. Change new pipette when pipette gets sticky.
	Too much medium was injected or nuclei was not injected properly	Inject nuclei carefully with minimal medium.
Precipitate formed in activation medium	$SrCl_2$ stock added to unequilibrated medium	Equilibrate Ca^{2+}-free CZB-G solution in CO_2 incubator for 15 to 20 minutes before adding $SrCl_2$ stock solution.
Poor fusion rate with fusion method	Donor cell lysed	Pick only healthy donor cells with good morphology.
	Donor–oocyte was not aligned well	Handle only a few reconstructed oocytes (3–4 oocytes per batch) when doing electrofusion. Apply electropulses when donor–oocyte pair align well. Remove polar body and its debris completely to prevent confusion with donor cell during alignment.
Reconstructed oocytes do not form pronuclei after activation	Activation medium contains Ca^{2+}	Make sure stock solution or activation medium does not contain Ca^{2+}.
	Failed to introduce donor nuclei into enucleated cytoplasm	Do not break donor cell membrane. Do not pierce cytoplasm membrane.
Reconstructed oocytes lyse after activation	Stock solution or tubes contain toxic material (when most or all oocytes lysed)	Ensure all tubes or the Dimethyl Sulfoxide (DMSO) used to make the stock solutions are not toxic (embryo culture test).
	Too much damage during nuclei injection (when some of oocytes lysed)	Inject donor nuclei extra carefully. Even though oocytes do not lyse immediately after injection, they will lyse during activation if injection was too harsh.

Problem	Explanation	Potential Solutions
Poor embryo development or arrest at two-cell stage	Many reasons: Cell cycle not properly synchronized Too much PVP solution or medium injected Medium too old Culture conditions not good	A total of 10 nM TSA for 10 hours after activation can improve embryo development dramatically. Synchronize donor cell cycle by culturing to confluence and serum starvation. Do not pick cells that are too large (usually, G2 phase cells are bigger). Inject nuclei with minimal solution, and dissolve PVP solution completely before use (dissolve PVP with CZB-G at 4°C for a few days). Make all medium biweekly. Weekly, check water and CO_2 levels of incubator.
Poor term development	Many reasons and highly dependent on donor cell types; exclude the reasons listed earlier: Surrogate mother not synchronized Poor embryo transfer skill	Do not manipulate for too long because oocytes will get old. Start activation no later than 20 hours after hCG injection. Properly synchronize surrogate mother (better with 12- to 14-week-old females) at day 2.5 for blastocyst transfer. Get more practice.

1.8 Summary Points

1. Nuclear transfer is technically demanding. Much practice is needed.
2. Choose your method of nuclear transfer (fusion or direct injection) based on the size and characteristics of the donor cell.
3. The use of TSA during activation for a total of 10 hours significantly increases development to the blastocyst stage and, therefore, the number of embryos available for ntES cell derivation.

Acknowledgments

The authors thank Dr. Shaorong Gao for his direction and technical support in establishing the mouse nuclear transfer protocol.

References

[1] Byrne, J. A., et al., "Producing Primate Embryonic Stem Cells by Somatic Cell Nuclear Transfer," *Nature*, 2007, pp. 450, 497–502.
[2] French, A. J., et al., "Development of Human Cloned Blastocysts Following Somatic Cell Nuclear Transfer with Adult Fibroblasts," *Stem Cells*, Vol. 26, 2008, pp. 485–493.
[3] Wakayama, T., et al., "Full-Term Development of Mice from Enucleated Oocytes Injected with Cumulus Cell Nuclei," *Nature*, Vol. 394, 1998, pp. 369–374.
[4] Brambrink, T., et al., "ES Cells Derived from Cloned and Fertilized Blastocysts Are Transcriptionally and Functionally Indistinguishable," *Proc. Natl. Acad. Sci. U S A*, Vol. 103, 2006, pp. 933–938.
[5] Wakayama, S., et al., "Equivalency of Nuclear Transfer-Derived Embryonic Stem Cells to Those Derived from Fertilized Mouse Blastocysts," *Stem Cells*, Vol. 24, 2006, pp. 2023–2033.
[6] Wakayama, T., et al., "Differentiation of Embryonic Stem Cell Lines Generated from Adult Somatic Cells by Nuclear Transfer," *Science*, Vol. 292, 2001, pp. 740–743.
[7] Rideout, W. M., 3rd, et al., "Correction of a Genetic Defect by Nuclear Transplantation and Combined Cell and Gene Therapy," *Cell*, Vol. 109, 2002, pp. 17–27.
[8] Gao, S., et al., "Cloning of Mice by Nuclear Transfer," *Cloning Stem Cells*, Vol. 5, 2003, pp. 287–294.
[9] Ogura, A., et al., "Birth of Mice after Nuclear Transfer by Electrofusion Using Tail Tip Cells," *Mol. Reprod. Dev.*, Vol. 57, 2000, pp. 55–59.

[10] Kishigami, S., et al., "Significant Improvement of Mouse Cloning Technique by Treatment with Trichostatin A after Somatic Nuclear Transfer," *Biochem. Biophys. Res. Commun.*, Vol. 340, 2006, pp. 183–189.

[11] Sung, L. Y., et al., "Differentiated Cells Are More Efficient Than Adult Stem Cells for Cloning by Somatic Cell Nuclear Transfer," *Nat. Genet.*, Vol. 38, 2006, pp. 1323–1328.

[12] Chang, C. C., et al. "Derivation of Embryonic Stem Cells by Nuclear Transfer using Cryopreserved Eggs," *Biology of Reproduction*, Vol. 69 (Society for the Study of Reproduction. 41st Annual Meeting Special Issue).

CHAPTER
2

Derivation of Mouse Parthenogenetic Embryonic Stem Cells

Akiko Yabuuchi,[1] Paul H. Lerou,[2] and George Q. Daley[3-6]

[1]Division of Pediatric Hematology/Oncology
Children's Hospital Boston
Harvard Medical School
Boston, MA

[2]Division of Newborn Medicine
Brigham & Women's Hospital and Children's Hospital Boston
Harvard Medical School
Boston, MA

[3]Division of Hematology/Oncology
Brigham & Women's Hospital
Boston, MA

[4]Department of Biological Chemistry and Molecular Pharmacology
Harvard Medical School
Boston, MA

[5]Harvard Stem Cell Institute
Boston, MA

[6]Howard Hughes Medical Institute
Chevy Chase, MD

Abstract

Parthenogenesis affords tremendous insight into oocyte biology and preimplantation embryonic development. Parthenogenetic activation can be performed at various stages of meiosis, yielding genetically distinct types of parthenogenetic embryonic stem cells. When parthenogenetic activation includes prevention of polar body extrusion, the resulting embryos will be genetically heterozygous. The pattern of heterozygosity in the embryonic stem cells derived from such embryos can be predicted by whether extrusion of the first or second polar body is blocked. In addition to their utility as research tools, parthenogenetic embryonic stem cells may also hold therapeutic potential. Heterozygous parthenogenetic embryonic stem cells can retain the full complement of major histocompatibility complex antigens of the oocyte donor and therefore could serve as a potential source of histocompatible cells and tissues for transplantation therapy. In this chapter, we describe detailed protocols for the generation of parthenogenetic embryos and derivation of parthenogenetic embryonic stem cells.

Key Terms Parthenogenesis
embryonic stem cells
mouse embryos

2.1 Introduction

Parthenogenesis (Greek for "virgin birth") is the process by which an oocyte develops into an embryo in the absence of fertilization. Many animal species, including certain plants, insects, fish, amphibians, reptiles, and birds, can reproduce by parthenogenesis. Parthenogenetic diploid mouse embryos were first reported in 1976, by Balakier and Tarkowski [1], who used heat shock to activate ovulated oocytes in the presence of cytochalasin, an inhibitor of microfilament production, which resulted in failure to extrude the second polar body. Embryonic stem (ES) cells were first derived from the inner cell mass (ICM) of blastocyst-stage fertilized embryos by Evans and Kaufman [2] in 1981. Interestingly, only 2 years later, these same authors demonstrated that parthenogenetically activated mouse oocytes can yield both diploid and "haploid" parthenogenetic embryonic stem (pES) cells [3, 4]. When injected into fertilized blastocysts, mouse pES cells contribute to nearly all tissues, but only rarely to the germline. When injected subcutaneously into immunodeficient mice, they generate tumors that contain tissues comprising all three germ layers [5]. Mouse parthenogenetic embryos fail to develop beyond the early limb bud stage as a result of the lack of paternal imprints in such embryos [6]. Recently, however, Kono et al. [7] and Kawahara et al. [8] generated live-born pups from mouse parthenogenetic embryos via nuclear transfer and altered expression of imprinted genes.

For protocols in which polar body extrusion is blocked, the timing of parthenogenetic activation relative to meiosis will determine the heterozygosity of the resultant pES cell line. pES cells derived from oocytes that were activated at meiosis I and in which first polar body extrusion is blocked are termed p(MI)ES cells [5, 9]. Because parental chromosome pairs fail to segregate, p(MI)ES cells retain pericentromeric heterozygosity. Because of recombination during early meiosis I, there will be increasing homozygosity with increasing distance from the centromere [Figures 2.1(b) and 2.2(a)]. Activation of oocytes during meiosis II along with blockage of extrusion of the second polar body will yield p(MII)ES cells. In these cells, there is pericentromeric homozygosity with distal heterozygosity [Figures 2.1(a) and 2.2(b)] [5]. pES cells derived from a haploid oocyte—termed *p(hap)ES cells*—contain a duplicated set of haploid chromosomes and so harbor the normal 2n DNA content, but are genetically homozygous at all loci [Figures 2.1(c) and 2.2(c)] [3]. In this chapter, we describe detailed protocols for creating parthenogenetic embryos and deriving pES cells.

2.2 Materials

These materials and formulations will be used for the generation of embryos and the derivation of ES cells from parthenotes.

2.2.1 Reagents

- Pregnant mare serum gonadotropin (PMSG; Calbiochem, 367222)
- Human chorionic gonadotropin (hCG; SIGMA, CG5)
- KSOM+AA (Millipore, MR-121-D)
- FHM (Millipore, MR-025-D)
- Acid tyrode solution (Millipore, MR-004-D)
- Dimethyl sulfoxide (DMSO; SIGMA, D2650)
- Cytochalasin B (SIGMA, C6762)
- Cytochalasin D (SIGMA, C8273)

2.2 Materials

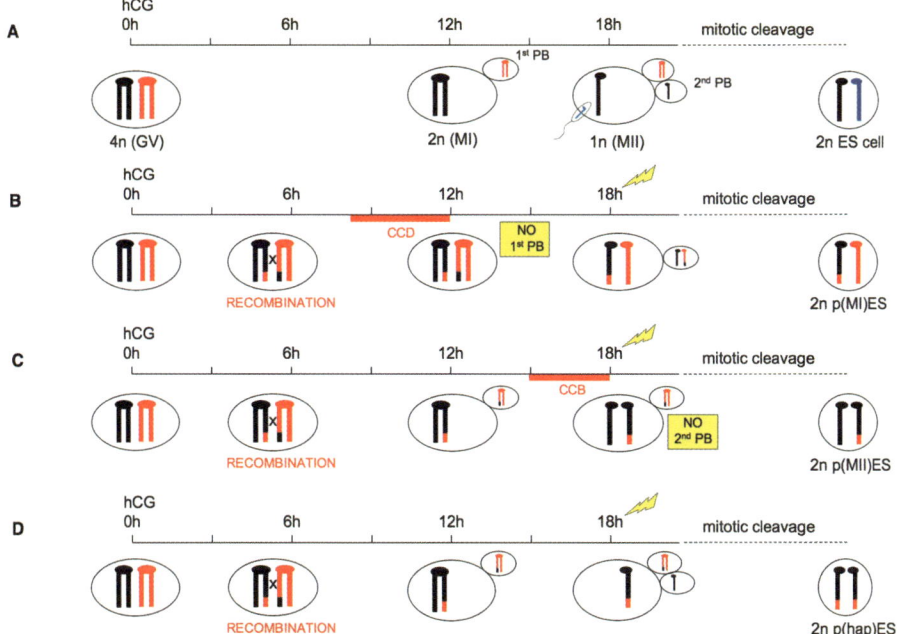

Figure 2.1 Chromosome dynamics, murine fertilization, and parthenogenetic oocyte activation. (a) Normal fertilization. Immature oocytes arrested at the first meiotic prophase contain 20 sets of paired homologous chromosomes. During meiosis I (MI), crossing over occurs as a function of distance from the centromere and, subsequently, the maternal or paternal chromosomes segregate into the first polar body (1st PB). At fertilization, half the chromosomes are extruded via the second polar body (2nd PB), and the incoming sperm restores the diploid chromosome complement. Blastocysts derived by fertilization yield fertilized embryonic stem cells (fES cells). (b) MI-arrested oocytes are activated in cytochalasin D, blocking extrusion of the 1st PB. Recombination events produce p(MI)ES cells with pericentric heterozygosity and distal homozygosity. (c) MII-arrested oocytes are activated in cytochalasin B, blocking extrusion of the 2nd PB. Recombination events produce p(MII)ES cells with pericentric homozygosity and distal heterozygosity. (d) Parthenogenetic activation in the absence of microtubule inhibitors results in a haploid pseudo-zygote. From the resultant blastocyst, homozygous diploid p(hap)ES cells can be derived.

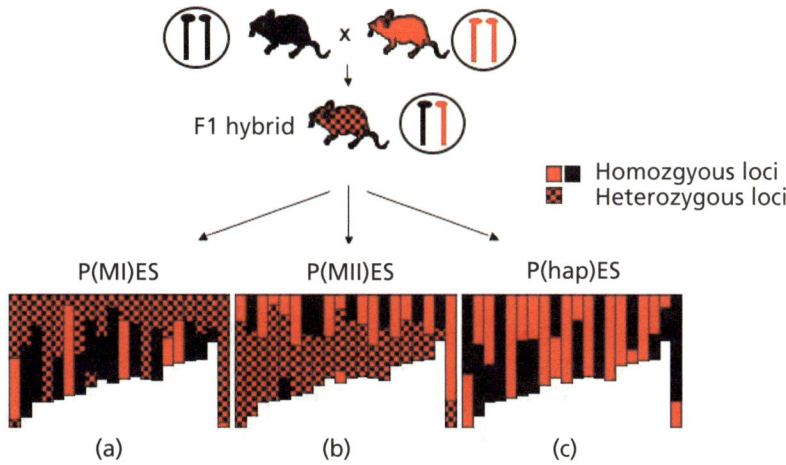

Figure 2.2 Diagram of heterozygosity by SNP analysis. (a) p(MI)ES: pericentromeric heterozygosity, distal homozygosity. (b) p(MII)ES: pericentromeric homozygosity, distal heterozygosity. (c) p(hap)ES: homozygous diploid, but the genomic content will be a mosaic of both parental genomes of the oocyte donor.

- Calcium ionophore (SIGMA, C7522)
- 6-Dimethylaminopurine (6-DMAP; SIGMA, D2629)
- Strontium chloride (SIGMA, 204463)
- Puromycin dihydrochloride, ready-made solution (SIGMA, P9620)
- Mineral oil (Fisher Scientific, O121-1)
- Hyaluronidase (SIGMA, H4272)
- Dulbecco's modified Eagle's medium (DMEM; Mediatech, 10-017-CV)
- Knockout serum replacement (Invitrogen, 10828-028)
- GlutaMax (Invitrogen, 35050-061)
- Penicillin–streptomycin (Invitrogen, 15070-063)
- ESGRO (Millipore, ESG1107)
- MEM nonessential amino acid solution (Invitrogen, 11140-050)
- 2-Mercaptoethanol (Invitrogen, 21985-023)
- Fetal bovine serum (FBS; GeminiBio, 100-106)
- Trypsin 0.25% ethylenediaminetetraacetic acid (EDTA) 0.04% (Invitrogen, 25200-072)
- Phosphate Buffered Saline (PBS)(–) (Mediatech, 21-040-CV)
- 0.1% Gelatin solution (Millipore, ES-006-B)
- 4% Paraformaldehyde (PFA; Electron Microscopy Sciences, 15710)
- Mouse anti-SSEA-1 immunoglobulin (Ig)M (Chemicon, MAB4301)
- Rabbit anti-Nanog IgG (Abcam, ab21603)
- Rabbit anti-Oct4 IgG (Abcam, ab19857)
- Alkaline phosphatase detection kit (Chemicon, SCR004)
- Alexa Fluor 594 goat antimouse IgM (Invitrogen, A-21044)
- Alexa Fluor 488 goat antirabbit IgG (Invitrogen, A-11034)
- ProLong Gold antifade reagent with DAPI (Invitrogen, P-36931)
- Triton X (Supelco, 21123)
- Tween 20 (SIGMA, P7949)
- Bovine collagen solution (StemCell technologies, 4902)
- Matrigel (SIGMA, E1270)

Mouse Strain

- B6CBA F1 female mice (The Jackson Laboratory, stock no. 100011, 4–6 weeks old)
- Immunodeficient mice: NOD SCID mice (Charles River Laboratories, strain code: 394, up to 42 days old)

2.2.2 Equipment

- Forceps (FST, 11002-13, 11050-10)
- Scissors (FST, 14058-11, 14060-09)
- No. 5 Dumont forceps (FST, 11295-10)
- 27G needle (BD, 305109)
- 1-mL syringe (BD, 309602)
- Mouth pipette (SIGMA, A5177)
- Drummond glass pipette (Sutter Instruments, B100-75-10)
- 35-mm Petri dish (Falcon, 351008)
- 96-well plate (Falcon, 353072)

- 24-well plate (Falcon, 353047)
- P200 pipette (Denville Scientific, P1122)
- P1000 pipette (Denville Scientific, P1123)
- Syringe filter (VWR, 28144-040)
- Bottle top filter (0.22 μm: Corning, 531096; 0.45 μm: VWR, 87006-070)
- Incubator
- Stereomicroscope
- Inverted microscope

2.2.3 Media recipe

Embryonic Stem Cell Derivation Media (100 mL)[a]

Component	Unit
DMEM	82 mL
Knockout serum replacement	15 mL
Nonessential amino acid solution	1 mL
GlutaMax (200-mM stock)	1 mL
Penicillin–streptomycin	1 mL
2-Mercaptoethanol	100 μL
ESGRO (10^7 U)	20 μL

[a]Filter and store at 4°C.

Embryonic Stem Cell Culture Media (100 mL)[a]

Component	Unit
DMEM	82 mL
Fetal bovine serum[b]	15 mL
Nonessential amino acid solution	1 mL
GlutaMax (200-mM stock)	1 mL
Penicillin–streptomycin	1 mL
2-Mercaptoethanol	100 μL
ESGRO (10^7 U)	10 μL

[a]Filter and store at 4°C.
[b]Heat inactivate (treat at 56°C for 30 minutes) and store at −20°C.

Mouse Fetal Fibroblast Media (100 mL)[a]

Component	Unit (mL)
DMEM	87
Fetal bovine serum[b]	10
Nonessential amino acid solution	1
GlutaMax (200-mM stock)	1
Penicillin–streptomycin	1

[a]Filter and store at 4°C.
[b]Heat inactivate (treat at 56°C for 30 minutes) and store at −20°C.

Strontium Solution (1M Stock)[a]

Component	Unit
Strontium chloride	266 mg
Double-distilled water	1 mL

[a]Filter and store at 4°C.

Hyaluronidase (0.1%)[a]

Component	Unit
Hyaluronidase	10 mg
FHM	10 mL

[a]Filter and store at –20°C.

Cytochalasin B (1-mg/mL Stock)[a]

Component	Unit
Cytochalasin B	1 mg
DMSO	1 mL

[a]Store at –20°C.

Cytochalasin D (1-mg/mL Stock)[a]

Component	Unit
Cytochalasin D	1 mg
DMSO	1 mL

[a]Store at –20°C.

Calcium Ionophore (Ionomycin, 5-mM Stock)[a]

Component	Unit
Calcium ionophore	1 mg
DMSO	267.6 μL

[a]Store at –20°C.

DMAP (200-mM Stock)[a]

Component	Unit
6-DMAP	100 mg
PBS(–)	3.06 mL

[a]Dissolve in 90°C water bath and store at –20°C for up to 6 months.

Mineral Oil

1. Filter by bottle top filter (0.45-μm pore size).
2. Store at room temperature and protect from light.

Pregnant Mare Serum Gonadotropin (100 IU)[a]

Component	Unit
PMSG	1,000 IU
PBS(–)	10 mL

[a]Store at –20°C.

Human Chorionic Gonadotropin (100 IU)[a]

Component	Unit
hCG	5000 IU
PBS(–)	50 mL

[a]Store at –20°C.

Calcium Free KSOM+AA Media (500 mL)[a]

Component	Catalog No.	mM	Unit
NaCl	Sigma S5886	95	2.775g
KCl	Sigma P9333	2.5	0.093g
KH_2PO_4	Sigma P5655	0.35	0.0238g
$MgSO_4\,7H_2O$	Sigma M5921	0.2	0.025g
Sodium lactate (60% syrup)	Sigma L7900	10	1.18 mL
Sodium pyruvate	Sigma P4562	0.2	0.011g
Glucose	Sigma G6152	0.2	0.018g
L-glutamine (200-mM stock)	Invitrogen25030-081	1	2.5 mL
BSA	Sigma A3311	—	0.5g
EDTA 4 Na (10-mM stock)	Sigma E5391	0.01	0.5 mL
$NaHCO_3$	Sigma S5761	25.4	1.05g
MEM amino acid (×50)	Invitrogen11130-051	—	10 mL
Nonessential amino acid (×100)	Invitrogen11140-050	—	5 mL
Penicillin–streptomycin (×100)	Invitrogen15070-063	—	5 mL
Phenol red (0.5%)	Sigma P3532	—	1 mL

[a]Filter and store at 4°C for up to 2 weeks or store at −20° for up to a month.

2.3 Methods

For the following experiments, the most convenient lighting cycle for the mouse facility is darkness from 7 pm to 5 am and light from 5 a.m. to 7 p.m. To prepare the culture media, make the drops of culture media and cover them with mineral oil. Equilibrate them in an incubator (37°C, 5% CO_2, 95% air) at least 3 hours to overnight (Figure 2.3).

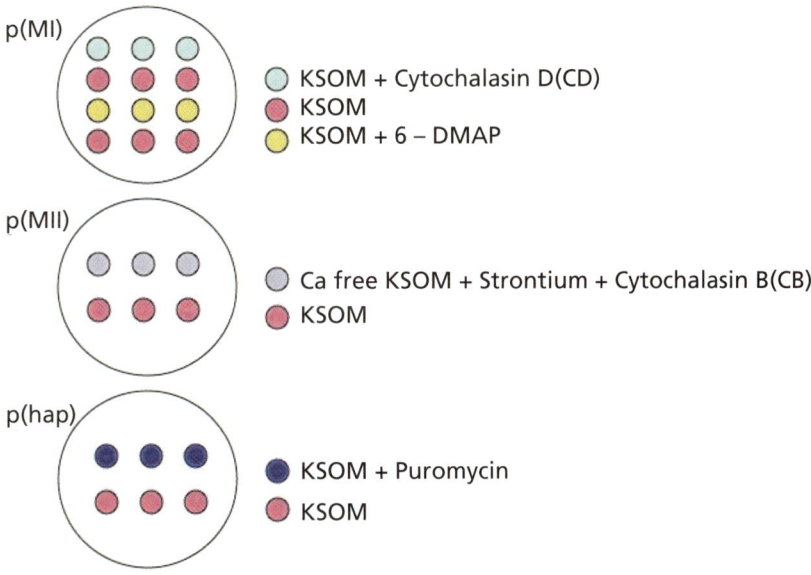

Figure 2.3 Diagram of culture drops.

2.3.1 Generation of p(MI) embryos

1. Give 5 IU (50 μL 100 IU stock) PMSG via intraperitoneal injection into each B6CBA F1 female.
2. Give 5 IU (50 μL 100 IU stock) hCG via intraperitoneal injection 48 hours after PMSG.
3. Collect ovaries 7 to 9 hours after hCG injection and place them in a 35-mm Petri dish with FHM media. Puncture the expanded follicles [Figure 2.4(a)] using a 27G needle to collect oocytes [Figure 2.4(b)].
4. Treat oocytes with hyaluronidase for 2 minutes. Agitate gently by aspirating up and down carefully until nearly all the cumulus cells are dispersed from the oocytes [Figure 2.4(c)].
5. Wash oocytes three times with FHM.
6. Culture oocytes in KSOM+AA containing 5 μg/mL cytochalasin D for 3 hours in incubator (37°C, 5% CO_2, 95% air).
7. Wash oocytes three times with FHM.
8. Culture oocytes in KSOM+AA for 6 hours in incubator (37°C, 5% CO_2, 95% air).
9. Activate oocytes in FHM containing 10 μM calcium ionophore for 5 minutes followed by culturing in KSOM+AA supplemented with 2 mM DMAP for 3 hours in incubator.
10. Wash oocytes three times with FHM.
11. Culture activated oocytes in KSOM+AA in incubator (37°C, 5% CO_2, 95% air) for 4 days.
12. Assess blastocyst formation.

2.3.2 Generation of p(MII) embryos

1. Give 5 IU (50 μL 100 IU stock) PMSG via intraperitoneal injection into each B6CBA F1 female.
2. Give 5 IU (50 μL 100 IU stock) hCG via intraperitoneal injection 48 hours after PMSG.
3. Collect oviducts 16 to 18 hours after hCG injection and place them in a 35-mm Petri dish with hyaluronidase.
4. Puncture the oviduct at the ampulla, take out the oocytes with the cumulus cells, and culture them in hyaluronidase for 1 to 2 minutes until cumulus cells partially fall off (Figure 2.5).

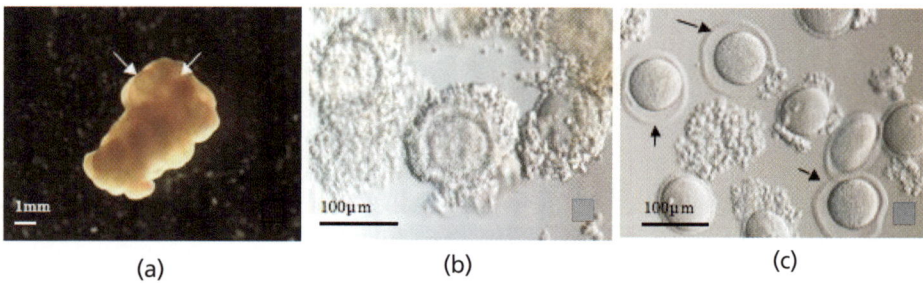

(a)   (b)   (c)

Figure 2.4 Collection of MI oocytes. (a) Ovary with expanded follicles (white arrows). (b) Oocytes with cumulus cells. (c) MI oocytes (black arrows).

2.3 Methods

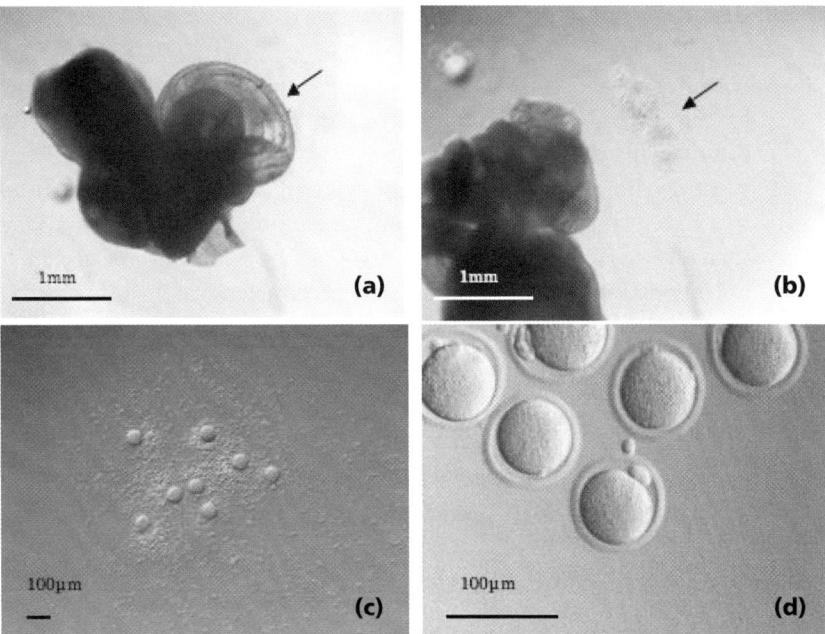

Figure 2.5 Collection of MII oocytes. (a) Oviduct with swollen ampulla (black arrow). (b) Oocytes with cumulus cells after puncturing the ampulla (black arrow). (c) Oocytes in hyaluronidase. (d) MI oocytes.

5. Transfer the oocytes into fresh FHM in a 35-mm Petri dish.
6. Denude the oocytes by pipetting gently.
7. Wash the oocytes two times with FHM.
8. Transfer the oocytes into calcium-free KSOM supplemented with 10 mM strontium solution and 5 μg/mL cytochalasin B, and culture them for 5 hours in an incubator (37°C, 5% CO_2, 95% air).
9. Wash the oocytes three times with FHM.
10. Culture the oocytes in KSOM+AA in an incubator (37°C, 5% CO_2, 95% air) for 4 days.
11. Assess blastocyst formation.

2.3.3 Generation of p(hap) embryos

1. Give 5 IU (50 μL 100 IU stock) PMSG via intraperitoneal injection into each B6CBA F1 female.
2. Give 5 IU (50 μL 100 IU stock) hCG via intraperitoneal injection 48 hours after PMSG.
3. Collect oviducts 16 to 18 hours after hCG injection and place them in a 35-mm Petri dish with hyaluronidase.
4. Puncture the oviduct at the ampulla, take out the oocytes with cumulus cells, and culture them in hyaluronidase for 1 to 2 minutes until cumulus cells partially fall off.
5. Transfer oocytes into another 35-mm Petri dish with FHM.

6. Denude oocytes by pipetting gently.
7. Wash oocytes two times with FHM.
8. Activate oocytes in FHM containing 10-μM calcium ionophore for 5 minutes followed by culturing in 10 μg/mL puromycin diluted in KSOM (1:1,000 from ready-made solution) in an incubator (37°C, 5% CO_2, 95% air) for 4 hours.
9. Wash two times in FHM. Observe oocytes using inverted microscope and select those that have two polar bodies and only one pronucleus, which should represent more than 80% of the population. The first polar body may not be visible, but the second polar body is quite large and only one pronucleus can be visualized [Figure 2.6(b)]. Some oocytes may have failed to extrude the second polar body and will have two pronuclei [Figure 2.6(a)].
10. Culture oocytes in KSOM+AA in an incubator (37°C, 5% CO_2, 95% air) for 4 days.
11. Assess blastocyst formation.

2.3.4 Derivation of p(MI), p(MII), and p(hap) ES cells

The following techniques should be performed in a sterile environment.

Day 1 (1 Day before Embryos Reach Blastocyst Stage)

1. Treat 96-well plate with 100 μL per well 0.1% gelatin for 20 minutes at room temperature.
2. Aspirate gelatin solution and plate mitotically inactivated mouse embryo fibroblast cells (MEF) at a density of 0.6×10^5 cells/200 μL.

Day 2 (Embryos at Blastocyst Stage, Ready to Plate)

3. Aspirate MEF media in a 96-well plate and add 200 μL ES cell derivation media.
4. Treat blastocyst embryos with acid tyrode solution until zona pellucida dissolves (<1 minute) in a 35-mm Petri dish (Figure 2.7).
5. Wash embryos two times with FHM.
6. Plate each blastocyst into a single well of a 96-well plate.
7. Culture in an incubator (37°C, 5% CO_2, 95% air) for 10 days.

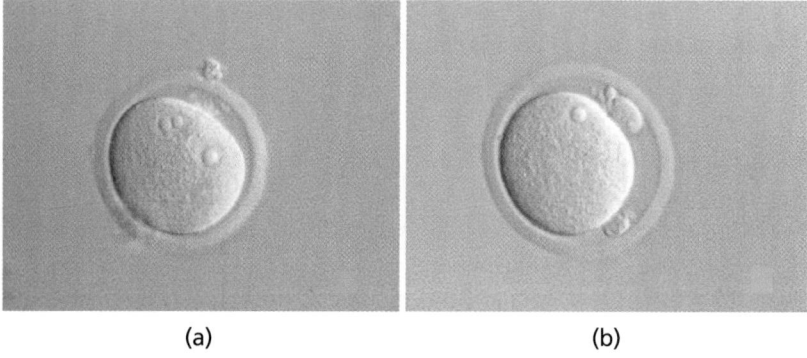

(a)   (b)

Figure 2.6 Parthenogenetically activated oocytes. (a) p(MII) oocytes after activation. (b) p(hap) oocytes after activation.

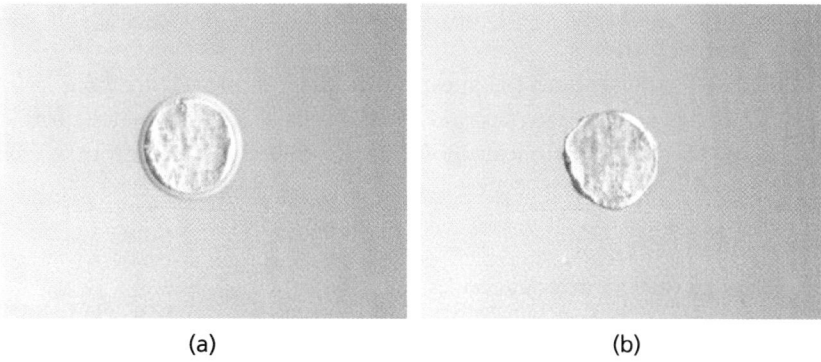

Figure 2.7 Blastocyst from parthenogenesis. (a) Blastocyst before treatment in acid tyrode solution. (b) Blastocyst after treatment in acid tyrode solution.

Day 11

8. Treat a 24-well plate with 1 mL 0.1% gelatin for 20 minutes at room temperature.
9. Aspirate gelatin solution and plate inactivated mouse fetal fibroblast cells on the plate.

Day 12

10. Aspirate MEF media in a 24-well plate and add 2 mL ES cell derivation media.
11. Aspirate ES cell derivation media from 96 wells and wash with PBS(−) once.
12. Add 40 μL trypsin EDTA.
13. Let them sit until individual cells can be recognized in the ICM outgrowth [Figure 2.8(c)].

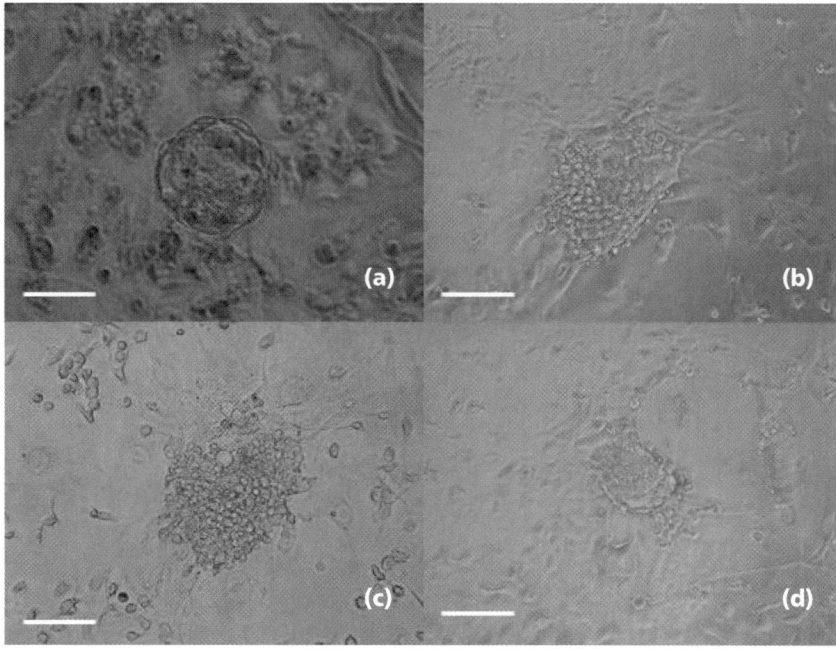

Figure 2.8 Derivation of parthenogenetic ES cells. (a) Blastocyst. (b) ICM outgrowth 10 days after plating. (c) Trypsinization of ICM outgrowth. (d) ES cell colony passes from (c). Scale bar = 100 μm.

14. Pipette ICM outgrowth with 100 μL MEF media and transfer into a single well of a 24-well plate.
15. ES cell colonies start to appear 2 days after plating [Figure 2.8(d)].
16. Change media every day and expand cells as previously described [2]. We usually use ES cell derivation media for two to three passages and then change to ES cell culture media.

2.3.5 ES cell characterization

2.3.5.1 Alkaline phosphatase staining

1. Fix ES cells with 4% PFA in PBS for 1 to 2 minutes.
2. Wash cells three times with PBS(–) containing 0.05% Tween 20.
3. During third washing, prepare reagent [mix fast red violet with naphthol AS-BI phosphate solution and water in a 2:1:1 ratio (all reagents are in the kit)].
4. Add stain solution and incubate in dark at room temperature for 15 to 20 minutes.
5. Wash wells with PBS(–) containing 0.05% Tween 20 two times and cover wells with PBS(–).

Alkaline phosphatase staining is also described in the kit data sheet (Chemicon, SCR004).

2.3.5.2 Immunohistochemistry

1. Fix ES cells with 4% PFA in PBS for 30 minutes.
2. Wash three times with PBS.
3. Permeabilize ES cells with 0.2% triton X/PBS for 30 minutes.
4. Treat ES cells with blocking solution (3% BSA in PBS) for 2 hours.
5. Dilute antibodies to working concentrations in blocking solution (SSEA-1, 1:100; Oct4, 1:200; Nanog, 1:200) and incubate overnight at 4°C.
6. Wash three times with PBS.
7. Dilute secondary antibodies in PBS (1:500) and incubate in dark for 3 hours at 4°C.
8. Wash three times with PBS.
9. Dilute antifade solution in PBS (1:20) and cover the wells.
10. Observe via epifluorescence microscope.

2.3.5.3 Karyotyping and fluorescence in situ hybridization

This analysis can be performed by a service company such as Cell Line genetics (http://www.clgenetics.com).

2.3.6 Teratoma induction

1. Suspend 10^6 ES cells in 50 μL 1:1:2 mixture of bovine collagen, matrigel, and MEF media (keep mixture on ice).

2. Inject intramuscularly in quadriceps of hind leg of immunodeficient mouse.
3. Teratoma will appear as a firm mass in 6 to 8 weeks.
4. Dissect teratoma from mouse and fix with 4% PFA overnight. Change into 70% ethanol and store at 4°C.
5. Sectioning and histological staining can be performed by a service facility.

2.4 Data Acquisition, Anticipated Results, and Interpretation

Oocytes (at collection, and before and after treatment with hyaluronidase and calcium ionophore), blastocysts (before and after acidic tyrode treatment), blastocyst outgrowth, and early-passage ES cells are pictured earlier. Immunostaining can be done to confirm ES cell-specific protein and cell surface marker expression (Figure 2.9). Karyotyping data is also important for ES cell characterization. Normal karyotype is 2n = 40 in mouse. We consider it to be karyotypically normal if 80% of ES cells have the normal chromosome number.

2.5 Discussion and Commentary

Timing is critical for the success of parthenogenetic activation and subsequent preimplantation embryonic development. For example, MII oocytes begin to age within 24 hours after hCG injection as a result of decreasing cytostatic factor activity. As a result, activation efficiency will suffer dramatically. Oocytes and embryos are sensitive to ambient conditions, including light, heat, and physical stimulation. Work quickly to minimize time outside the incubator and be wary that exposure to chemicals adheres to the guidelines presented earlier. Equilibrate media in the

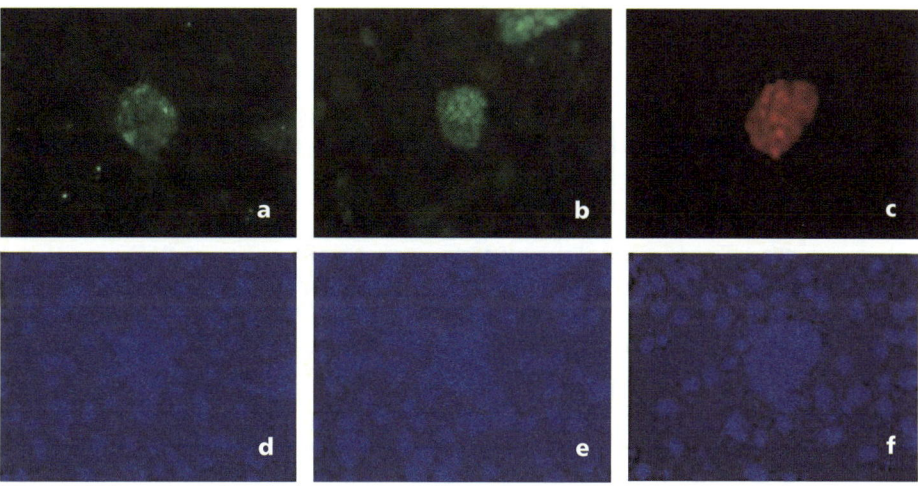

Figure 2.9 Immunohistochemistry of parthenogenetic ES cells. (a–f) SSEA-1 is stained cell surface (a), and Oct4 and Nanog are nucleus staining (b, c). DAPI is stained nucleus of both feeder cells and ES cells (d–f).

incubator at least 3 hours (or overnight) prior to use. The quality of mineral oil can affect embryo development and may vary from batch to batch. Mineral oil has to be tested by lot number and filtered prior to use. Mineral oil has a limited shelf life and should be used within 2 months after delivery from the supplier. Overall health and maintenance of the oocyte donor mice is also of importance to ensure good oocyte yield after superovulation.

The most common problem during ES cell derivation is differentiation after trypsinization of the ICM outgrowth. For the protocol described earlier, it is important that the ICM outgrowth is completely trypsinized to a single-cell suspension prior to replating. The trypsin must be adequately neutralized with serum-containing media after trypsin treatment. Thus, be sure to use the appropriate amounts of trypsin and media as described earlier.

Newly derived mouse ES cells must be characterized properly. It is imperative that the lines have a normal karyotype and differentiate appropriately (as determined by teratoma formation assay or blastocyst chimerism/complementation). We recommend that ES cells are karyotyped every 10 to 15 passages. Additional problems and suggested solutions are discussed in the troubleshooting table.

Troubleshooting Table

Problem	Explanation	Potential Solutions
Low oocyte yield	Poor-quality hormones	Make fresh hormones. Do not refreeze.
Poor oocyte activation	Oocytes are aged or were collected at an inappropriate time relative to ovulation	Follow the correct hormone administration and oocyte collection timing noted earlier. Consider altering oocyte collection by 1 to 2 hours to achieve better results.
	Activation media not appropriate	Prepare fresh media and calcium ionophore.
Oocyte death during activation	Media not equilibrated	Equilibrate media at least 3 hours to overnight prior to use. Prepare fresh.
ICM outgrowth is observed, but no ES cell colonies isolated	ICM outgrowth not adequately dissociated into single cells	Treat cells with trypsin until ICM is completely dispersed into single cells.
Differentiation observed in early-passage ES cells	Trypsin used to passage cells not adequately neutralized	Increase the amount of serum-containing media used to neutralize trypsin.
	MEF density too low	A total of 90% to 100% confluent MEFs are required.

2.6 Summary Points

1. Parthenogenesis and the resultant ES cells are powerful tools to study a myriad of biological processes, including meiosis, chromosomal segregation, cell cycle regulation, activation, preimplantation development, and ES cell derivation.
2. Timing of parthenogenetic activation with with respect to the meiosis will generate a distinct pattern of genetic heterozygosity.
    i. p(MI)ES: pericentromeric heterozygosity, distal homozygosity.
    ii. p(MII)ES: pericentromeric homozygosity, distal heterozygosity.
    iii. p(hap)ES: homozygous diploid, but the genomic content will be a mosaic of both parental genomes of the oocyte donor.

3. In this chapter, we described methods for deriving heterozygous and homozygous parthenogenetic mouse ES cells. Diploid human parthenogenetic ES cells have been derived and may offer therapeutic potential [11, 12].

Acknowledgments

The authors thank Dr. M. William Lensch, Dr. Kitai Kim, and Kerrianne Cunniff for help with the preparation of this manuscript. The experiments described were supported by grants from the Harvard Stem Cell Institute, Children's Hospital Boston, and Howard Hughes Medical Institute. G. Q. D. is a recipient of the Burroughs Wellcome Fund Clinical Scientist Award and the National Institutes of Health Director's Pioneer Award.

References

[1] Balakier, H., and A. K. Tarkowski, "Diploid Parthenogenetic Mouse Embryos Produced by Heat-Shock and Cytochalasin B," *J. Embryol. Exp. Morphol.*, Vol. 35, 1976, pp. 25–39.
[2] Evans, M. J., and M. H. Kaufman, "Establishment in Culture of Pluripotential Cells from Mouse Embryos," *Nature*, Vol. 292, 1981, pp. 154–156.
[3] Robertson, E. J., M. J. Evans, and M. H. Kaufman, "X-Chromosome Instability in Pluripotential Stem Cell Lines Derived from Parthenogenetic Embryos," *J. Embryol. Exp. Morphol.*, Vol. 74, 1983, pp. 297–309.
[4] Kaufman, M. H., et al., "Establishment of Pluripotential Cell Lines from Haploid Mouse Embryos," *J. Embryol. Exp. Morphol.*, Vol. 73, 1983, pp. 249–261.
[5] Kim, K., et al., "Histocompatible Embryonic Stem Cells by Parthenogenesis," *Science*, Vol. 315, 2007, pp. 482–486.
[6] Surani, M. A., S. C. Barton, and M. L. Norris, "Development of Reconstituted Mouse Eggs Suggests Imprinting of the Genome During Gametogenesis," *Nature*, Vol. 308, 1984, pp. 548–550.
[7] Kono, T., et al., "Birth of Parthenogenetic Mice That Can Develop to Adulthood," *Nature*, Vol. 428, 2004, pp. 860–864.
[8] Kawahara, M., et al., "High-Frequency Generation of Viable Mice from Engineered Bi-maternal Embryos," *Nat. Biotechnol.*, Vol. 25, 2007, pp. 1045–1050.
[9] Kubiak, J., et al., "Genetically Identical Parthenogenetic Mouse Embryos Produced by Inhibition of the First Meiotic Cleavage with Cytochalasin D," *Development*, Vol. 111, 1991, pp. 763–769.
[10] Nakasaka, H., et al., "Effective Activation Method with A23187 and Puromycin to Produce Haploid Parthenogenones from Freshly Ovulated Mouse Oocytes," *Zygote*, Vol. 8, 2000, pp. 203–208.
[11] Revazova, E. S., et al., "HLA Homozygous Stem Cell Lines Derived from Human Parthenogenetic Blastocysts," *Cloning Stem Cells*, Vol. 10, 2008, pp. 11–24.
[12] Revazova, E. S., et al., "Patient-Specific Stem Cell Lines Derived from Human Parthenogenetic Blastocysts," *Cloning Stem Cells*, Vol. 9, 2007, pp. 432–449.

CHAPTER

3

Generation of Mice from Embryonic Stem Cells Using Tetraploid Embryos as Hosts

Hiroshi Ohta and Teruhiko Wakayama

Laboratory for Genomic Reprogramming
Center for Developmental Biology, RIKEN
2-2-3 Minatojima-minamimachi, Chuo-ku, Kobe 650-0047, Japan

Abstract

Tetraploid (4n) embryos complemented with embryonic stem (ES) cells can develop into normal progeny, in which the embryonic lineages are derived entirely from the ES cells, and extraembryonic lineages arise largely from the tetraploid component (ES mice). ES mice can be used for the generation of gene-targeted mouse cell lines or for assessment of ES cell pluripotency, however low birth rates of ES mice limit their applicability. ES mice are typically produced by aggregating ES cells with four-cell stage 4n embryos or by injecting ES cells into 4n-embryo blastoceles. Recently, we improved the birthrate of ES mice by using multiple 4n embryos as hosts. Here we describe our procedure and compare the aggregation and injection methods using the same ES cell lines.

Key Terms Tetraploid complementation assay
embryonic stem cell
pluripotency

3.1 Introduction

Mouse chimeras are commonly used to establish genetically modified mouse strains. Chimeric mice are usually produced by injecting embryonic stem (ES) cells into diploid (2n) host preimplantation embryos [1] composed of modified donor cells and cells derived from the host embryo. The contribution of donor ES cells to the germline of chimeric mice allows the generation of mouse strains carrying the ES cell haplotype. The production of a mutant strain using this procedure is time intensive and may take more than 12 months before adult mutants can be analyzed. To accelerate the production of mutant mouse lines, a tetraploid (4n) embryo complementation assay has also been established [2, 3]. Because 4n embryos are incapable of completing normal development [4, 5], ES cells aggregated with 4n embryos develop into conceptuses in which embryonic lineages are derived entirely from ES cells, and extraembryonic lineages arise largely from the 4n component [2, 3]. Mice derived from ES cells (ES mice) show normal phenotypes, growth, and fertility [3], indicating that they can be used as founders to establish mouse lines. Because all germ cells in ES mice are derived from ES cells, germline transmission of ES cells is easier in ES mice than in 2n chimeric mice. Thus, producing ES $\leftrightarrow$ 4n embryos would be effective for analyzing gene function in vivo.

Although the methodology to produce ES mice derived from ES cell lines was described more than a decade ago [2, 3], its application remains limited because of a low recovery rate of viable mice [2, 3]. Technical improvement of the technique for producing ES mice was mainly carried out from the viewpoint of establishing ES cell lines (i.e., previous research focused on how to generate ES cell lines with higher potential for producing ES mice). This strategy significantly improved the technique through the discovery that ES cell lines derived from hybrid mouse strains support the development of viable ES mice at a higher degree than inbred ES cells [6]. Although the effect of donor ES cells on the production of ES mice has been well studied, the technique remains limited because ES mice can only be generated from specific ES cell lines [6] and cannot be applied to cell lines widely used for gene targeting.

Recently, we improved the technique by increasing the cell number of 4n host embryos to enhance production of ES mice [7]. Because this technique produces more functional 4n host embryos, it can be applied to any ES cell line. Here, we describe our procedure [7] and compare it with the blastocyst injection technique [8].

3.2 Experimental Design

ES cells were aggregated with three tetraploid (3 × 4n) embryos and transferred into pseudo-pregnant females. The birthrate with our technique varies from 0% to 14%, depending on the potential of the established ES cell line. Therefore, we recommend the preparation of 50 to 100 aggregated embryos per ES cell line. We also compared the birthrate of ES mice with that of the blastocyst injection technique. Both techniques can produce ES mice, but the 3 × 4n embryo technique is easier to perform, whereas the blastocyst injection technique is effective for assessing donor cell function, because micromanipulation allows the researcher to select donor cells.

3.3 Materials

3.3.1 Preparation of 4n embryos: Mice and reagents

- Mice: Any mouse strain can be used; however, hybrid strains (e.g., B6D2F1) or closed-colony mice (e.g., ICR) usually have more ovulations than inbred strains, which may produce embryos that are more difficult to culture. Mating or in vitro fertilization (IVF) can be used to obtain the embryos. In this study, we used B6D2F1 (C57BL/6 × DBA/2) and ICR females for oocyte collection. B6D2F1 oocytes were fertilized with B6D2F1 sperm by IVF. In some experiments fertilized embryos were collected from the oviducts of females after mating.
- Equine chorionic gonadotropin (eCG) or pregnant mare serum gonadotropin (PMSG, Sigma)
- Human chorionic gonadotropin (hCG; Sigma)
- Mineral oil (Sigma)
- Hyaluronidase (Specialty Media; Hyclone; ThermoScientific)
- 0.3M mannitol solution (Sigma)
- TYH medium for IVF [9]: 119.37 mM NaCl, 4.78 mM KCl, 1.71 mM $CaCl_2$, 1.19 mM $MgSO_4$, 1.19 mM KH_2PO_4, 1.00 mM sodium pyruvate, 5.56 mM d-glucose, 25.07 mM $NaHCO_3$, 50 µg/mL penicillin G, 70 µg/mL streptomycin, 0.1 mL phenol red (10 mg/mL solution in saline), and 4 mg/mL bovine serum albumin (BSA)
- CZB medium for oocyte culture [10]: 81.62 mM NaCl, 4.83 mM KCl, 1.70 mM $CaCl_2$ · $2H_2O$, 1.18 mM $MgSO_4$ · $7H_2O$, 1.18 mM KH_2PO_4, 0.11 mM ethylenediaminetetraacetic acid (EDTA) · 2 Na, 25.12 mM $NaHCO_3$, 31.3 mM sodium lactate, 0.27 mM sodium pyruvate, 5.55 mM d-glucose, 1.00 mM l-glutamine, 50 µg/mL penicillin G, 70 µg/mL streptomycin, 0.1 mL phenol red (10 mg/mL in saline), and 5 mg/mL BSA
- HEPES-CZB medium for embryo manipulation: CZB medium without BSA, with the 5 mM $NaHCO_3$, 20 mM HEPES sodium salt, and 0.1 mg/mL polyvinyl acetate

3.3.2 Preparation of 4n embryos: Equipment

- Stereomicroscope (Olympus)
- Transfer pipettes (80- to 100-µm internal bore diameter) for manipulating embryos.
- Electro cell fusion system (Model LF101; Nepagene)

3.3.3 ES cells and culture conditions

- ES cell lines: Two independent ES cell lines were used to generate the ES mice. The E14 ES cell line [11] was derived in 1985 from the 129/Ola inbred mouse strain by Dr. Martin Hooper in Edinburgh, Scotland, and obtained from Dr. Peter Mombaerts (Rockefeller University). 129B6F1G1 [12] is a nuclear transfer-derived ES (ntES) cell line previously established in our laboratory using Sertoli cells of 129B6F1 background with green fluorescent protein (GFP) as donor for nuclear transfer.
- ES cell medium (for maintenance): Knockout DMEM (Invitrogen) supplemented with 20% heat-inactivated fetal bovine serum (FBS; Sigma), 1,000 U leukemia inhibitory

factor/mL (Invitrogen), 1% penicillin–streptomycin (Invitrogen), 1% l-glutamine (Specialty Media), 1% nonessential amino acids (Specialty Media), 1% nucleosides (Specialty Media), and 1% β-mercaptoethanol (Specialty Media)
- Ca/Mg-free phosphate-buffered saline (Sigma)
- Trypsin/EDTA solution (GIBCO, Invitrogen)
- Acidic tyrode's solution (Specialty Media)

3.3.4 Micromanipulation system

- Inverted microscope (Olympus, IX 81)
- Microinjector (Narishige, IM-6-2)
- Piezo drive (Primetech, PMAS-01150)
- Microforge (Narishige, MF-900)
- Micropipette Puller Instrument (Shutter Instruments, P-97)
- Borosilicate glass (OD, 1 mm; ID, 0.75 mm; Shutter Instruments)

3.4 Methods

3.4.1 Preparation of host embryos

Females were injected with 5 IU eCG to induce superovulation (day 1 in Figure 3.1), followed by a second injection of 5 IU hCG 48 hours later (day 3 in Figure 3.1). The host 4n

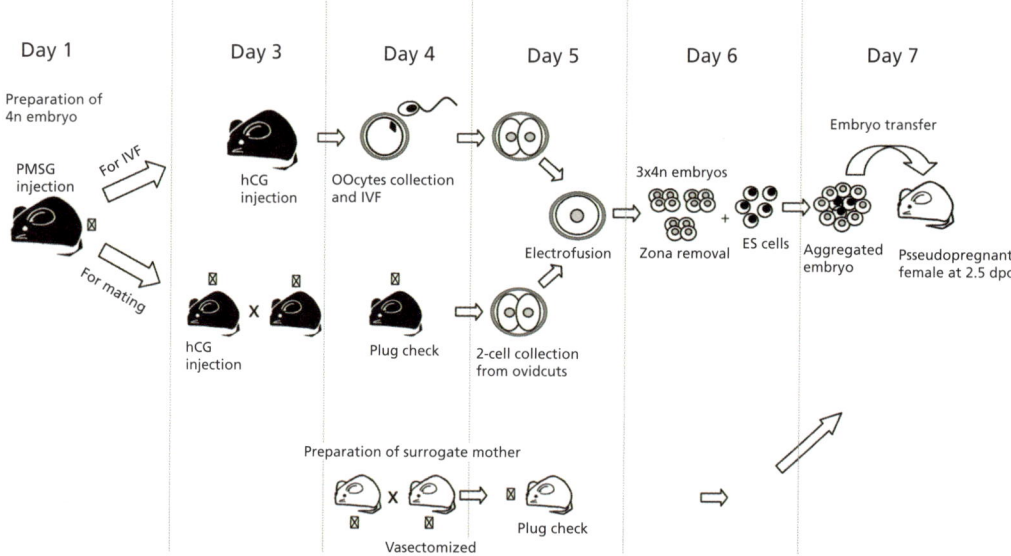

Figure 3.1 Time course for the 4n complementation assay using multiple 4n embryos. Day 1, females were injected with PMSG to induce superovulation in preparation for the 4n host embryos. Day 3, females were injected with PMSG on day 1 and injected with hCG on day 3 to prepare 4n embryos by IVF. To prepare 4n embryos by mating, females were injected with hCG and were mated with normal males. Day 4, IVF was performed. The plug was checked, and surrogate mothers were mated. Day 5, the two-cell stage embryos were collected and electrofused to induce 4n embryos. The plugs of females mated with vasectomized males were checked. Day 6, ES cells were aggregated with three 4n embryos. Day 7, aggregated embryos were transferred into the surrogate mother at 2.5 days postconception.

embryos can be prepared from either IVF or mating. For IVF, sperm were isolated from the cauda epididymis of mature males using the swim-up technique and were placed in TYH medium. Cumulus-intact, metaphase II-arrested oocytes were prepared from the females 14 hours after hCG injection and were inseminated with capacitated sperm (1 · 105 cells/mL; day 4 in Figure 3.1). Zygotes with two pronuclei were collected and cultured in CZB medium for 24 hours to obtain two-cell stage embryos (day 5 in Figure 3.1). For the preparation of embryos by mating, the superovulated females were mated with males (day 3 in Figure 3.1), and two-cell stage embryos were collected from the oviduct (day 5 in Figure 3.1). The two-cell stage embryos prepared by IVF and mating were used for electrofusion.

3.4.2 Electrofusion of two-cell stage embryos

The two-cell stage embryos were electrofused with an electrocell fusion system (model LF101, Nepagene). The two-cell stage embryos [Figure 3.2(a)] were transferred into a drop of 0.3M mannitol, and 10 to 20 embryos were placed single file between the electrodes. After charging the electrical pulse [20V alternating current (ac) at 2 MHz for 2 seconds followed by 60V direct current (dc) for 20 μsec], the embryos were cultured in CZB medium, and cell fusion was verified on day 5 [Figures 3.1 and 3.2(b)]. The fused embryos were cultured in CZB medium overnight at 37°C under 5% CO_2 until they developed to the two- to four-cell stage [Figure 3.2(c)].

3.4.3 Removal of the zona pellucida

The zonae pellucidae of the 4n embryos were removed with acidic Tyrode's solution (day 6, Figure 3.1). The two- to four-cell stage embryos were collected and transferred into HEPES-CZB medium. Then, 10 to 15 embryos were transferred into a drop of acidic tyrode's solution. The embryos were transferred into a new drop of acidic tyrode's solution and gently pipetted until the zonae pellucidae were removed [Figure 3.2(c)]. The embryos were then cultured in CZB medium.

3.4.4 Generation of ES ↔ multiple 4n embryos by aggregation

Three zona-free embryos were placed in small holes in a plastic dish (day 6, Figure 3.1). CZB drops covered with mineral oil were prepared in a 6-cm plastic dish [Figure 3.2(d)], and holes were created by pressing the tip of a pair of scissors into the bottom of the plastic dish [Figure 3.2(e–g)].

The ES cells were treated with a trypsin/EDTA solution and agitated mildly with a micropipette so as not to dissociate them into a single cell. ES medium was added to inactivate the trypsin, and the cells were transferred into a new tube. The ES cell suspension was then transferred into a drop of CZB [Figure 3.2(g)], and a clump of 8 to 15 ES cells [Figure 3.2(g, h)] was added to each hole that previously contained three 4n embryos [Figure 3.2(g, h)]. After a 24-hour incubation, the aggregates developed to the morula or blastocyst stage [Figure 3.2(h)], and 10 to 15 embryos were transferred to a pseudo-pregnant ICR-strain female [2.5 days postconception (dpc); day 7, Figure 3.1] and then analyzed at 18.5 or 19.5 dpc.

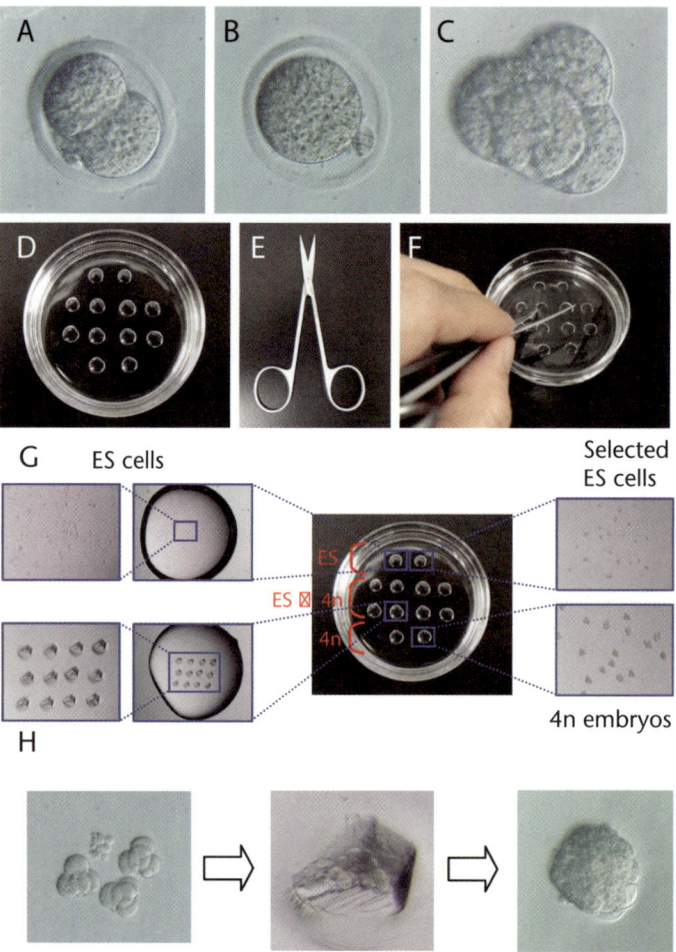

Figure 3.2 Procedure for generating ES ↔ 3 × 4n embryos. (a) A two-cell stage embryo before electrofusion. (b) An embryo after electrofusion. (c) A four-cell stage 4n embryo after 24 hours of culture. The zona pellucida was removed with acidified tyrode's solution. (d) CZB drops in a 6-cm plastic dish covered with mineral oil. (e) Scissors and a stereomicroscope were used to make (f) small holes on the bottom of the dish. (g, left) The ES cell suspension was placed in a drop of CZB, and a small clump of ES cells was selected. (g, middle) The small holes were used to aggregate the ES cells with the 3 × 4n embryos. (g, right) The 4n embryos were placed in a drop of CZB after removing the zona. (h) A small clump of ES cells and three 4n embryos (left) were placed in a hole of the plate (center). The aggregated embryos (ES ↔ 3 × 4n embryos) were generated (right) after a 24-hour culture.

3.4.5 Generation of ES ↔ 4n embryos by blastocyst injection

A micromanipulator system actuated with a piezo drive was used to microinject ES cells into the E3.5 or E4.5 4n blastocysts. After electrofusion, the 4n embryos were cultured for 48 hours (E3.5) or 72 hours (E4.5) to produce blastocysts. The ES cells were treated with trypsin/EDTA and agitated with a micropipette to obtain a single-cell suspension. ES medium was added to inactivate the trypsin, and the cell suspension was transferred into a new tube for blastocyst injection. The cell suspension was transferred into a drop of CZB [Figure 3.3(a)], and approximately 15 ES cells were injected into a blastocele with the micromanipulator [Figure 3.3(c)]. The zona pellucida and trophoblast layer were penetrated by the piezo pulse [Figure 3.3(b)].

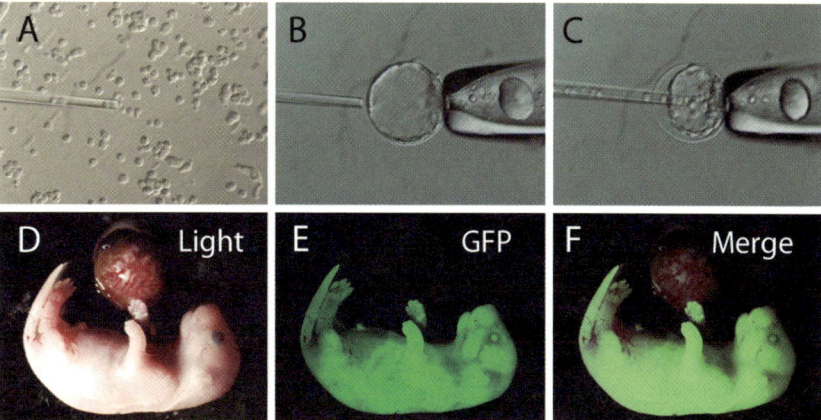

Figure 3.3 Generation of ES mice by blastocyst injection. (a) ES cells were loaded into an injection pipette. (b) The zona pellucida and trophoblast layer were penetrated by applying a piezo pulse. (c) Ten to 15 ES cells were injected into a blastocele. (d, e) ES mouse and placenta at 18.5 dpc delivered from 129B6F1G1 (GFP-expressing ES cell line) ↔ E4.5 4n embryos showing a light photograph (d) and its fluorescence image (e) [8]. (f) High-intensity green fluorescence was only found in the progeny.

3.4.6 Data acquisition

Cesarean section at 18.5 or 19.5 dpc is preferred over natural delivery to obtain ES mice. Abnormalities in ES mice, such as large-offspring syndrome and abdominal hernias [7], sometimes lead to cannibalism or the death of the surrogate mother resulting from complications during delivery. After the cesarean section, the progeny develop to adulthood with a foster mother. Figure 3.3(d–f) shows the normal ES mice at E18.5 derived from 129B6F1G1 (ES cells expressing GFP) ↔ 4n embryos.

3.5 Anticipated Results

The success rate of this procedure varies from 0% to 14.3% and depends on the ES cell line rather than the technique. The malformations in ES mice become problematic if the technique is used to propagate progeny.

3.6 Discussion and Commentary

Producing progeny directly from ES cells is an important technique for analyzing gene function in vivo. Although the methodology for producing ES mice from ES cell lines was described more than a decade ago [2, 3], its application remains limited because of extremely low viability. Previous improved methods required specific ES cell lines [6], but our technique can be applied to any ES cell line used for gene targeting. Thus, the use of multiple host 4n embryos is an effective procedure to generate genetically modified mouse lines because the germ cells in ES mice are all derived from ES cells.

Although we succeeded in improving the birthrate of ES mice [7], progeny resulting from the 4n complementation assay using ES cells often died just after birth as a result of respiratory failure or abdominal hernias [7]. In our previous study, approximately half the ES mice generated from 3 × 4n embryos died [7], indicating that the use of 3

× 4n embryos cannot rescue the abnormalities of ES mice. Because newborn mice lack differentiated gametes, it is impossible to establish mouse lines directly from gametes. Nevertheless, reproductive organ transplantation techniques can be applied. Our previous study showed that spermatogenesis can be induced from dead cloned mice by transplanting the testis into recipient nude mice [12], resulting in normal progeny by intracytoplasmic sperm injection [12].

In a previous study, we determined that using three 4n embryos was more efficient than one or two 4n embryos to obtain ES mice efficiently, and there was no improvement in the results using four or five 4n embryos [7], suggesting that a functional plateau was reached with three 4n embryos. When the birthrates of ES mice were compared based on the number of 4n embryos used, a total of five (0.8%) ES mice were delivered from 613 tetraploid embryos using the one 4n embryo method, whereas 12 (1.4%) ES mice were produced from 852 tetraploid embryos using the two 4n-embryo method [7]. However, using the three 4n-embryo method we produced 33 ES mice (2.4%) from 1386 tetraploid embryos [7], indicating that using three 4n embryos is the more efficient procedure even if it requires additional embryos.

In general, ES mice can be produced using two methods [1]: by injecting ES cells into 4n blastocysts [13] or by aggregating ES cells with 4n four-cell stage embryos [2, 3]. We recently compared these two techniques using the same ES cell lines. The birthrate of ES mice using three 4n embryos from the E14 and 129B6F1G1 strains was 14.3% and 9.3%, respectively (Table 3.1, [7]). Because this frequency was calculated from the number of transferred ES ↔ 3 × 4n embryos, the estimate from the actual number of embryos used was 4.8% for the E14 and 3.1% for the 129B6F1G1 strains. Similarly, the birthrate of ES mice from E3.5 and E4.5 embryos using blastocyst injection was approximately 3.8% for the E14 and 1.6% for the 129B6F1G1 strains (Table 3.1, [8]). The selection of technique depends on the purpose of the research. Blastocyst injection is effective for assessing donor cell function because micromanipulation allows the researcher to select donor cells, whereas 3 × 4n embryos is effective for producing ES mice as result of the ease of the procedure.

Table 3.1 Comparison of Birthrates of ES Mice by Different Procedures

ES Cell Line	Aggregation Using 3 × 4n Embryos		Blastocyst Injection	
	No. of Experiments	No. of pups (%)	No. of Experiments	No. of pups (%)
E14	105	15 (14.3)	105	4 (3.8)
129B6F1G1	108	10 (9.3)	124	2 (1.6)

Troubleshooting Table

Problem	Explanation	Potential Solutions
Inefficient electrofusion of two-cell stage embryos	Inappropriate ac and dc voltage settings	For each device, the optimal ac and dc voltages are necessary.
Loss of embryos in the acidic tyrode's solution used for zona removal	Increased stickiness of the embryos	Careful embryo control is required during the procedure. The attachment of embryos to the bottom of the plastic dish causes the loss of embryos.
Low birthrate of ES mice	Potential of the ES cell line or technical problems with embryo transfer	Use an ES cell line confirmed to generate ES mice as a positive control. Check the birthrate of normal embryos after zona removal.
Low blastocele formation at E3.5	Delayed in vitro development	E4.5 4n blastocysts can also be used as a host.

3.7 Application Notes

Because almost all the cells in ES mice are derived from ES cells, this technique can be applied to analyze gene-modified mouse phenotypes without the necessity for germline transmission (i.e., F0 assay). Although this application would be very effective for the prompt analysis of genetically modified mice, it is highly dependent on the ES cell lines used, because the production of ES mice varies among ES cell lines. In addition, investigators must pay attention to the presence of host 4n cells within the ES mice. Several studies have indicated that 4n host cells contributed to the ES mice, although their frequency was very low [8, 14], and their presence may affect some experiments. Furthermore, ES mice have abnormalities such as abdominal hernia, open eyelids, and large-offspring syndrome [7, 8]. These phenotypes should be considered as ES mouse phenotypes. If these problems can be solved, then the generation of ES mice for this type of application will become more efficient.

Recently, Dr. Yamanaka's group established a pluripotent cell line (which functions and behaves like ES cells) directly from somatic cells (referred to as *induced pluripotent stem* [iPS] *cells*) [15]. There are no ethical concerns with this procedure because it does not require oocytes for reprogramming [15]. Thus, iPS cells may be a candidate for use in human regenerative medicine. However, the effects of viral vectors and the problems of introducing oncogenic genes must be investigated before iPS cells can be used in humans. Because our technique can be applied to any pluripotent cell line, iPS cells can also be functionally evaluated. Producing and characterizing progeny derived from iPS cells using our procedure may provide valuable information regarding the safety of iPS cells in vivo.

ES mice derived from ntES cells [16] may also be used to generate progeny as an alternative to cloned mice. Animal cloning is still an inefficient technique, and the birthrate of cloned mice is usually only a few percent [17]. Although we have reported that somatic cell nuclear transfer can be improved with trichostatin A treatment [18], this method is limited because it requires fresh somatic cells as donors for nuclear transfer. However, establishing ntES cell lines has a higher success rate than the birthrate of cloned mice, and these cell lines have proliferation and differentiation abilities similar to those of normal ES cell lines [16, 17], thereby providing a sufficient source of donor cells. We previously demonstrated that ntES cells originally derived from Sertoli (129B6F1G1) and tail-tip (BDmt2) cells can be used to generate ntES mice using the techniques described here [7]. Therefore, reconstructing ntES cells ↔ multiple 4n embryos will enable the stable production of individuals from somatic cells.

3.8 Summary Points

1. The progeny from ES cell lines with genetic modifications obtained using our technique could be used as founder mice for germline transmission.
2. Use of 3 × 4n embryos is an effective way to produce ES mice even if it requires additional host embryos to reconstruct one ES ↔ 4n embryo.
3. The 4n complementation assay using multiple host 4n embryos can be used with any pluripotent cell line, such as ES, ntES, and iPS. This technique allowed us to assess the functional ability of newly established pluripotent cell lines.

4. ES mice can also be produced by injecting ES cells into 4n blastocysts. Donor ES cells can be selected under a microscope by their morphology or fluorescence.

Acknowledgments

This work was supported by grants for Scientific Research in Priority Areas and the Project for the Realization of Regenerative Medicine (research field: technical development of stem cell manipulation) to T. W. from the Ministry of Education, Culture, Sports, Science, and Technology of Japan.

References

[1] Nagy, A., et al., "Production of Chimeras," In A. Nagy et al. (eds.), *Manipulating the Mouse Embryo: A Laboratory Manual*, 3rd ed., New York: Cold Spring Harbor Laboratory Press, 2003, pp. 453–506.
[2] Nagy, A., et al., "Embryonic Stem Cells Alone Are Able to Support Fetal Development in the Mouse," *Development*, Vol. 110, 1990, pp. 815–821.
[3] Nagy, A., et al., "Derivation of Completely Cell Culture-Derived Mice from Early-Passage Embryonic Stem Cells," *Proc. Natl. Acad. Sci. USA*, Vol. 90, 1993, pp. 8424–8428.
[4] Kaufman, M. H., and S. Webb, "Postimplantation Development of Tetraploid Mouse Embryos Produced by Electrofusion," *Development*, Vol. 110, 1990, pp. 1121–1132.
[5] Eakin, G. S., and R. R. Behringer, "Tetraploid Development in the Mouse," *Dev. Dynamics*, Vol. 228, 2003, pp. 751–766.
[6] Eggan, K., et al., "Hybrid Vigor, Fetal Overgrowth, and Viability of Mice Derived by Nuclear Cloning and Tetraploid Embryo Complementation," *Proc. Natl. Acad. Sci. USA*, Vol. 98, 2001, pp. 6209–6214.
[7] Ohta, H., et al., "Increasing the Cell Number of Host Tetraploid Embryos Can Improve the Production of Mice Derived from Embryonic Stem Cells," *Biol. Reprod.*, Vol. 79, 2008, pp. 486–492. *Effect of 3 × 4n embryos in producing ES mice was described.*
[8] Ohta, H., Y. Sakaide, and T. Wakayama, "Generation of Mice Derived from Embryonic Stem Cells Using Blastocysts of Different Developmental Ages," *Reproduction*, Vol. 136, 2008, pp. 581–587. *ES mice were generated by blastocyst injection technique.*
[9] Toyoda, Y., M. Yokoyama, and T. Hosi, "Studies on the Fertilization of Mouse Eggs in Vitro. I. In Vitro Fertilization of Eggs by Fresh Epididymal Sperm," *Jap. J. Anim. Reprod.*, Vol. 16, 1971, 147–151.
[10] Chatot, C. L., et al., "An Improved Culture Medium Supports Development of Random-Bred 1-Cell Mouse Embryos in Vitro," *J. Reprod. Fertil.*, Vol. 86, 1989, pp. 679–688.
[11] Hooper, M., et al., "HPRT-Deficient (Lesch-Nyhan) Mouse Embryos Derived from Germline Colonization by Cultured Cells," *Nature*, Vol. 326, 1987, 292–295.
[12] Ohta, H., and T. Wakayama, "Generation of Normal Progeny by Intracytoplasmic Sperm Injection Following Grafting of Testicular Tissue from Cloned Mice That Died Postnatally," *Biol. Reprod.*, Vol. 73, 2005, pp. 390–395. *We succeeded in generating progeny from dead mice by testicular tissue transplantation.*
[13] Wang, Z. Q., et al., "Generation of Completely Embryonic Stem Cell-Derived Mutant Mice Using Tetraploid Blastocyst Injection," *Mech. Dev.*, Vol. 62, 1997, pp. 137–145.
[14] Li, J., et al., "Non-equivalence of Cloned and Clonal Mice," *Curr. Biol.*, Vol. 15, 2005, pp. R756–R757.
[15] Takahashi, K., and S. Yamanaka, "Induction of Pluripotent Stem Cells from Mouse Embryonic and Adult Fibroblast Cultures by Defined Factors," *Cell*, Vol. 126, 2006, 663–676.
[16] Wakayama, T., et al., "Differentiation of Embryonic Stem Cell Lines Generated from Adult Somatic Cells by Nuclear Transfer," *Science*, Vol. 292, 2001, pp. 740–743.
[17] Wakayama, T., "Production of Cloned Mice and ES Cells from Adult Somatic Cells by Nuclear Transfer: How to Improve Cloning Efficiency?," *J. Reprod. Dev.*, Vol. 53, 2007, pp. 13–26.
[18] Kishigami, S., et al., "Significant Improvement of Mouse Cloning Technique by Treatment with Trichostatin A after Somatic Nuclear Transfer," *Biochem. Biophys. Res. Commun.*, Vol. 340, 2006, pp. 183–189.

CHAPTER

4

Bioreactor Design and Implementation

G. Delbert Antwiler,[1] Kim T. Nguyen,[2] and Ian K. McNiece[2]

[1]CaridianBCT
Lakewood, CO 80215

[2]Interdisciplinary Stem Cell Institute
University of Miami
Miami, FL 33136

Abstract

A number of clinical applications of mesenchymal stem cells (MSC) are currently being evaluated and include the inhibition of graft-versus-host disease in bone marrow (BM) transplant patients and the regeneration of cardiac tissue in patients following a myocardial infarction. The large numbers of MSC that are required in some protocols (>200 million per patient) make standard culture conditions problematic and expensive, resulting from the need for extensive personnel resources and the high potential of contamination. To meet such clinical demand, a fast, robust, and sterile closed-loop MSC expansion method is optimal. In this chapter, we present a method for the ex vivo expansion of MSC from both BM mononuclear cells and whole BM using an automated, hollow-fiber bioreactor system. The bioreactor culture system is comprised of a synthetic hollow-fiber bioreactor connected to sterile closed-looped, computer-controlled media and gas exchangers. In experimental studies, therapeutic dosages of MSC have been grown from single 12- to 25-mL BM aspirates within 14 to 29 days.

Key Terms

Mesenchymal stem cell
bone marrow mononuclear cell
whole bone marrow
ex vivo expansion
dynamic cell culture
bioreactor
hollow fiber
closed-loop fluid circuit

4.1 Introduction

In the emerging field of stem cell therapeutics, there exists an ever-increasing demand for clinical-scale quantities of stem cells to be efficiently produced ex vivo. A number of clinical applications of mesenchymal stem cells (MSC) are currently being evaluated and include the inhibition of steroid-refractory graft-versus-host disease in bone marrow (BM) transplant patients and the regeneration of cardiac tissue in patients with myocardial ischemia. The large numbers of MSC that are required in some clinical protocols (>200 million per patient) make traditional flask and incubator culture methods problematic and expensive, because of the need for extensive personnel resources and the high potential of contamination. To meet such clinical demand, a bioreactor-based MSC expansion method is optimal. Bioreactors have been routinely used to transform laboratory-based experimental cell biology approaches into clinical or pharmaceutical production processes.

A bioreactor is defined as any device that provides the physiological requirements of a cell (e.g., pH, temperature, pressure, nutrient supply, and waste removal) for the scaling production of cells and their products. In the case of MSC ex vivo expansion for cellular therapy applications, four formidable engineering challenges exist in the design and implementation of a bioreactor-based system. First, the enhancement of mass transport is one of the major challenges in the engineering of bioreactors for cell proliferation; it must be ensured that there is continuous nutrition of cells and removal of waste products. Second, because MSC products for cellular therapy applications need to be individualized and tissue matched to avoid graft rejection, economies of scale such as those used in the production of protein-based pharmaceutical therapeutics deploying massive stainless steel bioreactors is not tenable; a bioreactor for MSC growth must be relatively compact to reduce incubator space required, disposable, and economical. Third, because MSC reach confluence at approximately $5 \cdot 10^3$ cells/cm^2 and maximal expansion relies on seeding at relatively low density (1–50 cells/cm^2), a large surface area of volume ratio is required in the bioreactor design. Last, the growth and differentiation of MSC are complex and tightly regulated, often requiring the addition of scarce and/or expensive components to the media, such as growth factors and serum components; a media-sparing bioreactor system design is optimal.

In this chapter we present the design and implementation of a hollow-fiber, bioreactor-based cell expansion system (CES) for the ex vivo expansion of MSC. The CES is a closed, automated, self-contained culture incubator system intended for the purpose of growing adherent and/or suspension cells for applications ranging from laboratory to good manufacturing practice (GMP)-compliant large-scale manufacturing. Being a closed system, it is especially suitable for clinical applications. It is intended as a general tool capable of replacing traditional culture flask and incubator systems. For adherent cell growth, a surface area of 1.7 m^2 is provided and is sufficient to grow up to 300 million MSC. For suspension cells, the system provides a chamber growth volume of approximately 120 mL and could manage significantly larger chamber volumes. The CES has a user interface designed to facilitate the development of protocols for growing a large variety of adherent cells, suspension cells, or cocultures.

The CES is designed to meet a number of user needs:

1. A growth environment free of contaminating events;
2. Ability to grow a variety of both adherent and suspension cells, which includes maintaining all required environmental conditions required for growing the cell

of interest, such as gas concentration, pH, media, temperature, management of nutrients, waste products, and required additives;
3. Physical compatibility—the size, weight, electrical needs, heat dissipation, and required facilities must be compatible with current research labs, GMP cell manufacturing facilities, and high-volume cell manufacturing;
4. CES workflow must be compatible or facilitate GMP while not hindering the routine use in non-GMP facilities;
5. Compliance with conventional U.S. and European laboratory equipment standards;
6. Reliability similar to or better than traditional flask and incubator systems;
7. Ease of use and training consistent with general laboratory technician skills;
8. A cost–benefit ratio, including all aspects of facilities, labor, supplies, time, and cell quality, greater than current flask and incubator systems.

4.2 Experimental Methods and Materials

Here, we will describe the assembly and operation of an automated bioreactor for the expansion of bone marrow-derived MSCs. These methods can be considered adopted for the growth of other adherent cell types, as well.

4.2.1 General system description

The CES is an integrated cell culture system intended as an alternative to the conventional culture flask and incubator means of growing cells. Both adherent and suspension cells can be grown, including cocultures of these cells. To meet the demanding cell culture need of preventing contamination, the CES is designed with a closed, sterile fluid compartment. Automation of the process is added to reduce labor, increase reliability, increase process control, reduce the affect of human variability, allow for automatic data collection, and facilitate a GMP cell growth/production environment. Bags of media, reagents, and solution remain attached to the system so that feeding schedules, waste removal, and general cell culture environment can be replaced, controlled, and optimized as desired. The CES is packaged so that it can be used as a benchtop unit in a laboratory or racked and stacked for a manufacturing facility. Figure 4.1 shows a picture of a prototype CES without fluid bags attached. It dimensions are $18 \times 18 \times 20$ inch deep.

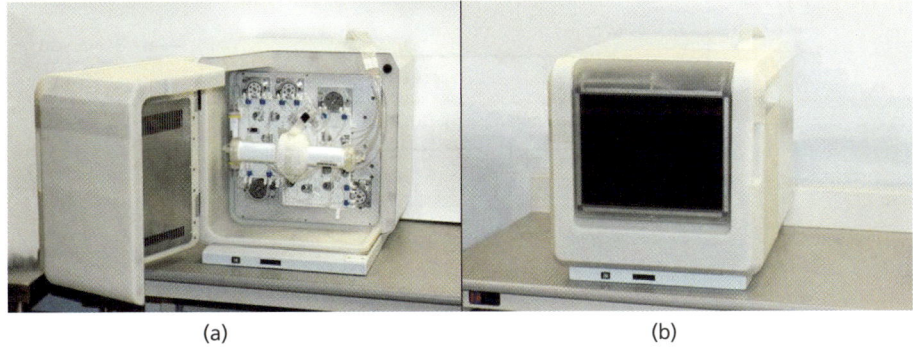

Figure 4.1 CES prototype showing unit with the door open (a) and with the door closed (b). Prototype developed and produced by CaridianBCT, Lakewood, Colorado.

4.2.2 Closed system

A crucial element for cell cultures is avoiding contaminating events. To accomplish this, the CES is a closed system. In the CES, traditional culture flasks or cell factories have been replaced with a hollow-fiber bioreactor. With hollow-fiber devices, cells can be grown inside the hollow fibers (intracapillary [IC]), outside the fibers (extracapillary [EC]), or simultaneously on both sides. The CES uses the inside of the fibers for the incubation space. The hollow-fiber bioreactor design allows for direct connection using plastic disposable tubing, which can then be routed through appropriate peristaltic pumps, pinch valves, and other system elements so that one can make a totally closed system with no open events that may allow system contamination. The CES fluid circuit is illustrated in Figure 4.2.

Gas control in the system is managed using a hollow-fiber oxygenator. The liquid side of the oxygenator is connected to the previously described disposable tubing set, thus maintaining the closed, sterile fluid path. The gas side of the oxygenator is protected from contamination using sterile barrier filters on both the gas inlet side and the gas outlet side of the oxygenator. The gas is supplied from a user-provided tank. After passing through the oxygenator, the gas exits the tubing and floods the incubator space, ensuring a similar gas environment outside the bioreactor as is maintained inside the bioreactor. By choosing a tank with the desired oxygen percentage, the desired carbon dioxide percentage, and with the remainder being nitrogen (or other gases as desired), users can grow cells at their desired gas concentration.

The system must also accommodate the ability to add and harvest cells, to replace media, to add reagents (e.g., trypsin for releasing adherent cells), to add special solutions (e.g., a phosphate-buffered saline solution with ethylenediaminetetraacetic acid for binding all Ca^{++} and Mg^{++} prior to adding trypsin), and to house a storage container for waste solutions. To perform these steps while maintaining a closed system, bags are used for all fluids, and the bag connections/disconnections all use sterile connecting technology.

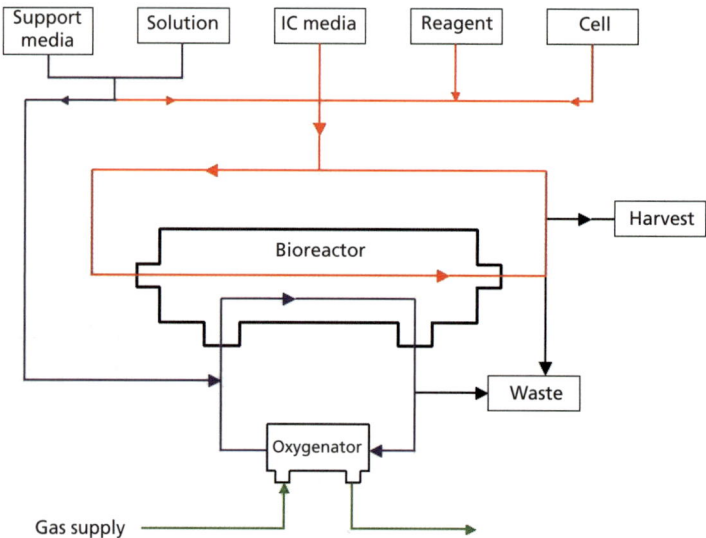

Figure 4.2 CES fluid circuit showing block diagram of system and all bag connections.

4.2.3 Hollow-fiber bioreactor

Hollow-fiber devices come in a large assortment. For a good bioreactor design, there are many parameters that must be considered, including the following:

- *Biocompatibility and stability:* The biocompatibility and stability of the hollow fiber material, the housing materials, and the potting materials must all be verified for the intended application. Depending on the cell type and the expansion desired, a hollow-fiber bioreactor may be in use for durations ranging from a week to a month. This requires that biocompatibility and stability of materials be appropriately tested over extended durations.
- *Hydraulic permeability:* The hydraulic permeability affects the freedom of water movement between the IC and EC sides of the fibers. If the fluid movement is excessive, concentration or dilution of solutes can occur, which in turn can negatively affect growth conditions. Cell expansion systems must consider these events and manage fluid movement accordingly.
- *Membrane sieving coefficient as a function of molecular size:* A membrane pore structure small enough to retain in the IC space growth factors, proteins, or other expensive reagents required for cell growth could allow a system design that optimizes the use of IC media. Likewise, having mass transfer characteristics that allow lactate, glucose, salts, and other small molecules allows feeding (and waste removal) to take place from the EC side across the membrane.
- *Number, diameter, wall thickness, and length of fibers:* These parameters affect the device surface area, the volume inside the fibers, and pressure changes down and across the fibers resulting during fluid flow conditions. The diameter of the fiber may also be important relative to cell size, how the cells arrange themselves on a curved surface, and diffusion distances from the edge to the fibers to the center. In general, although large fibers will give lower pressure drops and a flatter surface for adhesion of adherent cells or settling of suspension cells, they will also provide a lower surface area for the same volume and a longer diffusion distance for molecules to reach the center of the fiber.
- *Fiber bundle packing density:* The fiber packing density will affect the uniformity of flow through the EC space. This is especially important to minimize fluid flow shunting through a small selected area and thus not adequately perfuse all fibers. Hollow-fiber devices can also incorporate mechanical means (pleating of the fibers or inserted barriers) to help prevent shunting on the EC side.
- *Cell surface adhesion:* For expanding suspension cells, low-cell surface adhesion would be the first choice. This could be either no adhesion or adhesion forces that are easily broken using fluid flow shear. There may be an occasion when the adhesion of unwanted cells is desired or, in the case of a coculture, suspension cells may be grown over a bed of adherent cells. For adhesion cells, the surface must attach the cells of interest. Yet, the binding needs to be weak enough that the cell can be released either by chemicals (e.g., trypsin), by physical means (e.g., shear, reverse flow into the fiber lifting the cells, temperature), or by a combination of effects.
- *Gas permeability:* Gas permeability of most hollow-fiber bioreactors should usually not be an issue; however, it must be considered in any design.

The CES uses a hollow-fiber bioreactor that is still under final development by CaridianBCT. The unit, which has produced the applications results described herein, has the following parameters: good biocompatibility with no cell growth inhibition, the unit is stable over long use, has a low hydraulic permeability, and has a low permeability to large molecules such as albumin. Its physical characteristics are surface area, 1.7 m^2; length, 295 mm; internal diameter (ID), 215 μm; IC volume, 104 mL; EC volume, 330 mL; and number of fibers, 9,000. The unit is designed to give a high packing density with no shunting on the EC side. For the flow conditions used in the CES, gas permeability is high, resulting in gas equilibrium across the membrane at all times. For growing suspension cells, unmodified membranes with minimal surface binding are used. For growing adherent cells, the surface is fibronectin coated to give adhesion similar to standard tissue culture flasks.

4.2.4 CES fluid circuit

The CES fluid circuit is designed around two loops: one loop each for the IC and EC sides (Figure 4.2). All fluid bags (support media, solution, IC media, reagent, and cell bags) are connected to the IC loop. The user may chose to add fluid from any selected bag to the IC loop at a flow rate and volume that may also be chosen by the user.

- *Support media:* Use a base media composed of required salts, buffers, glucose, and possibly other small-molecular weight compounds that can pass through the hollow-fiber membrane and provide the basic elements to support cell growth. Larger molecular weight components, including serum, can be included in the base media, but may only be included in the IC media as desired.
- *Solution:* Use buffers or other solutions that may be required during the growth phase, such as a phosphate-buffered saline solution used to flush away the media before adding trypsin.
- *IC media:* Typically IC media is the same as base media plus serum or other proteins required to support cell growth. Large-molecular weight growth factors may be added to the IC media only.
- *Reagents:* Use any reagent required during the growth cycle (e.g., a concentrated source of glucose to feed the cells, a trypsin solution used to release adherent cells).
- *Cell:* Although designed to be the location from where cells are loaded into the system, this bag is almost identical to a reagent bag and may alternatively be used as a second reagent bag.

The support media and solution bags are the only fluid bags typically connected to the EC loop. For the EC loop, the user may select the rate of addition and the volume added. The user may chose to add fluid to the EC loop simultaneously with IC loop fluid additions, or independently. As a practical matter, the contents of these five bags are completely at the discretion of the user. As such, the design of the system allows a wide range of user options and thus the ability to tailor the CES operation to fit a wide assortment of cell growth needs.

As shown in Figure 4.2, fluid may exit the system to either the waste bag or the harvest bag. Given that the system has a constant volume, all additions of fluid result in an equal volume of fluid leaving the system. With the exception of cell harvest, the system always operates with an open fluid path to the waste bag. This bag is elevated slightly above the bulk of the system, which provides a constant, small, positive system pressure at all times. Thus, under standard conditions, all volume additions to the system result in an equal volume flowing from the system into the waste bag. At harvest, the path to the waste bag is clamped and the harvest bag is opened, resulting in the overflow volume going to the harvest bag.

4.2.5 Oxygenator design

In designing the gas transfer mechanism for a bioreactor, consideration must be given to system requirements. Flasks are usually placed in incubators containing the desired gas mixture, and simple diffusion through the liquid layer suffices to manage the concentration of gases. Gas transfer in bioreactors may be managed by a variety of methods, ranging from passive means (e.g., diffusion through a culture bag) to using active control of gas concentration.

In the CES, the system requirements are the following:

- Ability for the user to set the gas concentrations as desired. Typically, expected ranges are oxygen 1% to 20% and carbon dioxide 5% (however, this, too, may be set over a wide range).
- Maintain gas concentrations throughout all growth phases.
- Maintain gas concentrations during all fluid flow conditions, including those occasions when both the IC and EC fluids may be replaced with new unconditioned media.

These requirements mandate the design of a hollow-fiber oxygenator directly into the system. Figure 4.3 shows an ultrastructural view of a hollow fiber and adherent MSCs. The chosen oxygenator has excess capacity during steady-state growth and thus ensures that the gas concentration in the media will be in equilibrium with the source gas flowing on the gas side of the hollow fibers. This overcapacity design also provides the extra capacity needed to manage gas concentration during large-volume IC or EC exchanges. This oxygenation design allows for a very straightforward control of gas in the CES—specifically, the concentration of gas in the tank connected to the system sets the concentration of gas in the bioreactor. As previously mentioned, to maintain sterility

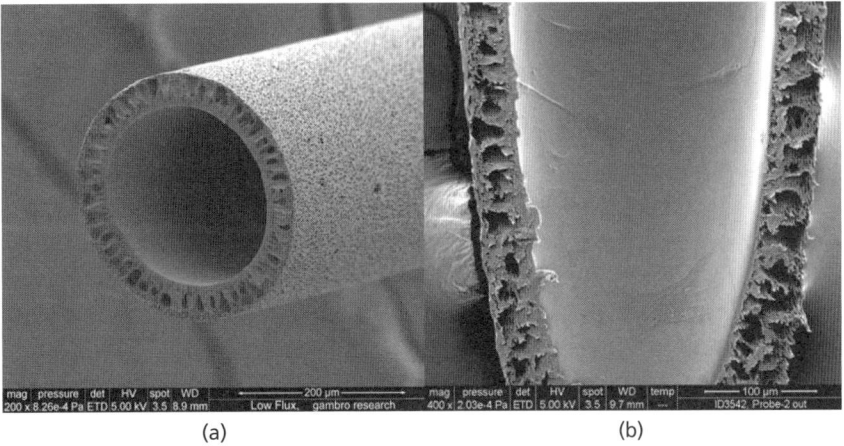

Figure 4.3 Scanning electron micrographs of a cross-section of a hollow fiber showing the porous membrane structure (a) and a sectional view showing several MSC attached to the interior wall of the hollow fiber (b).

of the CES closed system, the gas flows from the tank through a sterile barrier filter provided on the CES disposable set. After passing through the gas side of the hollow-fiber oxygenator, the gas then exits the disposables through another sterile barrier filter and into the incubator space, filling the incubator space with the same gas, also ensuring that there is no significant transfer of gas through the disposable plastic walls.

4.2.6 Monitoring

The CES has a number of monitors. Temperature monitors are placed at multiple locations in both the incubator and the fluid path. These are used both to control and to monitor the temperature. Pressure is monitored in both the IC and EC fluid paths and can be used to control processes. Sterile closed sample ports are provided in both the IC and EC loops, allowing the user to obtain both fluid samples and cellular samples. This allows monitoring a range of parameters, including metabolites, media composition, gases, cell counts, cell quality, phenotype, and so forth. This ability should allow a user to optimize desired conditions for the cell of interest.

4.2.7 User interface

The CES can perform operations ranging from a manual mode to full automation of specified sequences. The user selects the functions to be performed from the 15-inch embedded monitor (Figure 4.1). These functions operate pumps and valves to perform specific tasks. In all cases, the user may accept the default values or may use the monitor to input different parameters. Current functions include the following:

- *Manual:* The operator can activate individual pumps and valves.
- *Prime:* The system performs an automatic priming sequence.
- *Cell load:* The system supports an automatic function to transfer cells from the cell bag into the bioreactor.
- *IC/EC media exchange:* There is an automatic function to exchange fluid in the IC and/or EC loops. The user may select the fluid source, its destination, the rate of exchange, and the exchange volume.
- *Grow:* There is an automatic function to provide maintenance feeding on either the IC and/or EC sides.
- *Harvest:* There is an automatic function to move suspended cells from the bioreactor into the harvest bag.

These functions can be used in operator-defined sequences to define protocols for specific procedures and they can be combined to form complete expansion procedures from cell load to cell harvest.

4.3 Anticipated Results

MSC are adherent cells that must first be distributed across the entire membrane surface; then, the cells must be allowed to attach. In some cases, the initial colonies formed must be released, followed by their redistribution over the membrane surface and subsequent reattachment. Good cell distribution across the entire surface is especially important to achieve a uniform layer at confluence and thus to maximize total cell growth. A lack of good cell distribution could easily cause localized high-cell density clusters and possibly lead to undesired cellular effects. After adherent cells have grown, they must be released. If cells are overexposed to release agents, cellular damage may occur.

In the laboratory, MSC from three sources have been successfully loaded into the CES:

- *MSC source 1:* Whole BM, unprocessed except for gross filtration to remove bone chips and small clots that may have occurred during collection, would be loaded directly into the CES. Typically, 50-mL aspirates were obtained from donors. These BM aliquots may have been used as single loading doses or may have been further divided into smaller aliquots (i.e., four 12-mL BM samples).
- *MSC source 2:* A second source of MSC was derived from plating a small volume of BM onto standard tissue culture plates and subsequently growing and collecting the plastic adherent cells. These collected MSC were then loaded into the CES.
- *MSC source 3:* The third source of MSC, used for the following experiments, was the harvested product from procedures described earlier. In other words, the harvest (or a portion of the harvest) from a CES run has often been used as the starting cells for a subsequent CES procedure.

For sources 2 and 3, in some procedures the MSC were frozen, stored in liquid nitrogen, and later used in a CES procedure. No differences between using previously frozen MSC or never frozen MSC has been observed. Whole BM was never frozen. All CES procedures reported herein used α-mem as the base media. Protein sources varied between MSC-qualified fetal bovine serum (FBS) and human platelet lysate. For the gas concentration, carbon dioxide was always set at 5% and oxygen was set at either 5% or 20%. No major differences were attributed to any of these variations.

The following three tests were used to identify harvested cells as MSC:

1. *Morphology:*
   a. Day 0: Load 10,000 cells per well in a 24-well plate.
   b. Day 1: Check for cell attachment and spindle shape.
   c. Day 4: Check for growth. A typical day 4 plate is shown in Figure 4.4.

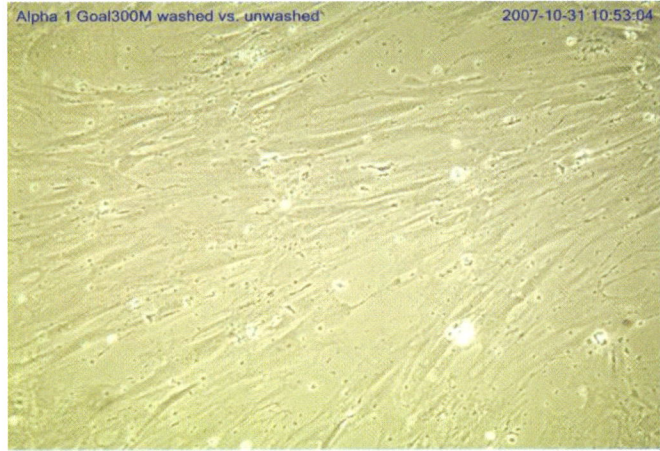

Figure 4.4 Typical day 4 morphology plate showing MSC growth.

Table 4.1 Standard Biomarkers Used for Identification of MSC

Growth Phase	CD34+ <2%	CD45+ <2%	HLA-DR+ <2%	CD73+ >95%	CD90+ >95%	CD105+ >95%
Primary (n = 8)	5.57% (±6.3)	14.7% (±4.6)	17.3% (±2.7)	78.1% (±30.1)	76.3% (±26.6)	75.9% (±26.7)
Secondary (n = 3)	0.73% (±0.3)	1.82% (±1.1)	1.5% (±0.9)	98.1% (±0.7)	95.5% (±5.3)	96.1% (±2.1)
Tertiary (n = 3)	0.40% (±0.3)	0.65% (± 0.3)	0.9% (±0.3)	98.4% (±0.6)	97.6% (±0.3)	97.1% (±1.3)

2. *Flow cytometry:* Table 4.1 shows the standard biomarkers (first row with acceptance limit shown as a percentage) that were used to determine whether the cells are MSC. It should be noted that with each successive growth phase, the purity of the product improved. This is because of three reasons: (1) automated CES wash cycles purged the bioreactor of nonattached cells and (2) with time some of the contaminating cells die, whereas (3) the MSC simply outgrow other cell types.
3. *Differentiation:* Harvested MSC must also show the characteristic trilineage differentiation typical of MSC. In all cases, the MSC harvested from the CES met these criteria. Typical results are shown in Figure 4.5.

4.3.1 MSC source 1: Loading whole BM marrow into the CES

Figure 4.6 shows data for 26 CES procedures whereby whole unprocessed BM was loaded into the CES. The average MSC doubling time (i.e., the bar height) is shown as a function of the volume of loaded BM plotted. For the first three bars, the data allowed calculation of a sample standard deviation and is shown as a bracket at the top of the corresponding bar. The number of procedures (n) at each condition is shown along with the number of days the cells grew (i.e., the time between loading the BM and harvesting the cells). As shown in Figure 4.6, the first three bars represent data with growth durations ranging from 12 to 14 days; the average time was 13 days. This data shows substantially similar MSC doubling times regardless of the volume of BM loaded. However, for the last two bars (the two bars on the right side of the graph) the extended culture times gave sig-

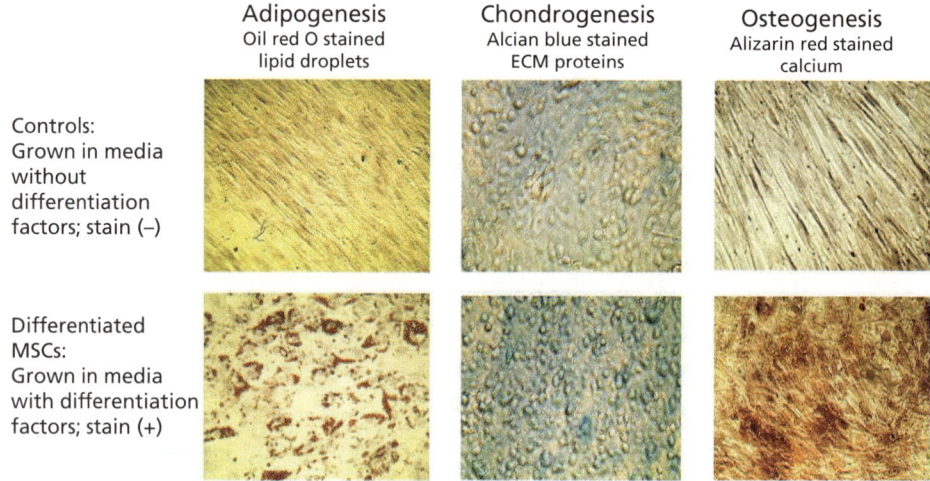

Figure 4.5 Typical differentiation results.

4.3 Anticipated Results

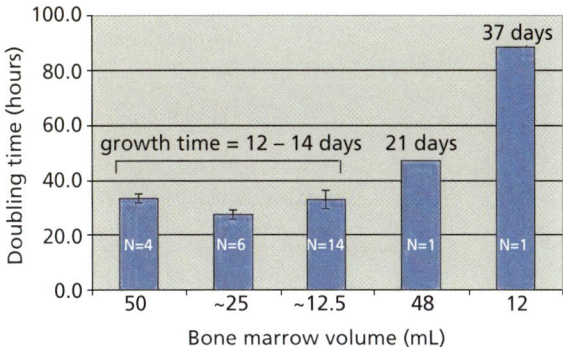

Figure 4.6 Cell doubling time in the CES as a function of loaded BM volume and growth time in the CES.

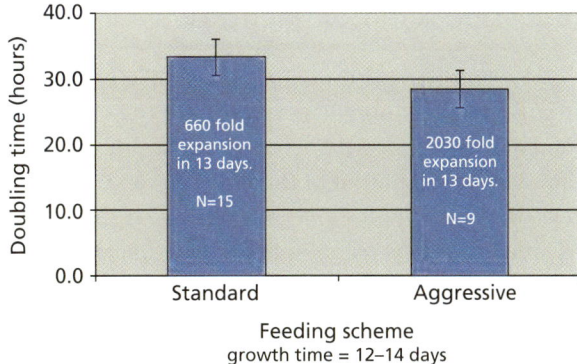

Figure 4.7 Results showing the effect of two feeding schemes.

nificantly increased MSC doubling time. This data is consistent with an MSC growth model predicting that, as individual colonies grow larger, MSC growth slows.

Figure 4.7 shows the results of using two different feeding schemes on the MSC doubling time. The first bar shows data for a standard feeding scheme in which media were exchanged in the CES simulating a standard, twice-weekly tradition plate media exchange. The second bar used a more aggressive feeding scheme, with continual addition of both glucose and FBS. Although, most users may chose the options that grow MSC the fastest, the primary point here is not the growth rate, but the fact that automated cell expansion systems, like the CES, provide easy, automated closed-system approaches so that a number of variables can be easily examined in a controlled, reproducible environment.

4.3.2 MSC source 2 or 3: Loading preselected MSC into the CES

Similar results can be shown when MSC (MSC sources 2 or 3) are loaded directly into the CES. Figure 4.8 shows data for 23 runs with culture times from 7 to 13 days. As the culture time increases beyond 9 days, the MSC doubling time increases and is consistent with large cell colonies, resulting in slower MSC growth.

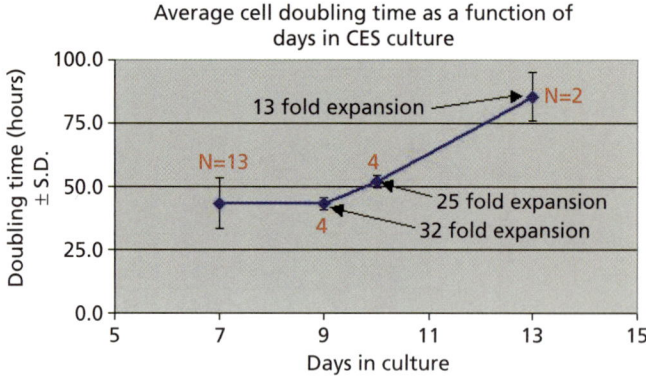

Figure 4.8 Effect of culture time on MSC growth rate for MSC loaded directly into the CES.

4.4 Discussion and Commentary

Experimental results demonstrate that robust MSC ex vivo expansion is possible using a fully automated hollow-fiber-based bioreactor system. Of particular significance, there is the potential to generate MSC from whole unprocessed BM in the CES, eliminating the need for density separation of the BM aspirate. Expansion of other types of mononuclear cells of clinical interest may be possible, including the expansion of cord blood mononuclear cells in suspension in the hollow-fiber bioreactor both with and without a feeder layer of adherent MSC.

However, there are some significant bioengineering hurdles to overcome as well those associated with the hollow-fiber growth of adherent cells. Because adherent cells grow in colonies, they must first be distributed across the entire membrane surface. Good cell distribution across the entire surface is especially important to achieve a uniform layer at confluence and thus maximize total cell growth. A lack of good cell distribution could easily cause localized high-cell density clusters and possibly lead to undesired cellular effects. In traditional laboratory cultures, technicians routinely observe when the cells have reached confluence and when they have released from the membrane. Observation inside a hollow fiber is not routine using today's technology.

Automated cell expansion systems like the CES may have degrees of automation ranging from single steps in a process to fully automated protocols to grow cells from loading to harvest. Yet, it will always be the responsibility of the biologist or researcher to define the appropriate cell growth process. The CES is not designed to tell one how to grow a cell type. Some users may want to grow their cells using a standard feeding schedule, whereas others may want to use an aggressive feeding schedule. Some will use a bioreactor provided for suspension cell growth; others will use a bioreactor with a surface designed for adherent cells. A manufacturing site may run the same exact protocol for years, whereas a researcher may run a different protocol each day. To meet these varied needs, the CES must have the types of functions defined previously: the ability to load and harvest cells, wash out contaminating cells, and control cell feeding, gas, temperature, and waste removal. In addition, the CES must provide a platform that is closed, easy to use, automated, yielding reproducible and predictable results. The CES is a tool to be used to manage the cellular environment as dictated by the biologist.

Troubleshooting Table

Problem	Explanation	Potential solutions
Adherent cells do not attach to the hollow fibers in the bioreactor	Inadequate deposition of fibronectin on the hollow fiber walls	Incubate the fibronectin solution for a longer period of time (i.e., overnight) in the bioreactor before flushing the fibronectin solution out and seeding adherent cells into the bioreactor.
Adherent cells do not detach adequately from the hollow fibers in the bioreactor upon harvest	Cells were not exposed to the trypsin solution for an adequate length of time for full cell detachment prior to running the cell harvest function	The cells remaining on the hollow fibers can be trypsinized a second time and the harvest function can be run again to collect all cells not harvested during the first trypsinization.
MSC doubling time increases as length of time cells are in culture increases	Large cell colonies inside the bioreactor result in slower MSC growth	Trypsinize and harvest the cells inside the bioreactor and reseed the cells inside the bioreactor. This allows for the dissociation of the large colonies.

4.5 Application Notes

4.5.1 Therapeutic dose of MSC grown from a whole BM sample

Table 4.2 shows a typical expansion process that resulted in more than a therapeutic dose (100 million cells) of MSC. This particular run started with 11.8 mL whole BM loaded into a CES. On day 13, 6.8 million MSC were harvested from the initial primary growth. In a second growth cycle, 3.8 million MSC were loaded, resulting in a harvest of 79.2 million MSC after 9 days of culture. This was repeated using 20 million MSC in a third growth cycle, resulting in 226 million MSC 7 days later—more than two therapeutic doses. The 62 million cells unused from the primary and secondary growths could be used for assays, additional tertiary growth cycles, or frozen and saved.

4.5.2 Nonadherent cell culture: Kg1a cells grown in suspension

Kg1a cells (an acute myelogenous leukemia cell, American Type Culture Collection (ATCC) cat. no. 30-2020) have been used for evaluating growth of suspension cells. These cells do not require special growth factors nor are the conditions for loading, growing, and harvesting challenging. Data for a representative set of runs is shown in Figure 4.9, presenting the Kg1a average cell concentrations in the IC loop immediately after loading the cells at time zero and the increasing cell concentration as a function of culture time. Also given for each curve is the average cell doubling time (i.e., the culture time required for the number of cells to double). Doubling time was calculated

Table 4.2 Therapeutic Dose of MSC Grown from a BM Sample

Parameter	BM Primary Growth	Secondary Growth	Tertiary Growth
Loaded	11.8 mL	$3.8 \cdot 10^6$	$20 \cdot 10^6$
Incubation time	13 days	9 days	7 days
Harvest number	$6.8 \cdot 10^6$	$79.2 \cdot 10^6$	$226 \cdot 10^6$
Feeding	Traditional	Traditional	Aggressive

Note: Harvest number for the primary growth phase is diluted to become the loaded amount for the secondary growth phase. Correspondingly, the secondary growth phase harvest number is diluted to become the loaded amount for the tertiary growth phase.

Bioreactor Design and Implementation

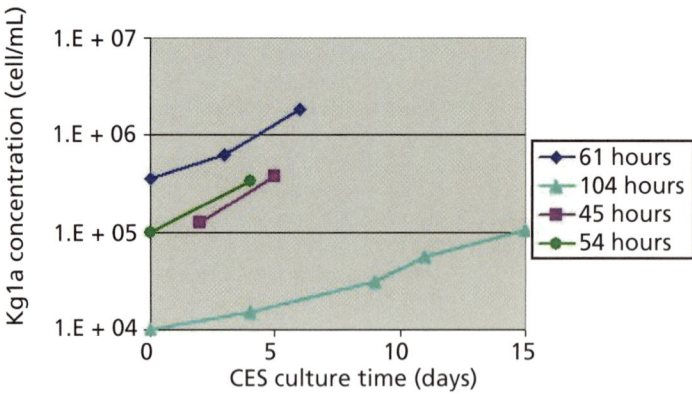

Figure 4.9 Growth of Kg1a cells.

as $0.693\ (t_2 - t_1)/\ln(n_2/n_1)$, where t is the culture time, n is the number of cells, and the subscripts 1 and 2 represent the initial and final time points, respectively. Media used were Iscove's Modified Dulbecco's Media plus 20% FBS. Gas concentrations used were 5% carbon dioxide and 20% oxygen.

4.6 Summary Points

1. The CES is an automated, closed-loop, sterile bioreactor system that is capable of generating MSC for clinical applications from both isolated MSC and whole BM.
2. The instrument is a complete incubation, cell culture medium, and fluid management system designed to grow both adherent and suspension cells.
3. The closed-loop design of the bioreactor system allows for the seeding, growth, feeding, and harvesting of cells under completely sterile conditions.
4. This hollow-fiber bioreactor-based system for rapid MSC expansion shows significant promise for clinical applications currently under evaluation that require large numbers of MSC, such as the inhibition of graft-versus-host disease in BM transplant patients and the regeneration of cardiac tissue in patients following a myocardial infarction.

CHAPTER 5

Extracellular Matrix Microarrays and Stem Cell Fate

Gregory H. Underhill,[1] Christopher J. Flaim,[2] and Sangeeta N. Bhatia[1,3]

[1]Laboratory for Multiscale Regenerative Technologies
Division of Health Sciences and Technology/
Electrical Engineering and Computer Science
Massachusetts Institute of Technology
Cambridge, MA 02139

[2]Departments of Bioengineering and Medicine
University of California-San Diego
La Jolla, CA 92093

[3]Division of Medicine
Brigham & Women's Hospital
Boston, MA 02115

Abstract

We present procedures for an extracellular matrix microarray platform, which was designed for the analysis of cell responses to combinatorial mixtures of matrix components. This array approach enables simultaneous investigation of the role of numerous matrix environments in parallel, and requires approximately 1,000 times less protein than conventional strategies to investigate extracellular matrix interactions. We have utilized this system in several experimental contexts, including the investigation of factors influencing early hepatic differentiation of mouse embryonic stem cells. Here, we outline key aspects of the fabrication process for this versatile platform.

Key Terms Extracellular matrix
microarray
robotic spotting
stem cell

5.1 Introduction

Stem cell fate and function are regulated by a combination of intrinsic determinants and signals from the local cellular microenvironment, or niche. Microenvironmental influences include distinct cell–cell and cell–extracellular matrix (ECM) interactions, localized soluble factors and gradients of soluble stimuli, and the three-dimensional architecture of the niche itself. Such specialized niches have been identified for many adult stem cell populations, and niche elements have been demonstrated to modulate proliferation, control differentiation, and protect stem cells from physiological insults [1, 2]. In addition, embryonic development proceeds through a highly ordered sequence of differentiation and patterning of events in which inductive extracellular signals play a critical role. Pluripotent embryonic stem (ES) cells derived from the early embryo represent a model system for investigating early developmental events, such as self-renewal and differentiation induction. Recent work has highlighted the autocrine regulation that ES cells exhibit within colonies, as well as the influence of niche composition and size on ES cell functions [3, 4]. Overall, as a means to probe systematically mechanisms of both embryonic and adult stem cell function, platforms in which stem cell microenvironmental interactions can be tightly manipulated and evaluated in a high-throughput manner have begun to be developed.

To decouple the complex spatiotemporal cues that cells experience in vivo, microfabrication technologies have been applied to in vitro cell culture models and have found great utility [5], particularly as a result of the highly controlled regulation of environmental signals that these systems afford. Another key feature of microfabricated systems, broadly applicable to numerous cell types, including stem cells, is the capacity to miniaturize cell culture platforms for parallel analysis. These high-throughput systems enable the systematic screening of cellular processes on a large scale, including an ability to examine the effects of combinations of extracellular signals [6]. One such system recently applied to investigate explicitly microenvironmental regulation of stem cell differentiation is cell microarrays.

Cell microarrays consist of printed spots of biomolecules onto which cells are seeded [7, 8]. These spots normally include adhesive factors to retain the seeded cells, as well as other elements for influencing cellular function or detection of specific cellular processes. Notably, a key benefit to utilizing high-throughput cell microarrays is the ability to begin to analyze mechanistically the responses of cells to complex environmental stimuli, including often conflicting signals. One particular interest in our laboratory is to examine and understand more fully the combinatorial role of ECM molecules in regulating cellular processes. For example, ECM components have been suggested to be involved in retaining stem cells within anatomic niches and regulating stem cell signaling and proliferation [9–13]. Thus, to investigate the effect of combinations of these factors, we developed an ECM microarray platform with broad utility for diverse cell types, including stem cells [14]. In this chapter, we describe methods for fabricating these ECM microarrays and highlight general points to consider in the development of high-throughput array platforms.

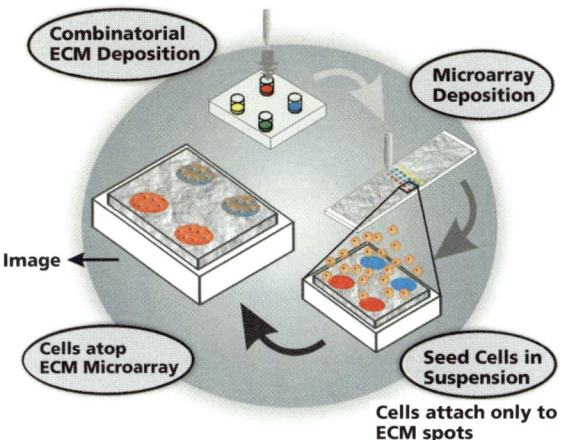

Figure 5.1 Schematic illustrating fabrication and implementation of ECM microarrays. Defined ECM mixtures are deposited on a hydrogel slide using a standard DNA microarrayer. Cells are seeded in suspension, cultured for several hours to allow for attachment, and the excess cells are rinsed away. The cell arrays can be stained for an in situ phenotypic marker, imaged, and quantified for further analysis. (Figure adapted from [14].)

5.2 Experimental Design

The ECM microarray platform was designed to facilitate the systematic investigation of the combinatorial effect of ECM molecules on cellular function (Figure 5.1). This platform did not require any custom-built equipment and is not dependent on photolithography-based cell micropatterning tools. Furthermore, miniaturization into an array format drastically reduced the amount of protein required per experimental condition (approximately 10 pg), enabling an extensive range of ECM combinations to be assessed in parallel, with numerous replicates for improving statistical analysis. Among the key developments in this procedure were the identification of an array substrate that sufficiently immobilized ECM proteins while maintaining the fidelity of the cellular islands, as well as modifications to a protein printing buffer for efficient and reproducible ECM deposition.

5.3 Materials

- Standard DNA microarray spotter
- SMP 3.0 spotting pins
- Glass microscope slides, 75 × 25 × 1 mm (VWR)
- Acetone (Sigma)
- Methanol (Sigma)
- NaOH (Sigma)
- 3-(Trimethoxysilyl)propyl methacrylate (Sigma)
- Toluene (Sigma)
- Acrylamide (Sigma)
- Bis-acrylamide (Sigma)
- Irgacure-2959 (I-2959) photoinitiator (Ciba)
- Glass coverslips, no. 1, 22 × 60 mm or 22 × 22 mm (VWR)

- Ultraviolet (UV) light sources: 365-nm source for polyacrylamide gel polymerization; 254-nm germicidal source for sterilization
- Printing buffer (2×): 100 mM sodium acetate, 5 mM ethylenediaminetetraacetic acid (EDTA), 20% glycerol, and 0.25% triton X-100; adjusted to pH 4.8 with glacial acetic acid
- Collagen type I (rat tail), concentration approximately 1 mg/mL
- Human collagen III (Becton Dickinson)
- Mouse collagen IV (Becton Dickinson)
- Human fibronectin (Becton Dickinson)
- Mouse laminin (Sigma)
- Spotting pin cleaning solutions (Telechem)
- QuadriPERM cell culture vessels (Sigma)
- Multiwell gasket system (e.g., ProPlate system from Grace Bio-Labs)
- Hank's balanced salt solution (HBSS; Sigma)
- Paraformaldehyde (Sigma)
- Sodium chloride (Sigma)
- Phosphate-buffered saline (PBS; Invitrogen)
- 150 mM phosphate buffer (pH, 7.2)
- Blocking buffer for immunostaining: 3% bovine serum albumin (BSA), 50 mM glycine, in Tris-EDTA (pH, 8.0)

5.4 Methods

5.4.1 Preparation of substrates for arrays

5.4.1.1 Cleaning glass slides

1. Detergent-clean glass microscope slides (75 × 25 × 1 mm) in slide chamber on an orbital shaker for 30 minutes, followed by five rinses in deionized water.
2. Wash slides in Millipore water (MQH_2O, 18 M-ohm/cm^2) for 30 minutes, followed by 30-minute washes with 100% acetone, then 100% methanol, and then thorough washing with MQH_2O.
3. Etch slides for 1 hour in 0.05N NaOH solution, followed by thorough washing with MQH_2O, then blow dry with filtered compressed air and further dry in a vacuum oven for 1 hour.

5.4.1.2 Silanization treatment

1. Prepare a 2% solution of 3-(trimethoxysilyl)propyl methacrylate in 100% anhydrous toluene and stir for 5 minutes prior to use.
2. Add this solution to cleaned slides and treat for 30 minutes in an orbital shaker.
3. Rinse briefly with 100% toluene, then dry with compressed air and bake for at least 15 minutes in a vacuum oven.

5.4.1.3 Acrylamide gel substrate fabrication

1. Prepare stock solutions of acrylamide/bis-acrylamide and photoinitiator. Specifically, prepare a solution of 10.55% acrylamide and 0.55% bis-acrylamide in MQH_2O. Vortex

and/or sonicate to solubilize, followed by 0.2-μm syringe filtration. Prepare a 10× photoinitiator stock of I-2959 at 200 mg/mL in 100% methanol.

2. Prepare the working polymer solution by combining nine parts acrylamide stock solution with one part photoinitiator stock solution at room temperature, and degas in a vacuum chamber for 15 minutes. This final solution consists of 10% acrylamide, 0.5% bis-acrylamide, 20 mg/mL I-2959, in 90% MQH$_2$O, 10% methanol.
3. To fabricate one continuous gel surface, immediately after degassing, place 120 μL prepolymer solution onto a silanized slide and cover with a 22 × 60-mm no. 1 coverslip. The coverslips should not be aggressively cleaned (compressed air is sufficient). Alternatively, three individual pads can be fabricated by individually overlaying 40 μL prepolymer solution with three separate 22 × 22-mm coverslips.
4. Expose the slide to 365 nm UVA (approximately 1.5–2.0 mW/cm^2) for 10 to 15 minutes. Acrylamide polymerization can be greatly affected by UV spectrum and intensity, and therefore must be optimized for the particular UV bulb setup utilized.
5. After UV exposure, immerse slides in MQH$_2$O for 2 minutes prior to removing the coverslip gently with a razor blade. The coverslip should be able to be removed easily. If UV intensity is too high, the coverslip will adhere too strongly to the gel. If UV intensity or duration is not sufficient, pads will not be fully gelled. After removing the coverslips, soak the slides in MQH$_2$O for 72 hours, with daily changes of MQH$_2$O.

5.4.2 Fabrication of ECM arrays

5.4.2.1 Preparation of printing buffer and ECM protein mixtures

1. Prepare the following 2× printing buffer. For 10 mL printing buffer, add 164 mg sodium acetate and 37.2 mg EDTA to MQH$_2$O. After solubilization, add 50 μL warmed triton X-100 and 4 mL glycerol. Then add approximately 40 μL glacial acetic acid, adding incrementally to adjust the pH to 4.8.
2. ECM stock solutions are typically prepared at 1 mg/mL and stored as appropriately indicated. Add an equal volume of 2× printing buffer to each ECM stock solution and mix thoroughly with pipetting. Mix individual ECM components as desired in a 384-well polypropylene plate for array spotting. It is recommended to mix the proteins and spot them on the same day if possible.

5.4.2.2 Arraying ECM proteins

1. Prepare SMP 3.0 spotting pins according to manufacturer directions. Sonicate in 5% microclean solution (Telechem) for 10 minutes, then rinse and sonicate in MQH$_2$O for 10 minutes. Lightly dry pins with a Kimwipe, including gently touching pin tip with an unsupported Kimwipe to remove excess water from the tip. Clean shaft of pin with a 100% ethanol-soaked Kimwipe to prevent pin sticking in print head.
2. Prepare gel substrates for arraying by dehydrating on a 40°C hot plate for 15 minutes.
3. Print ECM combinations at room temperature with humidity controlled to approximately 65% relative humidity using a platform compatible with contact arraying. In our studies, we have used both the SpotArray 24 (Perkin Elmer) and SpotBot 2 (Telechem) systems. Although the described protocol is adaptable for use with most ECM preparations and array configurations, one typical array layout that we have

utilized is a 100-spot (10 × 10) array, consisting of 20 combinations of five ECM molecules (rat collagen I, human collagen III, mouse collagen IV, mouse laminin, and human fibronectin), with five replicates and 450-µm spacing. After printing, arrays should be stored dry at 4°C within a sealed box humidified with a solution of saturated sodium chloride for approximately 48 hours.

5.4.3 Cell culture on ECM arrays

1. Sterilize array slides with exposure to UVC germicidal (254 nm) radiation.
2. For "ungasketed" seeding of an entire array slide with a single cell type, quadriPERM cell culture vessels (Sigma-Aldrich) are well suited. Approximately 4 mL cellular suspension is required for seeding in this configuration. Cells can be added to the array after two washes and hydration in culture medium for 10 to 15 minutes. In our previous studies utilizing ES cells as well as primary liver cell types, densities ranging from $0.5 \cdot 10^6$ to $1.0 \cdot 10^6$ cells/mL result in well-populated arrays after an 18-hour attachment period. Attachment time and cell density must be optimized for each individual cell type and experiment of interest. Cell culture can then proceed on the arrays as required.

(*optional*) To adapt the microarrays to a multiwell format, several commercial well/gasket systems have been explored and can work well for this purpose. Recent studies in our laboratory have utilized the ProPlate system from Grace Bio-Labs. Such multiwell gaskets can be sterilized by germicidal UV exposure in parallel with the array slides, then assembled and washed prior to introducing cells. Typically 100 µL cell suspension is added to each well/array for cell attachment.

5.4.4 Staining, imaging, and data acquisition

5.4.4.1 Fixation and immunostaining

1. For immunostaining of cellular microarrays, the following multistep procedure can be utilized. First, slides should be rinsed briefly in cold HBSS.
2. Fix slides using a chilled 4% paraformaldehyde solution freshly prepared in 150 mM phosphate buffer (pH, 7.2). Fix slides for 5 minutes at 4°C, followed by 10 minutes at room temperature.
3. Wash slides 3× with HBSS and then transfer to −20°C 100% methanol for 6 minutes as a secondary fixation step.
4. Wash with cold HBSS and store at 4°C.
5. Permeabilize cells with 0.1% triton X-100 in PBS for 8 minutes, followed by several washes with PBS.
6. Block arrays for 1.5 hours at room temperature with 3% BSA, 50 mM glycine in Tris-EDTA buffer (pH, 8.0).
7. Immunostaining can be performed according to specific antibody protocols. Each individual array on the slide can be stained for distinct readouts in parallel using multiwell gaskets, analogous to their use during the culture phase. In general, the ECM microarrays are compatible with both fluorescent and enzyme-based detection strategies. Mounting of the array slides with coverslips can be done with mounting mediums such as Fluoromount-G (Southern Biotechnology).

5.4.4.2 Imaging and quantification

1. Microscope images can be acquired manually or with various automation strategies. Previously, we have acquired images at 10× using an Olympus IX81 motorized microscope with a Prior Proscan stage, ORCA-ER 12-bit cooled-CCD camera (Hammamatsu) and an image acquisition journal written in Metamorph 6.2r3 (Universal Imaging).

2. Alternatively, array spot intensities can be quantified using a microarray scanner-based approach. In previous studies, we have utilized a confocal DNA microarray scanner (Scanarray 4000) designed for dual detection of Cy-3 and Cy-5 signals to image array slides at 5-μm pixel resolution. Nucleic acid staining with POPO-3 (similar to Cy-3) was imaged using 543-nm laser excitation and a 570-nm emission filter. GFP expression was detected using a Cy-5 converted signal, by labeling with anti-GFP-Alexafluor 647 (Cy-5 equivalent), and imaging using 633 nm excitation and a 670-nm emission filter. Each well array should be imaged using a focus height that provides the maximum signal for each channel at the center of the array.

3. Microscope montaged images or scanner images can be analyzed and quantified with numerous different software packages. We have quantified arrays using Metamorph or GenePix software. Array features can be autoaligned according to the array feature size and dimension. Spot identification can be adjusted manually if incorrectly identified spots are present. In our studies, only spots in which more than 70% of pixels were above local background in both channels were used during subsequent analysis.

5.4.5 Data analysis

A broad spectrum of cellular readouts can be processed from the ECM microarrays. For instance, average (±standard deviation) spot intensity values can provide quantitative measures of collective cell growth, differentiation, or functional alterations in response to the arrayed environmental stimuli. Numerical transformation and normalization across multiple arrays can be used to assess distribution and variance, and to compare multiple data sets. Factorial analysis is a powerful tool for the assessment of combinatorial effects within an array context. In previous studies, we have analyzed array data with a 2^5 full factorial design with four blocks (for four replicate microarrays) using Minitab statistical software [14]. Main effects, as well as two-factor, three-factor, and four-factor interactions, including the statistical significance of each of these properties, were calculated using standard factorial analysis methods.

5.5 Anticipated Results

Utilizing these procedures, the fabricated ECM arrays should be robust and reproducible. Although it is typical that cell adhesion, survival, and function can be highly dependent on cell types and ECM components used. Thorough kinetic analysis achieved by incorporating live cell fluorescent reporters or by fixation and immunostaining at multiple time points has proved to be very useful in examining cellular responses in the array context. Furthermore, in addition to overall quantitative measurements for each spot within the array, individual cell measurements and high content assessment can be achieved through integration of image analysis modalities with cytometric and subcellular analysis capabilities.

5.6 Discussion and Commentary

The ECM microarrays are a versatile platform appropriate for studies with a wide range of cell types. During initial experiments, our laboratory explored the role of ECM components and combinations in primary hepatocyte survival and functional stabilization [14]. Through this approach, collagen IV was identified as a factor that exhibits a significant positive effect on hepatocyte function (measured by intracellular albumin staining), contrasting with laminin and collagen III, which each demonstrated a negative effect. Of note, factorial analysis illustrated intriguing interactions between components. For example, the combination of laminin and collagen III exhibited a positive influence on function despite their negative affects individually.

As highlighted in this chapter, this platform also exhibits particular utility for investigating the growth and differentiation of stem cells. Previously, we have examined ES cells containing a β-galactosidase reporter for the fetal liver-specific gene *Ankrd17* in the presence of 32 different combinations of collagen I, collagen III, collagen IV, laminin, and fibronectin [14]. An approximately 140-fold difference in β-galactosidase signal was observed between the least and most efficient conditions, suggesting that environmental matrix composition can influence early hepatic lineage specification (Figure 5.2). Further investigations of ES cell differentiation in response to spotted microenvironmental stimuli continue in our laboratory, as well as the analysis of various adult stem cell populations. In addition, because soluble factors are also important components of the stem cell microenvironment, and soluble factor/ECM cross-talk has been suggested in many settings [15, 16], our group has recently extended this matrix array platform into a multiwell format with a 96-well plate footprint to investigate stem cell differentiation simultaneously in 1,200 parallel experiments representing 240 unique soluble factor/ECM environments [17].

Another approach for exploring stem cell differentiation with arrays of signaling molecules was demonstrated by Soen et al. [18], and utilized printed combinations of ECM molecules, growth factors, and other signaling proteins. In this work, the proliferation and differentiation of human neural precursor cells toward a neuronal or glial fate was examined by quantitative image analysis in response to these various exogenous stimuli. Some of the key findings from this work include a dose responsive role of the Notch ligand, Jagged-1, in shifting differentiation toward the glial fate, and the observation that simultaneous stimulation of the Notch and Wnt signaling pathways resulted in the proliferation of cells exhibiting undifferentiated characteristics. Furthermore, the presence of bone morphogenetic protein 4 induced the acquisition of a hybrid phenotype, with cells expressing markers of both neurons and glial cells. Overall, numerous complementary approaches for enhancing the throughput and efficacy of cellular microarray platforms continue to be explored, and these systems should ultimately aid in the further understanding of microenvironmental regulation.

5.6 Discussion and Commentary

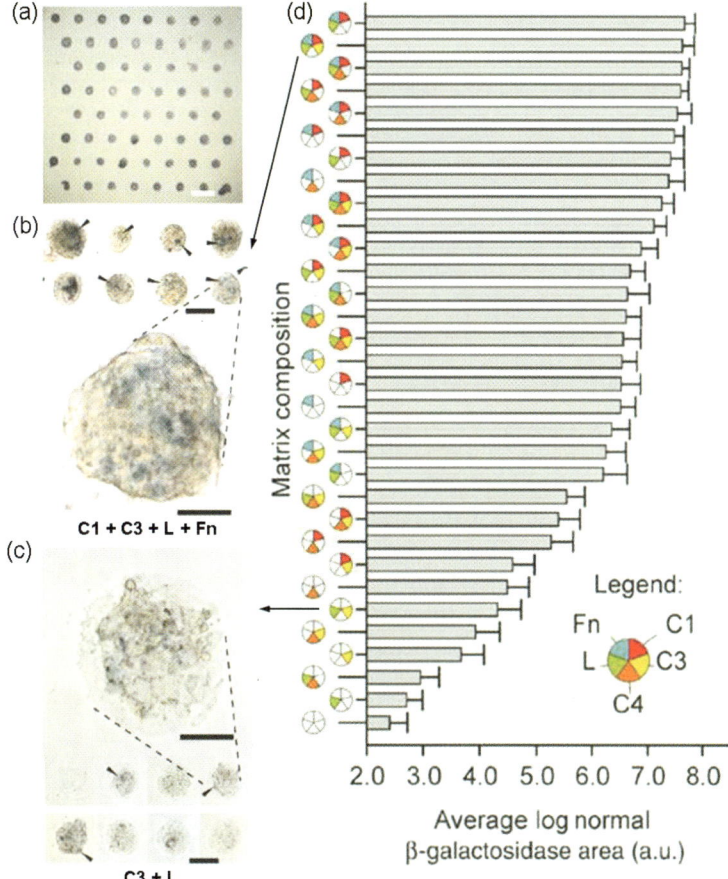

Figure 5.2 ECM microarray utilized to investigate ES cell differentiation toward an early hepatic lineage. (a) Alkaline phosphatase staining of day 1 ES cultures on ECM microarrays (scale bar = 1 mm). (b, c) Bright-field micrograph of selected X-gal-stained conditions after 3 days of culture in retinoic acid. Collagen I (C1) + collagen III (C3) + laminin (L) + fibronectin (Fn) (b) induced higher reporter activity (arrowheads) for *Ankrd17*, a fetal liver-specific gene, than was seen in cells cultured on C3 + L (c). Scale bars = 250 µm. Magnified views of reporter activity: scale bars = 50 µm. (d) Hierarchical depiction of "blue" image area (pooled data from four microarrays) for each of the matrix mixtures. Error bars, standard error of mean (n = 32). The C1 + C3 + L + Fn culture condition induced an approximate 27-fold more reporter positive image area than the C3 + L cultures. (Figure adapted from [14].)

Troubleshooting Table

Problem	Explanation	Potential Solutions
Lack of cell attachment	Inadequate deposition of ECM material	Increase concentration of ECM solution. Confirm spotting parameters using fluorescently tagged material. Check for pin clogging or ECM aggregation.
Aggregation of ECM molecules in printing buffer/pin clogging	Printing buffer is not optimal; pin not sufficiently clean	Check pH of printing buffer. Generally, the printing buffer is made fresh after 1 month at 4°C. Clean pins thoroughly prior to the print run according to manufacturer guidelines. Also, cleaning cycles within the print run can be increased.

(continues)

Problem	Explanation	Potential Solutions
Detachment of polyacrylamide gel substrate from slide	Long-term culture in serum media can occasionally cause partial detachment of the gel substrate, particularly if entire slide is hydrated (ungasketed).	Make certain that the glass is hydroxylated prior to silanization. Other approaches could be to use alternative silane coupling regimes or a highly porous glass surface [19–22].
Reduction in cell viability	Some cell types can exhibit profound sensitivity to certain contaminating agents.	Ensure acrylamide gel pads are adequately washed after polymerization. Confirm that multiwell gaskets, if utilized, are biocompatible.

5.7 Application Notes

The ECM microarrays outlined in this chapter represent a method for parallel analysis of cell responses to a multitude of ECM conditions. This system is compatible with standard and widely available robotic spotting technology. Included among the important parameters is the choice of microarray substrate. In initial experiments, our laboratory tested a range of potential substrates, identifying a custom polyacrylamide surface as optimal for retention of spotted ECM molecules while still resisting adsorption of serum proteins and maintaining localized cell adhesion. Although current studies suggest that this acrylamide substrate can immobilize a wide range of spotted factors (unpublished results), potential chemical modifications could be used to tailor the surface functionality further. In addition, polyacrylamide hydrogel substrates have been broadly utilized as means to manipulate surface stiffness and to examine the effects of elastic properties on cell behavior [23, 24]. As a result of the fact that mechanical cues have been implicated in stem cell differentiation [24, 25], and mode of presentation can modulate the function of some ligands [26, 27], systems that incorporate surface chemistry or material modifications to explore these additional issues systematically will likely be key extensions of cellular array platforms in the future. Additional precedence for such material-based systems has been demonstrated by Anderson et al. [28], who described a synthetic polymer array consisting of 1,700 cell–biomaterial interactions that was utilized to identify biomaterial compositions influencing human ES cell attachment, growth, and differentiation.

5.8 Summary Points

1. We have developed an ECM microarray platform for analyzing the combinatorial effect of ECM molecules on cell fate. The modular nature of this system is compatible with an extensive range of ECM components, and the layout of the array can be easily tailored to specific experimental requirements.
2. A dehydrated polyacrylamide gel substrate was determined to be optimal for this platform by efficiently trapping and presenting spotted ECM molecules while still preventing cell migration and nonspecific attachment. Additionally, a printing buffer was modified to prevent ECM aggregation and pin clogging, as well as enable efficient and reproducible deposition of material.

3. The ECM microarray platform is compatible with a wide selection of cellular assays such as the fixation and immunostaining procedures described here.
4. We have also adapted the array platform to a multiwell format to investigate interactions between ECM components and soluble stimuli. Current studies in our laboratory continue to explore additional modifications to this system to expand functionality and improve throughput further.

Acknowledgments

This work was supported by the National Institutes of Health, the National Science Foundation, and the David and Lucille Packard Foundation.

References

[1] Scadden, D.T., "The Stem-Cell Niche as an Entity of Action," *Nature*, Vol. 441, 2006, pp. 1075–1079.
[2] Fuchs, E., T. Tumbar, and G. Guasch, "Socializing with the Neighbors: Stem Cells and Their Niche," *Cell*, Vol. 116, 2004, pp. 769–778.
[3] Davey, R. E., and P. W. Zandstra, "Spatial Organization of Embryonic Stem Cell Responsiveness to Autocrine gp130 Ligands Reveals an Autoregulatory Stem Cell Niche," *Stem Cells*, Vol. 24, 2006, pp. 2538–2548.
[4] Peerani, R., et al., "Niche-Mediated Control of Human Embryonic Stem Cell Self-Renewal and Differentiation," *EMBO J.*, Vol. 26, 2007, pp. 4744–4755.
[5] Folch, A., and M. Toner, "Microengineering of Cellular Interaction," *Annu. Rev. Biomed. Eng.*, Vol. 2, 2000, pp. 227–256.
[6] Underhill, G. H., and S. N. Bhatia, "High-Throughput Analysis of Signals Regulating Stem Cell Fate and Function," *Curr. Opin. Chem. Biol.*, Vol. 11, 2007, pp. 357–366.
[7] Castel, D., et al., "Cell Microarrays in Drug Discovery," *Drug Discov. Today*, Vol. 11, 2006, pp. 616–622.
[8] Chen, D. S., and M. M. Davis, "Molecular and Functional Analysis Using Live Cell Microarrays," *Curr. Opin. Chem. Biol.*, Vol. 10, 2006, pp. 28–34.
[9] Jones, P. H., and F. M. Watt, "Separation of Human Epidermal Stem Cells from Transit Amplifying Cells on the Basis of Differences in Integrin Function and Expression," *Cell*, Vol. 73, 1993, pp. 713–724.
[10] Campos, L. S., et al., "Beta1 Integrins Activate a MAPK Signalling Pathway in Neural Stem Cells That Contributes to Their Maintenance," *Development*, Vol. 131, 2004, pp. 3433–3444.
[11] Garcion, E., et al., "Generation of an Environmental Niche for Neural Stem Cell Development by the Extracellular Matrix Molecule Tenascin C," *Development*, Vol. 131, 2004, pp. 3423–3432.
[12] Stier, S., et al., "Osteopontin Is a Hematopoietic Stem Cell Niche Component That Negatively Regulates Stem Cell Pool Size," *J. Exp. Med.*, Vol. 201, 2005, pp. 1781–1791.
[13] Nilsson, S. K., et al., "Osteopontin, a Key Component of the Hematopoietic Stem Cell Niche and Regulator of Primitive Hematopoietic Progenitor Cells," *Blood*, Vol. 106, 2005, pp. 1232–1239.
[14] Flaim, C. J., S. Chien, and S. N. Bhatia, "An Extracellular Matrix Microarray for Probing Cellular Differentiation," *Nat. Methods*, Vol. 2, 2005, pp. 119–125.
The ECM microarray platform developed in our laboratory was first described here, with several examples of its utility.
[15] Sastry, S. K., and A. F. Horwitz, "Adhesion–Growth Factor Interactions During Differentiation: An Integrated Biological Response," *Dev. Biol.*, Vol. 180, 1996, pp. 455–467.
[16] Comoglio, P. M., C. Boccaccio, and L. Trusolino, "Interactions between Growth Factor Receptors and Adhesion Molecules: Breaking the Rules," *Curr. Opin. Cell Biol.*, Vol., 15, 2003, pp. 565–571.
[17] Flaim, C. J., et al., "Combinatorial Signaling Microenvironments for Studying Stem Cell Fate," *Stem Cells Dev.*, Vol. 17, 2008, pp. 29–40.
[18] Soen, Y., et al., "Exploring the Regulation of Human Neural Precursor Cell Differentiation Using Arrays of Signaling Microenvironments," *Mol. Syst. Biol.*, Vol. 2, 2006, p. 37.
The authors utilized a microarray platform to explore the effects of combinations of ECM, growth factors, and other signaling proteins on neural precursor differentiation. This work is an excellent example of the benefits of high-throughput microarray approaches for examining stem cell responses.
[19] Revzin, A., et al., "Fabrication of Poly(Ethylene Glycol) Hydrogel Microstructures Using Photolithography," *Langmuir*, Vol. 17, 2001, pp. 5440–5447.

[20] Koh, W. G., A. Revzin, and M. V. Pishko, "Poly(Ethylene Glycol) Hydrogel Microstructures Encapsulating Living Cells," *Langmuir*, Vol. 18, 2002, pp. 2459–2462.
[21] Kim, C. O., et al., "Modification of Indium–Tin Oxide (ITO) Glass with Aziridine Provides a Surface of High Amine Density," *J. Colloid Interface Sci.*, Vol. 277, 2004, pp. 499–504.
[22] Timofeev, E., et al., "Regioselective Immobilization of Short Oligonucleotides to Acrylic Copolymer Gels," *Nucl. Acids Res.*, Vol. 24, 1996, pp. 3142–3148.
[23] Pelham, R. J., Jr., and Y. Wang, "Cell Locomotion and Focal Adhesions Are Regulated by Substrate Flexibility," *Proc. Natl. Acad. Sci. USA*, Vol. 94, 1997, pp. 13661–13665.
[24] Engler, A. J., et al., "Matrix Elasticity Directs Stem Cell Lineage Specification," *Cell*, Vol. 126, 2006, pp. 677–689.
[25] McBeath, R., et al., "Cell Shape, Cytoskeletal Tension, and RhoA Regulate Stem Cell Lineage Commitment," *Dev. Cell*, Vol. 6, 2004, pp. 483–495.
[26] Varnum-Finney, B., et al., "Immobilization of Notch Ligand, Delta-1, Is Required for Induction of Notch Signaling," *J. Cell Sci.*, Vol. 113, 2000, pp. 4313–4318.
[27] Hicks, C., et al., "A Secreted Delta1–Fc Fusion Protein Functions Both as an Activator and Inhibitor of Notch1 Signaling," *J. Neurosci. Res.*, Vol. 68, 2002, pp. 655–667.
[28] Anderson, D. G., S. Levenberg, and R. Langer, "Nanoliter-Scale Synthesis of Arrayed Biomaterials and Application to Human Embryonic Stem Cells," *Nat. Biotechnol.*, Vol. 22, 2004, pp. 863–866.

CHAPTER

6

Microfluidic Culture Platform for Investigating the Proliferation and Differentiation of Stem Cells

Hyung Joon Kim,[1] Bong Geun Chung,[1] Hwa-Sung Shin,[1] Aixu Sun,[2] Ken W. Y. Cho,[2] and Noo Li Jeon[1]

[1]Department of Biomedical Engineering
[2]Department of Developmental and Cell Biology
3120 Natural Science II
University of California Irvine
Irvine, CA, 92697

Abstract

This chapter describes microfluidic culture platforms for the differentiation and proliferation of stem cells and neural stem cells. Stem cells have enormous therapeutic potential to derive transplantable cells for various human diseases. This potential is contingent on finding ways to control their proliferation and differentiation into specific types of cells. We developed several microfluidic culture platforms to provide the delivery of growth factors to stem cells in a controlled manner to direct cell proliferation and differentiation. The role of bone morphogenic protein and growth factors in regulating proliferation and differentiation of stem cells was investigated by utilizing these microfluidic culture platforms that are designed for introducing dynamically controlled spatial and temporal gradients.

| Key Terms | Microfluidic
gradient
stem cells
differentiation
proliferation |

6.1 Introduction

The generation and maintenance of spatial and temporal gradients is crucial for investigating the proliferation and differentiation of stem cells in a controlled environment. Microfabrication and microfluidics are believed to open the gate for innovative approaches in stem cell biology. Here we describe several microfluidic culture platforms for studying the proliferation and differentiation of stem cells, including fluidic network-based microfluidic devices (known as *Christmas tree*) for chemotaxis of neutrophils [1, 2], and differentiation of human neural progenitor cells [3] as well as metastatic cancer cells [4]. This platform has a series of fluidic channels that generate a combinatorial mixture of soluble factors by repeatedly splitting and mixing fluid streams. At the observing area, one can easily verify the response of cells toward the spatial gradient of soluble molecules. However, it is difficult to plate stem cells uniformly inside the microfluidic chamber before each experiment and maintain them at near-confluence for a long time because of the fact that embryonic stem cells (ESCs), like neural precursor cells, are sensitive to environmental changes and often undergo apoptosis within hours after plating (unpublished data).

To clear this hurdle, we recently developed a new hybrid microfluidic platform that has fluidic channels embedded within a vacuum network to generate a gradient of soluble factors in a conventional culture platform [5]. It allows for the reversible application of microfluidic networks onto preplated cell culture surfaces, ensuring the survival of the cells within the chamber. In addition, the system can be easily assembled onto monolayer cells grown in a Petri dish, and therefore multiple experiments can be performed. This chapter reviews recent developments in the microfluidic culture platforms to monitor the proliferation and differentiation of stem cells in precisely controlled environments.

6.2 Experimental Design

6.2.1 Microfluidic platform for differentiation of human neural progenitor cells

Stem cells hold tremendous promise for cell-based therapies in human diseases [1,2], because they can be a source of differentiated cells, while continuing to self-renew [7]. The promise of stem cells also holds true for tissue-specific stem cells such as neural stem cells (NSCs). NSCs can be differentiated into the three major types of cells in the central nervous system [8–10] so that they can be one of the therapeutic candidates in neurodegenerative diseases [6, 11, 12]. One of the most important issues in this development is to control and optimize factors precisely in stem cell culture, such as manipulating their proliferation and differentiation into a specific cell type.

To control a cellular environment precisely for stem cell culture, microfluidic culture platforms have been recently developed [13] and used for studying proliferation and differentiation of human NSCs (hNSCs) [3]. Using this device, we cultured hNSCs isolated from the developing cerebral cortex in a continuous concentration gradient of known growth factors. These cells exhibited proliferation and differentiation responses that were concentration dependent and quantitatively similar to those seen in parallel control cultures. Figure 6.1(a) shows a schematic of the microfluidic culture device that consists of control and gradient chambers. A gradient profile of growth factors was confirmed

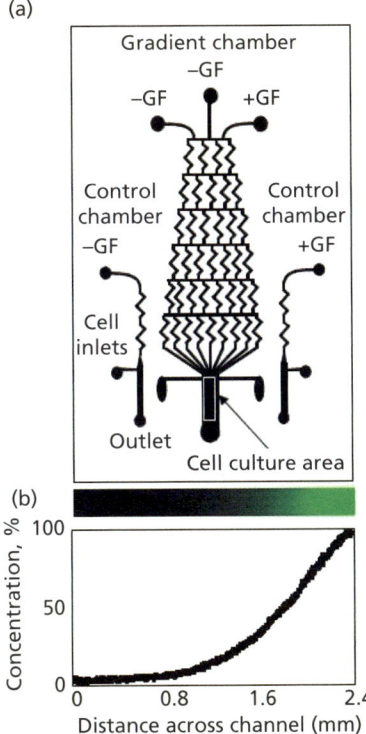

Figure 6.1 A gradient-generating microfluidic device for proliferation and differentiation of hNSCs. (a) Schematic design of the microfluidic device showing the gradient chamber and two control chambers. Cells were loaded into the chambers via inlet ports, and the entire device was placed on an inverted microscope for live cell imaging. GF, growth factor. (b) The gradient profile generated within the gradient chamber was visualized with the fluorescence profile of FITC–dextran.

by fluorescence imaging from fluorescein isothiocyanate (FITC)–dextran as shown in Figure 6.1(b). hNSCs exposed to gradients of growth factors were cultured for 7 days in vitro. hNSCs proliferated and differentiated into astrocytes in a graded, proportional fashion that varied directly with the concentration of growth factors.

6.2.2 A hybrid microfluidic platform for stem cell biology

This section describes the design and application of a versatile microfluidic device that can be directly interfaced with conventional cell culture platforms for stem cell biology applications. Microfluidic culture is an enabling platform that overcomes the current limitations in traditional culturing tools. However, it is difficult to work with stem cells and other sensitive cells that do not survive long-term culture inside microfluidic devices. We describe a new design that incorporates separate sets of fluidic and vacuum channels on a single device that allows gradient generation and reversible application of microfluidic networks on wet cell culture surfaces. This platform provides a simple yet highly adaptable tool for incorporating the advantages of a microfluidics approach to basic biological assays without any changes to well-established tissue culture protocols.

Figure 6.2(a) shows the schematic design of the hybrid microfluidic device. The key feature in this device was to place the fluidic channels in the center region, which is

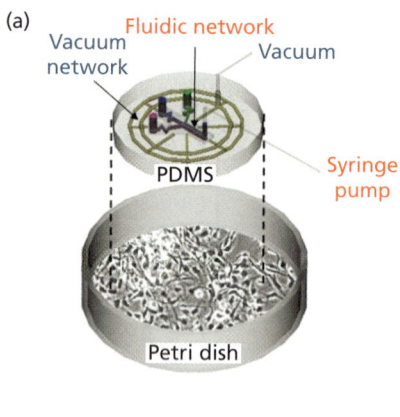

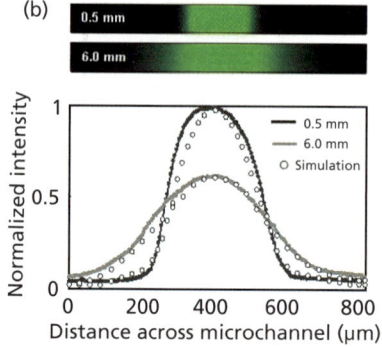

Figure 6.2 A hybrid microfluidic vacuum platform for interfacing with a Petri dish. (a) Schematic design of the microfluidic chamber integrated with vacuum and fluidic channels. Side reservoirs contain buffer, and buffer with FITC–dextran fills the middle reservoir. Parallel laminar flows from the three reservoirs can generate stable gradients by diffusion. The external vacuum source was connected to the vacuum inlet. (b) Steep and shallow gradients were generated at 0.5 mm and 6 mm downstream from the junction of the fluidic channel with a withdrawal rate of 1 µL/minute. Two different gradient profiles generated at 0.5 mm and 6 mm downstream were visualized with the fluorescence profile of FITC–dextran. Scale bars = 100 µm.

isolated with a vacuum network for interfacing with conventionally cultured tissues. The vacuum channels can be placed anywhere from 200 µm to 2 mm away from the fluidic channels. Because of the soft elastomeric property of polydimethysil-oxane (PDMS), microfluidic channels can be reversibly formed on any type of flat substrate by using vacuum channels. The bond between device and surface is maintained by applying a vacuum. Experimental setup can be performed simply when the cells are ready in the Petri dish. In sum, the hybrid microfluidic vacuum platform has advantages over previous microfluidic culture platforms: (1) it can be directly interfaced with cultured cells on Petri dishes, (2) it can be utilized for sensitive cells such as mouse neural progenitor cells, and (3) reversible bonding allows immunocytochemistry and further biochemical assay. Using a three-inlet design, we can generate various gradient profiles by controlling the flow rate and by designating various positions downstream of the fluidic channel. By withdrawing different soluble factors from the three reservoirs, continuous laminar flow can generate a stable gradient that is perpendicular to the flow. Multiple gradient profiles can be generated at different positions (e.g., a few millimeters apart) on a single device and controlled by adjusting different flow rates (0.1–1 µL/minute). Figure 6.2(b) shows two different gradient profiles at 0.5 mm and 6 mm downstream from the junction of fluidic channels that were generated by flowing a solution containing FITC–dextran (10 μM; molecular weight, 10 kDa) from the middle reservoir while the side reservoirs contained buffer. The gradients can be maintained for 6 to 24 hours, depending on the reservoir capacity (150–600 μL) and flow rates. Also, the gradient profile had agreement with simulation using an incompressible Navier-Stokes convection and diffusion model (COMSOL Multiphysics 3.2 FEMLAB software, COMSOL Inc.).

6.2.3 ESC response under dynamically controlled gradient condition

It is generally acknowledged that proper progression of stem cells into differentiated states is achieved step by step as stem cells gradually differentiate into more complex, specialized cell types after receiving various developmental cues [14]. An optimal condition for the combinations of factors must be addressed to recreate the process of targeted cell differentiation, because the biochemical environment (e.g., presence of extracellular matrix proteins, exposure to growth factors) surrounding the proliferating and differentiating stem cells changes at each stage of differentiation. Regardless of the rigor of such an approach, it may still be difficult to define unequivocally favorable differentiation conditions, because the conventional static cell culture system results in a soluble microenvironment with characteristics that drift over time as cells deplete nutrients from the media and secrete diffusible signals and wastes to surrounding cells. The issue becomes increasingly challenging as we start developing multistep procedures that involve a series of growth factor treatments and media changes, and each step creates an increasingly more heterogeneous cell population. An improved culture system that alleviates these issues and increases the efficacy of cell proliferation and differentiation is therefore a requirement if we wish to utilize stem cells as therapeutic agents. Ideally, this improved system should be able to regulate the microenvironment surrounding the cells by controlling the spatiotemporal exposure to growth factors. The hybrid microfluidic culture platform discussed earlier meets this requirement.

Mouse ESCs (mESCs) can be cultured with a layer of mouse embryonic fibroblast cells, which produce certain factors important for maintenance of mESCs. Leukemia inhibitory factor (LIF) is one factor produced by mouse embryonic fibroblast cells that can support mESC growth [15–18]. Although LIF alone has been shown to be insufficient for stem cell maintenance, bone morphogenic protein 4 (BMP-4) was found to coordinate with LIF to maintain mESC pluripotency in serum-free culture conditions [19]. BMPs are a subgroup of secreted dimeric signaling proteins within the larger transforming growth factor α superfamily, and are key players in regulating cell proliferation, differentiation, and apoptosis [20]. BMP signals are also well known for their ability to inhibit neural differentiation in various embryos and ESCs [19, 21], as well as to induce mesoderm, endoderm, and trophoblast lineages [19, 22–25]. In addition to BMPs, Wnt and fibroblast growth factor (FGF) signaling components are involved in ESC proliferation and differentiation. For instance, although controversy exists, Wnt–catenin signaling has been demonstrated to maintain pluripotency in ESCs under certain conditions and is critical for the expansion of progenitors [26–28]. Elevated concentrations of FGF2 permit the culture of human ESCs in the absence of fibroblasts or fibroblast-conditioned medium [29]. Currently, the precise roles of these growth factors in conjunction with BMPs on ESC proliferation and maintenance are still not well understood.

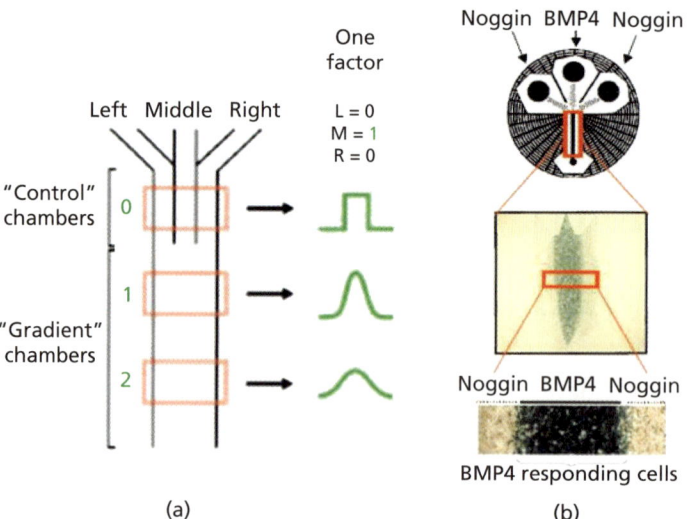

Figure 6.3 A hybrid microfluidic platform for monitoring the BMP responsiveness of mESCs. (a) Spatiotemporal concentration of a molecule in laminar flow is affected by convective flow and diffusion, resulting in multiple gradient profiles at different downstream positions along the cell culture chamber. (b) Three-inlet microfluidic system device is sealed onto tissue culture grown in a Petri dish by suctioning a vacuum through the vacuum port. Media enter via three inlets and exit via one outlet continuously. Noggin and BMP-containing media pass through the inlets and form a BMP gradient. Gradient formation was measured by mixing a fluorescent dye with Noggin and BMP. After 24 hours of exposure to BMP-4, ESC responses toward various BMP gradients were monitored.

Cells experience a nonsteady-state culture environment over time in a static culture, as they continuously deplete nutrients from the media and secrete diffusible signals and wastes to surrounding cells. Thus, any system with perfusion offers advantages because it provides better steady-state conditions. We incorporated a simple fluidic network composed of three inlet reservoirs and one outlet for gradient generation. For generating flow, a syringe pump connected to the channel outlet is operated in withdrawal mode to minimize pressurizing the channel, which could disrupt the seal between the device and substrate. ESC culture media supplemented with either BMP or Noggin are placed in the reservoirs and passed through the inlets at desired flow rates using a syringe pump-driven flow system. By changing the laminar flow rates, differential mixing occurs as solutions move across the chamber, resulting in the generation of a BMP gradient across a microchamber (Figure 6.3). Formation of a gradient was monitored by mixing fluorescent dyes (e.g., fluorescein) into the BMP solutions and then examining the distribution of dyes in the chamber using time-lapse fluorescence microscopy.

6.3 Materials and Methods

6.3.1 Fabrication of the microfluidic device

The microfluidic NSC culture device was fabricated in PDMS using rapid prototyping and soft lithography following published procedures [1, 12, 30, 31]. The master mold was fabricated by patterning 100-μm-thick negative photoresist (SU8 50, Microchem) by photolithography [32]. A positive replica with an embossed network of microchannels was fabricated by replica molding PDMS against the master [13, 30, 33, 34]. The surface of the PDMS and the glass slide were activated with reactive oxygen plasma (2 minutes at 30W; model PDC-001, Harrick Scientific) and brought together immediately to form an irreversible seal [1, 13]. The PDMS was attached to the glass slide such that the glass formed the bottom of the channels and provided a surface for cellular adhesion. The cell culture area (near the outlet, a 2.4-mm-wide channel in gradient devices) was covered with a glass slide during plasma treatment to prevent permanent bonding. This step allowed removal of the PDMS portion around the cell culture area for immunocytochemistry and fluorescence microscopy. After assembly, the device surface was coated with poly-L-lysine (0.5 mg/mL in 0.1M borate buffer at room temperature for 1 hour) [35, 36] and mouse laminin (0.5 mg/mL at 37°C for 8 hours). Microfluidic devices were connected to syringe pumps with base medium (left two inlets) or base medium with growth factors (right inlet) to generate a spatial concentration gradient (combinatorial mixture) of the growth factors perpendicular to the channel across the cell culture area [1, 34]. The stability and shape of the soluble growth factor gradient was confirmed by imaging fluorescence from FITC–dextran. FITC–dextran (10 μM; molecular weight, 10 kDa), which has a similar molecular weight to growth factors like epidermal growth factor (EGF; molecular weight, 6 kDa), was added to the growth factor-containing media to serve as an indirect indicator of the growth factor gradient inside the channel [37]. The observed gradient profile matched the mathematical prediction, as in previous works [13, 32].

6.3.2 Fabrication of a hybrid microfluidic platform

This device consists of a network of vacuum lines and a fluidic network. The vacuum lines are made with 250-μm-wide channels in 300-μm intervals. The external vacuum source was connected to the vacuum inlet of the device. A device can be directly applied to cells cultured in tissue culture plates when the vacuum lines are constantly aspirating. This allows a reversible bond between the PDMS device and tissue culture plate without a requirement for special equipment or processes (e.g., plasma treatment). The fluidic channel is divided into two regions: control and gradient. Each channel is separated by a 100-μm-wide barrier. The two physical barriers of the control region prevented diffusing to the other channels. Downstream of the control region, the three inlets combine into one channel, which forms the gradient region (800 μm wide). Buffer containing FITC–dextran (10 μM; molecular weight, 10 kDa; Sigma) flowed into the middle channel and buffer was placed in the other channels. Withdrawing at a rate 1 μL/minute, a gradient was generated. The soluble gradient profile was confirmed by imaging fluorescence from FITC–dextran and was compared with simulations (COMSOL Multiphysics 3.2 FEMLAB software, COMSOL Inc.).

6.3.3 Human neural stem cells

The hNSCs isolated from the developing cerebral cortex of premature human infants (SC23) [38, 39] were provided by the National Human Neural Stem Cell Resource at the Children's Hospital of Orange County and were grown as adherent cultures in fibronectin-coated flasks in a humidified incubator at 37°C with 5% CO_2. Cells were cultured in base medium consisting of Dulbecco's modified Eagle's medium–F12 nutrient mixtures (Invitrogen) supplemented with 20% BIT 9500 (Stem Cell Technologies) and 1% antibiotic/antimycotic (Invitrogen) [38, 39]. Growth medium was prepared from base medium by adding three human recombinant growth factors, each at 40 ng/mL: EGF (BD Biosciences), FGF2 (BD Biosciences), and platelet-derived growth factor (PeproTech) [38, 39].

6.3.4 Mouse neural stem cells

6.3.4.1 Mice

Wild-type (WT) CD1 mice were used for these studies. Noon of the vaginal plug date was day 0.5 in timed pregnancies between WT CD1 females and WT CD1 males. All animal studies were done in accordance with Institutional Animal Care and Use Committee guidelines.

6.3.4.2 NSC culture

Telencephalic NSC cultures were prepared from embryos harvested on gestational day 12.5. Briefly, telencephalic vesicles were isolated, and cells were dissociated for 20 minutes at 37°C in Hanks' balanced salt solution (Invitrogen) containing 0.05% trypsin with 0.02% ethylenediaminetetraacetic acid (Invitrogen), and 0.2% bovine serum albumin (BSA; ICN Biomedicals). Trypsinization was stopped by adding an equal volume of 1 mg/mL soybean trypsin inhibitor (Invitrogen) in phosphate-buffered saline (PBS). Tissue digests were dissociated using several rounds of trituration using a fire-polished Pasteur pipette. Cells were washed once with Hank's balanced salt solution containing 0.2% BSA and then were resuspended in Temple medium with 10 ng/mL FGF, 20 ng/mL EGF, and 2 μg/mL heparin. Cells were grown as neurospheres in six-well nontissue culture-treated plates at a density of 100,000 cells in a well. Cells were incubated at 37°C in humidified 5% CO_2/95% air atmosphere for 3 days. Neurospheres were then dissociated with the NeuroCult Chemical Dissociation Kit (Stem Cell Technologies). Dissociated cells were plated on poly-d-lysine/laminin-coated six-well tissue culture-treated plates (Corning) at 600,000 cells per well in Temple medium with 10 ng/mL FGF, 20 ng/mL EGF, and 2 μg/mL heparin for 24 hours before applying the microfluidic device.

6.3.5 Culturing cells inside the microfluidic chamber and time-lapse microscopy

The hNSCs were detached from the culture flask using cell dissociation buffer (Invitrogen), washed, and resuspended in culture medium. Cells (100 μL of a suspension of 500,000 cells/mL) were loaded into the microfluidic device via cell inlet ports on the side of the chambers using a micropipette tip. The microfluidic device containing adherent hNSCs was placed inside an environmental chamber (37°C and 5% CO_2) on an inverted microscope (Nikon). The microfluidic chamber was maintained with a constant perfusion of media at physiological pH. Polyethylene tubing was inserted into three inlets at the top of the gradient chamber to make fluidic connections [1]. The media with and without growth factor were injected into the gradient chamber using a syringe pump at a controlled rate of 0.1 μL/minute. Cells cultured inside the microfluidic gradient chambers were thus exposed to a growth factor gradient in a stable microenvironment.

A motorized stage was used to obtain images at multiple positions in the microfluidic device at 10-minute intervals.

6.3.6 Immunocytochemistry

After culturing the cells inside the microfluidic device for 7 days, they were fixed in 4% paraformaldehyde (Sigma) and permeabilized with 0.3% triton X-100 in PBS (Invitrogen). After washing with PBS, cells were blocked with 5% BSA (Sigma) in PBS and sequentially exposed to primary and secondary antibodies: antiglial fibrillary acidic protein (Chemicon International; overnight at 4°C) and FITC-conjugated AffiniPure donkey antirabbit immunoglobulin G (Jackson ImmunoResearch Laboratories; 2 hours at room temperature) [38, 39]. Cell nuclei were then counterstained with Hoechst 33342 (Molecular Probes) and device mounted with Vectashield mounting medium (Vector Laboratories). Immunostained cells were kept at 4°C until analyzed. Fluorescent images were obtained with a Nikon E800 upright microscope using a chroma standard filter (350 nm) for DAPI/Hoechst and a chroma high Q filter (480 nm) for FITC.

6.4 Data Acquisition, Anticipated Results, and Interpretation

6.4.1 hNSC proliferation in the gradient chamber

We then cultured cells in the gradient chamber of the microfluidic device. The gradient chamber had two barriers that limited cell migration and divided the continuous growth factor gradient into three compartments with low, intermediate, or high concentrations of growth factors: 0 to 2.8 ng/mL (0% to 7%), 3.2 to 14 ng/mL (8% to 35%), and 14.4 to 40 ng/mL (36% to 100%) for each growth factor. Soon after plating (on day 1), the cells had adhered to the glass surface, but were fairly sparse in all three compartments. After 4 days, the cells had elongated and undergone limited proliferation in the low growth factor compartment, some proliferation in the intermediate growth factor compartment, and more proliferation in the high growth factor compartment (Figure 6.4). This trend continued through day 7, when many more cells were evident in the high growth factor compartment. In addition to the effects on cell proliferation, the growth factor gradient within the intermediate and high growth factor compartments stimulated cell migration toward the higher growth factor concentrations. Quantification of total cell numbers revealed that the hNSCs proliferated in direct proportion to the growth factor concentration. The hNSCs plated in the control chamber without growth factors showed no increase in cell number at 4 or 7 days. However, cells in the low growth factor compartment of the gradient chamber (0–2.8 ng/mL each growth factor) showed a 1.8-fold increase at 4 days and a 2.6-fold increase by day 7 [Figure 6.4(b)]. Cells in the intermediate growth factor compartment (3.2–14 ng/mL) showed a 2.5-fold increase on day 4 and a 3.5-fold increase on day 7, whereas cell numbers in the high growth factor compartment (14.4–40 ng/mL) increased by 3.5-fold and 5-fold at 4 and 7 days, respectively [Figure 6.4(b)]. The control chamber with 100% growth factor concentration showed a 4-fold increase on day 4 and a 6.8-fold increase on day 7 [Figure 6.4(a)]. Therefore, by culturing hNSCs under a continuous gradient of growth factors, we showed that these cells respond in direct proportion to growth factor concentration, at least within the

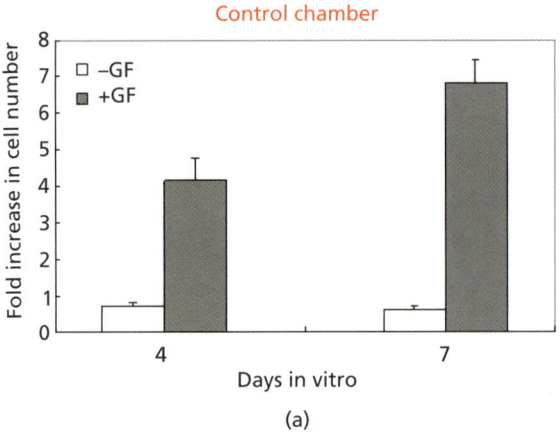

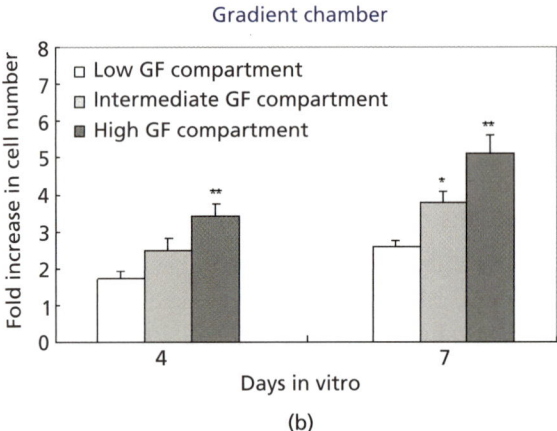

Figure 6.4 Quantitative analysis of hNSC proliferation in the control chamber (a) and gradient chamber (b) at 4 and 7 days. The three compartments of the gradient chamber are termed *low*, *intermediate*, and *high*. The increase in cell number represents cell numbers on day 4 or 7 divided by initial cell number on day 1. Note that cell numbers are directly proportional to growth factor (GF) concentration in each gradient compartment. Quantification within the subdivided intermediate GF compartment shows a strong positive correlation between cell number and GF concentration (*$P < 0.05$, **$P < 0.01$).

0- to 40-ng/mL range for EGF, FGF2, and platelet-derived growth factor, and that there is no threshold or "all-or-none" proliferation response in this concentration range.

6.4.2 Differentiation of hNSCs into astrocytes in the gradient chamber

Because growth factor concentration directed hNSC proliferation, we tested whether the growth factor gradient also regulated their differentiation [40]. Cells grown for 1 week in the growth factor gradient were fixed and stained with antibodies to astrocytes, one of the main cell types that differentiate from hNSCs. Cells in the low growth factor compartment showed increased astrocyte differentiation compared with cells in the high growth factor compartment (Figure 6.5). This pattern was similar to that of cells on coverslips in parallel conventional culture experiments. More important, the percentage of astrocytes across the three growth factor compartments in the gradient

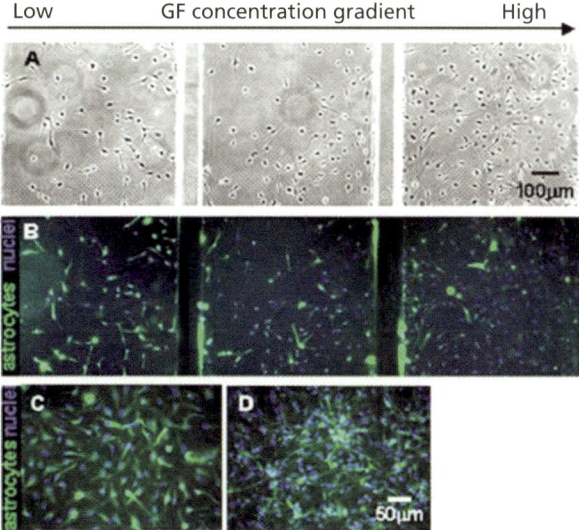

Figure 6.5 Differentiation of hNSCs into astrocytes in the gradient chamber. The hNSCs cultured in the gradient chamber (a, b) or on coverslips (c, d) for 7 days exhibit differentiation into astrocytes (stained by antibody against glial fibrillary acidic protein). Phase contrast images (a) and fluorescence micrographs (b–d) showing stained nuclei (Hoechst) identify all cells in the field. Note the significantly higher proportion of astrocytes in the low growth factor (GF) compartment compared with the other two compartments (b).

chamber decreased with increasing growth factor concentration. Astrocyte percentages in the gradient chamber were consistent with those seen in the control microfluidic chambers and on the coverslips in conventional cultures. We further analyzed the data after subdividing each compartment into eight equal bins to analyze total cell numbers. We continued to find strong correlations between astrocyte percentage and growth factor concentration in all three compartments. Thus, astrocyte differentiation was inversely proportional to growth factor concentration, whereas proliferation was directly proportional. Similar to the proliferation effect, no threshold response in astrocyte differentiation was seen at the population level over the growth factor concentrations used in these experiments.

6.4.3 ESC response to BMP signaling

We generated a mouse ESC line (BRE mESC) harboring a b-galactosidase (lacZ) gene under the influence of a BMP-responsive element (BRE). We examined the responses of the BRE mESCs toward BMP-4 under a conventional culture condition (Petri dish with noncirculating media) and in a hybrid microfluidic chamber where a stable growth factor gradient can be dynamically established. A significantly uniform response to BMP-4 treatment was observed in the microfluidic chamber, where cells are constantly perfused with a medium containing BMP-4. The amount of BMP-4 required to induce the expression of BRE-lacZ was significantly lower in the microfluidic condition than that of conventional culture condition, suggesting that the approach can be used to improve the differentiation of ESCs. Because it is possible to elicit a uniform response of ESCs toward BMP using the hybrid microfluidic device, we examined the role of BMP signaling on ESC proliferation in the presence and absence of LIF. BMP-4 was able to accelerate the overall rate of cell proliferation, suggesting a specific role of BMP-4 together with LIF in mESC proliferation. We first determined whether BMP-4 affects the rate of mESC cell proliferation by simply treating E14 mESCs with different concentrations of BMP-4 continuously in a Petri dish culture with LIF. Cells were isolated at various time intervals and counted to determine E14 mESC doubling time. The average doubling time was about 12 hours as previously reported (data not shown). Similar experiments were performed after E14 mESCs were stimulated with BMP-4 at 5 ng/mL and 20 ng/mL. In both cases, an average E14 mESC doubling time was shortened to approximately 8 hours (data not shown). Because mESCs grown in the Petri dish culture respond to BMP signaling heterogeneously, we also attempted to use a microfluidic device to examine the effect of BMP-4 on mESC proliferation. A stable BMP-4 gradient was generated using a microfluidic chamber, and the proliferation of mESCs was continuously monitored by time-lapse microscopy. The cell doubling time was determined over 16 to 24 hours, until ESCs reached saturation in the Petri dish. We found that E14 mESCs treated with BMP-4 proliferated in about 8 hours, a substantially faster rate than under the normal stem cell growth medium supplemented with LIF. We performed a similar analysis in the absence of LIF and found that the effect of BMP-4 on cell proliferation was not observed in the absence of LIF.

6.5 Discussion and Commentary

Stem cells are one of the most promising sources for transplantable cell therapy in human diseases. Despite their promise, conventional culture methods lack an ability to control cellular behaviors (e.g., stem cell growth, differentiation, purity). We verified that our microfluidic culture platforms could address these drawbacks over conventional culture methods. By using microfluidic culture platforms, one can monitor the proliferation and differentiation of stem cells under precisely controlled environments to understand better the underlying cellular mechanisms and to develop improved culturing processes. As we described in Section 6.3, a significantly improved uniform response to BMP-4 treatment was observed in the microfluidic chamber when steady levels of BMP-4 were continuously perfused over ESCs. This suggests that perfusion of a growth factor to ESCs may be an efficient way to direct the differentiation of ESCs, and this approach could be a significant technological improvement in current research to expand the population and uniformly steer the differentiation of stem cells.

Troubleshooting Table

Characteristics	Conventional Cell Culture Platform	"Christmas Tree" Microfluidic Device	Hybrid Microfluidic Culture Platform
Culturing sensitive cells	+	−	+
Precisely controlled cellular environment	−	+	+
Uniform delivery of serum and growth factors	−	+	+
Uniform response of stem cells toward growth factors	−	+	+

6.6 Application Notes

The microfluidic culture platform is a unique methodology application to stem cell research in multiple fields, such as transplantable cell therapy, regenerative medicine, and neurodegenerative disease. Its uniqueness originates from its ability to introduce a well-defined microenvironment to cultured cells. Using the microfluidic culture platform, one can investigate many developmental processes of stem cells so that optimized conditions for the proliferation and differentiation of stem cells can be systematically established in vitro to understand better the underlying cellular mechanisms and to develop improved culturing processes.

6.7 Summary Points

1. We verified that microfluidic-based cell culture (bioreactor) systems enable one to provide better control of cues and signals to influence ESC behavior in culture.
2. Microfluidic culture platforms can uniformly deliver serum and growth factors over the surface of stem cells to regulate the microenvironment.
3. We envision that a microfluidic device with multiple parallel inlets will allow high-throughput screening of multiple conditions in a single experimental setup.

Acknowledgments

We thank Roman Reed Spinal Cord Injury Research Fund of California.

References

[1] F. Lin, W. Saadi, S. W. Rhee, S. J. Wang, S. Mittal and N. L. Jeon, "Generation of dynamic temporal and spatial concentration gradients using microfluidic devices," *Lab Chip*, volume 4, 3 2004, pp. 164-7.
[2] S. K. Dertinger, X. Jiang, Z. Li, V. N. Murthy and G. M. Whitesides, "Gradients of substrate-bound laminin orient axonal specification of neurons," *Proc Natl Acad Sci U S A*, volume 99, 20 2002, pp. 12542-7.
[3] B. G. Chung, A. Manbachi, W. Saadi, F. Lin, N. L. Jeon and A. Khademhosseini, "A gradient-generating microfluidic device for cell biology," *J Vis Exp*, 7 2007, pp. 271.
[4] S. J. Wang, W. Saadi, F. Lin, C. Minh-Canh Nguyen and N. Li Jeon, "Differential effects of EGF gradient profiles on MDA-MB-231 breast cancer cell chemotaxis," *Exp Cell Res*, volume 300, 1 2004, pp. 180-9.
[5] B. G. Chung, L. A. Flanagan, S. W. Rhee, P. H. Schwartz, A. P. Lee, E. S. Monuki and N. L. Jeon, "Human neural stem cell growth and differentiation in a gradient-generating microfluidic device," *Lab Chip*, volume 5, 4 2005, pp. 401-6.
[6] C. N. Svendsen and A. G. Smith, "New prospects for human stem-cell therapy in the nervous system," *Trends Neurosci*, volume 22, 8 1999, pp. 357-64.
[7] T. D. Palmer, P. H. Schwartz, P. Taupin, B. Kaspar, S. A. Stein and F. H. Gage, "Cell culture. Progenitor cells from human brain after death," *Nature*, volume 411, 6833 2001, pp. 42-3.
[8] F. H. Gage and I. M. Verma, "Stem cells at the dawn of the 21st century," *Proc Natl Acad Sci U S A*, volume 100 Suppl 1 2003, pp. 11817-8.
[9] D. J. Anderson, A. Groves, L. Lo, Q. Ma, M. Rao, N. M. Shah and L. Sommer, "Cell lineage determination and the control of neuronal identity in the neural crest," *Cold Spring Harb Symp Quant Biol*, volume 62 1997, pp. 493-504.
[10] B. A. Reynolds and S. Weiss, "Generation of neurons and astrocytes from isolated cells of the adult mammalian central nervous system," *Science*, volume 255, 5052 1992, pp. 1707-10.
[11] C. T. Gregg, T. Shingo and S. Weiss, "Neural stem cells of the mammalian forebrain," *Symp Soc Exp Biol*, 53 2001, pp. 1-19.
[12] H. S. Keirstead, "Stem cell transplantation into the central nervous system and the control of differentiation," *J Neurosci Res*, volume 63, 3 2001, pp. 233-6.
[13] N. L. Kennea and H. Mehmet, "Transdifferentiation of neural stem cells, or not?," *Pediatr Res*, volume 52, 3 2002, pp. 320-1.

[14] N. L. Kennea and H. Mehmet, "Neural stem cells," *J Pathol*, volume 197, 4 2002, pp. 536-50.
[15] D. T. Chiu, N. L. Jeon, S. Huang, R. S. Kane, C. J. Wargo, I. S. Choi, D. E. Ingber and G. M. Whitesides, "Patterned deposition of cells and proteins onto surfaces by using three-dimensional microfluidic systems," *Proc Natl Acad Sci U S A*, volume 97, 6 2000, pp. 2408-13.
[16] C. M. Metallo, J. C. Mohr, C. J. Detzel, J. J. de Pablo, B. J. Van Wie and S. P. Palecek, "Engineering the stem cell microenvironment," *Biotechnol Prog*, volume 23, 1 2007, pp. 18-23.
[17] J. B. Bard and A. S. Ross, "LIF, the ES-cell inhibition factor, reversibly blocks nephrogenesis in cultured mouse kidney rudiments," *Development*, volume 113, 1 1991, pp. 193-8.
[18] N. M. Gough, R. L. Williams, D. J. Hilton, S. Pease, T. A. Willson, J. Stahl, D. P. Gearing, N. A. Nicola and D. Metcalf, "LIF: a molecule with divergent actions on myeloid leukaemic cells and embryonic stem cells," *Reprod Fertil Dev*, volume 1, 4 1989, pp. 281-8.
[19] A. G. Smith, J. K. Heath, D. D. Donaldson, G. G. Wong, J. Moreau, M. Stahl and D. Rogers, "Inhibition of pluripotential embryonic stem cell differentiation by purified polypeptides," *Nature*, volume 336, 6200 1988, pp. 688-90.
[20] R. L. Williams, D. J. Hilton, S. Pease, T. A. Willson, C. L. Stewart, D. P. Gearing, E. F. Wagner, D. Metcalf, N. A. Nicola and N. M. Gough, "Myeloid leukaemia inhibitory factor maintains the developmental potential of embryonic stem cells," *Nature*, volume 336, 6200 1988, pp. 684-7.
[21] Q. L. Ying, J. Nichols, I. Chambers and A. Smith, "BMP induction of Id proteins suppresses differentiation and sustains embryonic stem cell self-renewal in collaboration with STAT3," *Cell*, volume 115, 3 2003, pp. 281-92.
[22] J. Massague, "TGF-beta signal transduction," *Annu Rev Biochem*, volume 67 1998, pp. 753-91.
[23] V. Tropepe, S. Hitoshi, C. Sirard, T. W. Mak, J. Rossant and D. van der Kooy, "Direct neural fate specification from embryonic stem cells: a primitive mammalian neural stem cell stage acquired through a default mechanism," *Neuron*, volume 30, 1 2001, pp. 65-78.
[24] F. Li, S. Lu, L. Vida, J. A. Thomson and G. R. Honig, "Bone morphogenetic protein 4 induces efficient hematopoietic differentiation of rhesus monkey embryonic stem cells in vitro," *Blood*, volume 98, 2 2001, pp. 335-42.
[25] N. Nakayama, D. Duryea, R. Manoukian, G. Chow and C. Y. Han, "Macroscopic cartilage formation with embryonic stem-cell-derived mesodermal progenitor cells," *J Cell Sci*, volume 116, Pt 10 2003, pp. 2015-28.
[26] M. F. Pera, J. Andrade, S. Houssami, B. Reubinoff, A. Trounson, E. G. Stanley, D. Ward-van Oostwaard and C. Mummery, "Regulation of human embryonic stem cell differentiation by BMP-2 and its antagonist noggin," *J Cell Sci*, volume 117, Pt 7 2004, pp. 1269-80.
[27] R. H. Xu, X. Chen, D. S. Li, R. Li, G. C. Addicks, C. Glennon, T. P. Zwaka and J. A. Thomson, "BMP4 initiates human embryonic stem cell differentiation to trophoblast," *Nat Biotechnol*, volume 20, 12 2002, pp. 1261-4.
[28] G. Dravid, Z. Ye, H. Hammond, G. Chen, A. Pyle, P. Donovan, X. Yu and L. Cheng, "Defining the role of Wnt/beta-catenin signaling in the survival, proliferation, and self-renewal of human embryonic stem cells," *Stem Cells*, volume 23, 10 2005, pp. 1489-501.
[29] P. Lu, Y. Yu, Y. Perdue and Z. Werb, "The apical ectodermal ridge is a timer for generating distal limb progenitors," *Development*, volume 135, 8 2008, pp. 1395-405.
[30] L. Cai, Z. Ye, B. Y. Zhou, P. Mali, C. Zhou and L. Cheng, "Promoting human embryonic stem cell renewal or differentiation by modulating Wnt signal and culture conditions," *Cell Res*, volume 17, 1 2007, pp. 62-72.
[31] M. E. Levenstein, T. E. Ludwig, R. H. Xu, R. A. Llanas, K. VanDenHeuvel-Kramer, D. Manning and J. A. Thomson, "Basic fibroblast growth factor support of human embryonic stem cell self-renewal," *Stem Cells*, volume 24, 3 2006, pp. 568-74.
[32] J. C. McDonald, D. C. Duffy, J. R. Anderson, D. T. Chiu, H. Wu, O. J. Schueller and G. M. Whitesides, "Fabrication of microfluidic systems in poly(dimethylsiloxane)," *Electrophoresis*, volume 21, 1 2000, pp. 27-40.
[33] J. C. McDonald, S. J. Metallo and G. M. Whitesides, "Fabrication of a configurable, single-use microfluidic device," *Anal Chem*, volume 73, 23 2001, pp. 5645-50.
[34] N. Li Jeon, H. Baskaran, S. K. Dertinger, G. M. Whitesides, L. Van de Water and M. Toner, "Neutrophil chemotaxis in linear and complex gradients of interleukin-8 formed in a microfabricated device," *Nat Biotechnol*, volume 20, 8 2002, pp. 826-30.
[35] L. Yu, H. Huang, X. Dong, D. Wu, J. Qin and B. Lin, "Simple, fast and high-throughput single-cell analysis on PDMS microfluidic chips," *Electrophoresis*, volume 29, 24 2008, pp. 5055-60.
[36] M. Rhee and M. A. Burns, "Microfluidic assembly blocks," *Lab Chip*, volume 8, 8 2008, pp. 1365-73.
[37] H. Yu, Y. Lu, Y. G. Zhou, F. B. Wang, F. Y. He and X. H. Xia, "A simple, disposable microfluidic device for rapid protein concentration and purification via direct-printing," *Lab Chip*, volume 8, 9 2008, pp. 1496-501.
[38] S. Kaech and G. Banker, "Culturing hippocampal neurons," *Nat Protoc*, volume 1, 5 2006, pp. 2406-15.
[39] P. H. Schwartz, P. J. Bryant, T. J. Fuja, H. Su, D. K. O'Dowd and H. Klassen, "Isolation and characterization of neural progenitor cells from post-mortem human cortex," *J Neurosci Res*, volume 74, 6 2003, pp. 838-51.

CHAPTER 7

Analysis of Mouse Hematopoietic Stem and Progenitor Cells

Louise E. Purton[1,2] and David T. Scadden[3,4]

[1]Department of Medicine
St. Vincent's Hospital
University of Melbourne
Fitzroy, Victoria, 3065, Australia

[2]St. Vincent's Institute
Fitzroy, Victoria, 3065, Australia

[3]Center for Regenerative Medicine
Massachusetts General Hospital
Boston, MA 02114

[4]Harvard Stem Cell Institute
Cambridge, MA 02138

Abstract

Hematopoiesis (the process by which blood cell formation occurs) is a finely regulated process involving both self-renewal and differentiation decisions of hematopoietic stem cells. In this chapter we provide detailed instructions on how to perform some of the in vitro and in vivo methods routinely used to assess hematopoietic stem and progenitor cell content in the mouse model, which is the most commonly used small-animal model for hematopoiesis studies in research laboratories around the world.

Key Terms
Limiting dilution assay
competitive repopulating assay
colony-forming unit-spleen
colony-forming cells
HSC immunophenotype
HSC transplants

7.1 Introduction

Hematopoietic stem cells (HSCs) are the most primitive cells in the blood cell lineage. They are capable of sustaining hematopoiesis throughout the life span of an animal.

HSCs are a heterogeneous population identified predominantly by their functional potential [1]. There are two commonly referenced populations of HSCs in the mouse model: long-term repopulating HSCs, which are capable of giving rise to hematopoiesis for a minimum of 4 months, but generally more than 6 months [2, 3]; and short-term repopulating HSCs, which repopulate for more than 3 months and less than 6 months [3, 4].

HSCs are not the only widely studied populations of hematopoietic cells. There are also other immature progenitor cells that have early engrafting in vivo repopulating potential but are not HSCs [4, 5]. An example of such a cell population, colony-forming unit-spleen (CFU-S) [6], is given in this chapter.

Much of our knowledge of HSCs comes from studies in mice, which are the most widely used nonprimate model of hematopoiesis. The methods described in this section are therefore all mouse-based methods used to assay properties of hematopoietic stem and progenitor cells. We first describe a method routinely used to deplete whole bone marrow cells of relatively mature lineage-positive cells. This can be used to isolate HSCs and progenitor cells further using various different antibodies and fluorescent-assisted cell sorting (FACS).

Next we describe how to establish and count routinely used colony-forming cell (CFC) assays, which are clonogenic assays used to quantitate relatively mature progenitor cell populations. We then include methods for two different in vivo functional assays: one being the CFU-S assay; the other, the competitive repopulating units (CRU) assay, a long-term repopulating cell assay that is used to quantitate the number of HSCs in a given sample.

Note that there are many different assays that are used in analyzing the hematopoietic compartments of mice. The methods described here touch on some of the basics; many other methods can be easily modified from published literature. Our recent review [1] provides a more detailed explanation of the different types of assays if readers require more information on these assays.

All experiments should be performed with the approval of the animal ethics committee at the researcher's institute, and should be conducted in strict compliance with the regulatory standards of the institute country's code of practice for the care and use of animals for scientific purposes.

7.2 Experimental Design of Lineage Depletion of Whole Bone Marrow Cells

HSCs and progenitor cells comprise a small percentage of whole bone marrow. These cells are "lineage-negative/low" (i.e., they do not express any or express very low levels of the different hematopoietic differentiation markers) [7]. For methods involving stem and progenitor cell isolation, it is often best to first deplete the bone marrow of lineage-positive cells too enriched for this immature cell population. Note that mice that have been treated with substances (e.g., 5-fluorouracil [5-FU]), and some mutant mouse strains may have altered lineage expression. For example, it is known that HSCs in 5-FU-treated marrow express CD11b [8], hence the use of CD11b in the lineage cocktail for 5-FU marrow is not desirable because it would also deplete HSCs.

All reagents and tools should be sterile, especially if using the HSC/progenitor cells for procedures such as in vivo transplantation, cell culture, and isolation of RNA.

7.3 Materials for Lineage Depletion of Whole Bone Marrow Cells

7.3.1 Tools and plasticware

1. Mouse instruments (forceps, scissors, scalpel)
2. Mortar and pestle
3. Conical tubes, 50 mL, and holders
4. Mesh filters, 40-µm
5. Sterile FACS tubes (capped)

7.3.2 Reagents

6. Phosphate-buffered saline (PBS)/2% fetal bovine serum (FBS) (store at 4°C)
7. Turk's solution (3% acetic acid with a few crystals of gentian violet dissolved)
8. Ficoll-Hypaque (keep protected from light)
9. Pretitered saturating lineage depletion antibody mix (biotinylated antimouse TER-119, CD2, CD3, CD4, CD5, CD8, B220, CD11b, Gr-1) stored at 4°C
10. Fluorescent-labeled streptavidin stored at 4°C
11. Ice in a light-shielded container

7.3.3 Additional equipment and reagents required for method 1 (MACS beads method)

12. Degassed magnetic activated cell sorting (MACS) buffer (see manufacturer instructions)
13. Streptavidin microbeads (Miltenyi Biotec)
14. MACS column and magnet (Miltenyi Biotec)
15. Collection tubes

7.3.4 Additional equipment and reagents required for method 2 (Dynabeads method)

16. Streptavidin Dynabeads (Invitrogen Dynal AS)
17. Dynabeads magnet (Invitrogen Dynal AS)

7.3.5 Common protocols for both methods

1. Obtain femurs, tibias, and iliac crests from the mice. Clean all fat and muscle away using a scalpel.
2. Crush bones in mortar and pestle with PBS/2% FBS. Filter the retrieved cells into 50-mL conical tubes through 40-µm mesh filters. Continue to crush and retrieve

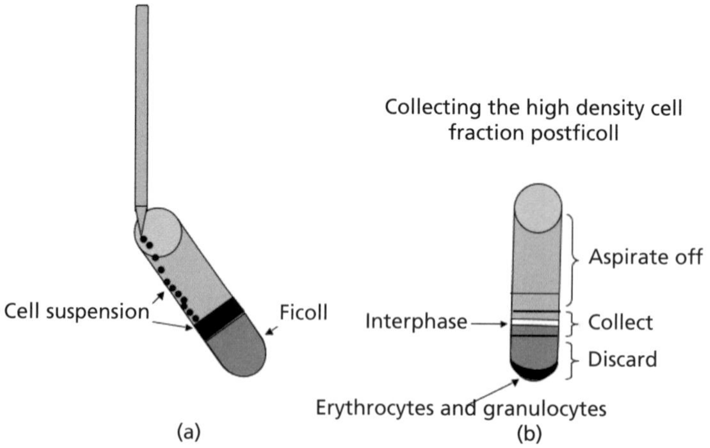

Figure 7.1 (a, b) Illustration depicting the loading of a Ficoll-Hypaque column and retrieval of high-density cells (containing HSCs) after centrifugation.

   the cells until the bone fragments are white in appearance for maximum retrieval of bone marrow cells.
3. Take an aliquot of cells to count (if manual counts are to be done, it is easiest to do this in Turk's solution, which contains acetic acid to hemolyze the erythrocytes, and gentian violet, which stains the nuclei of the other cells purple, which aids in visualizing the cells).
4. Centrifuge tubes at 1,400 rpm for 5 minutes.
5. Pool cells in PBS/2% FBS to be able to layer 4-mL cell suspension over 3-mL Ficoll-Hypaque gradients (in 15-mL conical tube) or 9-mL cell suspension over 10-mL gradients (in 50-mL tubes). As a general rule, use one small Ficoll-Hypaque gradient per two mice and one large gradient per five mice. Layer the cells very gently over the Ficoll-Hypaque gradient (you do not want the Ficoll-Hypaque and cells to mix together). The best procedure for this is to tilt the tube to the side (approximately 45-deg angle), and gently load the cells from the top of the tube such that the cells travel down the side of the tube and form a layer above the Ficoll-Hypaque (Figure 7.1).
6. Centrifuge Ficoll-Hypaque gradients at 1,800 rpm for 10 minutes at 4°C with brake off.
7. A band of cells (predominantly white) should be visible at the interphase (see Figure 7.1). Mark just above and just below this cell fraction using a waterproof marker for ease of cell retrieval. Aspirate the majority of the top (aqueous) phase.
8. Remove interphase fraction (high-density cells) into 50-mL conical tubes with excess PBS/2% FBS (to wash).
9. Take an aliquot of cells for counting.
10. Centrifuge at 1,400 rpm for 5 minutes.
11. Resuspend cells in lineage cocktail (50 μL per $5 \cdot 10^6$ cells). Incubate on ice or at 4°C for 20 to 30 minutes.

7.3.5.1 Method 1: Depletion using MACS beads

12. Wash cells with excess MACS buffer and centrifuge at 1,400 rpm for 5 minutes. Wash control samples with PBS/2% serum and spin down.
13. Resuspend cell pellet in MACS buffer and goat antirat microbeads or streptavidin microbeads per manufacturer instructions.
14. Incubate on ice for 15 minutes with constant agitation.
15. Wash the cells with excess MACS buffer and centrifuge at 1,400 rpm for 5 minutes. Decant supernatant and resuspend cells in MACS buffer [volume depending on which column is used (see manufacturer instructions)], avoiding bubbles.
16. Prepare and rinse the MACS column per manufacturer instructions.
17. Load cells onto column, collecting the lineage-negative cells.
18. Wash the column with MACS buffer per manufacturer instructions.
19. Take an aliquot of cells for counting. Centrifuge fractions at 1,400 rpm for 5 minutes.
20. *Optional* (if not staining for lineage cells in the sample being used for sorting/analysis): Stain an aliquot of the collected lineage-negative cells with fluorescent-labeled streptavidin to assess efficiency of lineage depletion (the cells will not be completely lineage negative, but will be lineage low; this is normal).

7.3.5.2 Method 2: Depletion using Dynabeads

Steps 1 through 11 are the same.

12. Wash the cells with excess PBS/2% FBS and centrifuge at 1,400 rpm for 5 minutes. Wash control samples with PBS/2% serum and spin down.
13. Transfer the cells into a 50-mL conical tube and add the Dynabeads (four to eight beads per cell) dropwise. Gently agitate the cells/Dynabeads, centrifuge the cells at 400 rpm (this slow speed is correct) for 3 minutes, decant supernatant, and resuspend the cells in 1 mL. Transfer to a sterile tube (one that fits in the magnetic force), place on the Dynal magnetic force, and remove the nonmagnetic fraction into another 50-mL tube. Repeat the Dynabead depletion step once on this nonmagnetic fraction, and retain the lineage-depleted nonmagnetic fraction.

The lineage-negative/low cells can be used for various methods of detection of HSCs (e.g., identification of HSC/progenitor cells by immunophenotyping). Some examples of HSC-containing populations routinely used by investigators are lineage-negative/low c-*Kit*+, Sca-1+ (LKS+) cells [9, 10]; LKS+ CD34 cells [11]; LKS+ CD34, Flt3, cells [4,5]; Hoescht 33342 side population and variations of this method [12, 13]; and the more recently identified SLAM "SLAM receptor fractionation method", which does not necessarily require lineage depletion for HSC identification and isolation [14].

7.3.6 Discussion and commentary

The procedure described here is a standard one for obtaining a population enriched in lineage-negative/low bone marrow cells. The efficiency of lineage depletion can be checked at each step for quality control (not necessary but recommended, especially for those new to the procedure). To do this, take a small sample of cells from whole bone marrow, post-Ficoll-Hypaque cells and lineage-depleted cells, and stain these populations for lineage antibodies.

The most difficult step described here is loading the Ficoll-Hypaque gradient. Care should be taken not to mix the Ficoll-Hypaque with the cell suspension (see Figure 7.1), otherwise the density separation will not work (see the Troubleshooting Table if this occurs). The Ficoll-Hypaque gradient step is optional, but it does help to remove erythrocytes and some granulocytes prior to staining with the lineage antibodies (hence, less antibodies and beads are required to stain post-Ficoll-Hypaque cells as opposed to whole bone marrow cells).

Supernatants obtained from antibody-producing cell lines can be used in place of purified antibodies (each batch has to be thoroughly tested). We prefer to use biotinylated antibodies because you can stain for any remaining lineage-positive cells together with the antibodies used for positive selection of HSCs/progenitors. In addition, purified CD3 is usually a hamster clone; hence, detecting lineage cells after using purified lineage antibodies would require both antirat and antihamster secondary antibodies. Note that if unconjugated lineage antibodies are used instead of biotinylated antibodies, this can create problems if staining the cells for both HSC/progenitor markers together with secondary antibodies to detect any remaining lineage-positive cells, because many of the ant-rat secondary antibodies can also bind to the rat antimouse HSC/progenitor antibodies (resulting in incorrect profiles when analyzing the cells).

MACS columns come in different sizes and each column has a specific maximum capacity of positively labeled cells. It is best to check with the information sheets that come with the columns (and are also available online) to determine which one is best for your use, depending on how many initial cells you are using. If high numbers of erythroid cells are present, they may use up many of the MACS beads and lead to a lower purity of lineage-negative/low cells. Usually the Ficoll-Hypaque procedure will help to deplete these cells (in addition to removing many granulocytes); however, the bone marrow sample can alternatively be treated with hemolytic buffer to remove the erythrocytes (this may lead to clumping of other cell types if left on for too long).

The use of Dynabeads provides a quicker method of depleting the lineage-positive cells, but is also more costly and sometimes not as efficient as depleting using MACS beads. It is very useful when processing multiple individual mice at the same time.

Troubleshooting Table for Lineage Depletion Method

Problem	Explanation	Potential Solutions
There is no visible band of cells at the Ficoll-Hypaque interphase	Mixing of the cells and Ficoll-Hypaque occurred	First check to make sure the cells cannot be seen (holding the tube up to the light may aid in seeing the band). If the band still cannot be seen, retrieve the cells (dilute the Ficoll-Hypaque/cells mix with a large volume of PBS/2% FBS and centrifuge at 1,400 rpm for 5 minutes) then prepare a new column and carefully load the cells (see Figure 7.1).
Many of the cells retrieved after depletion express high levels of lineage antibodies	The antibody depletion step did not work well	Check the titer of each of the antibodies. Make sure there are no bubbles in the MACS buffer (if MACS beads are used). If too many erythrocytes may have been left in the sample, deplete of erythrocytes by Ficoll-Hypaque or hemolysis prior to incubating the cells with lineage antibodies.
Few or no cells are retrieved after depletion using the MACS column	Too many cells were loaded into the MACS column	Load fewer cells per column. Make sure there are no bubbles in the MACS buffer (if MACS beads are used). If too many erythrocytes may have been left in the sample, deplete of erythrocytes by Ficoll-Hypaque or hemolysis prior to incubating the cells with lineage antibodies.

7.4 Methylcellulose-Based in Vitro Colony-Forming Assay

A common method used in hematopoietic cell biology is the assessment of colony-forming cells (abbreviated as CFCs or CFUs) from bone marrow or other organs. The first description of the clonal growth of hematopoietic bone marrow cells was by Ray Bradley and Don Metcalf in 1966. There are a few different clonogenic assays used to measure such progenitors. The assay described here is a methylcellulose-based one. The advantage of this method over some of the other CFC assays is that you can discriminate between different types of colonies—namely, granulocyte (CFU-G), granulocyte/macrophage (CFU-GM), granulocyte/erythroid/ macrophage/megakaryoctye (CFU-GEMM), and erythroid colonies (BFU-E and CFU-E).

7.4.1 Materials

7.4.1.1 Tools and plasticware

1. Sterile Petri dishes, 35 mm
2. Syringe, 10 mL, with 18G needle or sterile 10-mL pipettes

7.4.1.2 Reagents and cells

3. Methylcellulose medium (1.2% final concentration methylcellulose), supplemented with cytokines
4. Hematopoietic cell source (bone marrow cells, isolated HSC/progenitor cells)

7.4.1.3 Equipment

5. Inverted microscope or a dissecting microscope

7.4.2 Methods

1. Label your Petri dishes so that you can discriminate between groups. It is best to use triplicate plates per cell population.
2. Plate the hematopoietic cells in the bottom of the Petri dish (usually $5 \cdot 10^4$ nucleated unfractionated bone marrow cells per dish). Have a final volume of 100 μL cells (no more than this volume) per dish. It is recommended to prepare triplicate cultures per mouse.
3. Using the syringe and needle (the methylcellulose mix is usually very viscous) or pipette (if the methylcellulose mix is not viscous), plate 900 μL methylcellulose mix over the cells.
4. Mix the cells/methylcellulose mix together thoroughly by swirling the medium around the plate (gently but thoroughly).
5. Incubate at 37°C with 5% CO_2 in air atmosphere (make sure the dishes are well humidified so they do not dry out).
6. CFU-E can be monitored on day 3. These are very small colonies.
7. CFU-GM are counted on day 7.
8. BFU-E are counted on day 8.
9. CFU-GEMM are counted on day 12.

10. All colonies can be counted from the same plate, just remember to place them back in the incubator in between counting days.

7.4.3 Data acquisition, anticipated results, and interpretation

Count the colonies on the appropriate days and record numbers for each colony type enumerated in the dish. Excel spreadsheets can be used to determine the mean ±standard deviation or standard error of the mean (both of which are valid to use in these studies) for each colony type, and also to determine the total number of colonies (sum of all types of colonies) in each dish. Statistical analysis can be performed using Student's t-test comparing between the groups (if two groups) or using analysis of variance (ANOVA) if more than two groups.

The data can be presented as the number of colonies per number of cells plated; however, if there are significant differences between the numbers of cells per femur in the mice being assessed, it is more appropriate to present the data as the total number of colonies per femur. To do this, divide the number of colonies by the number of cells plated and multiply this by the total number of cells per femur for each respective mouse.

The average number of total colonies produced on day 12 of culture per 50,000 bone marrow cells from a wild-type C57BL/6 mouse is approximately 90, of which approximately eight will be mixed colonies. Note, however, that different types of cytokines, strains of mice and even sources of mice can produce different results.

7.4.4 Discussion and commentary

StemCell Technologies and R and D Systems are two companies that make methylcellulose solutions for CFC assays. There are options to buy the methylcellulose base (without anything else added) or methylcellulose with all cytokines, serum, and so forth, added. If buying the former, you will need to supplement the methylcellulose with cytokines and serum. Recombinant cytokines are best to use for reproducibility of the assays, but conditioned medium made by cell lines can be used as alternative growth factor sources (especially if made in large batches to ensure reproducibility). You will need to titrate each batch of conditioned medium to find the appropriate concentration to use. Different batches of FBS also need to be tested for optimal growth of colonies, especially erythroid colonies.

The colonies are best counted using a dissecting microscope, but some people prefer to use inverted microscopes. StemCell Technologies has a useful technical sheet available for free from their website that shows examples of the different types of colonies if you need help in identifying the different colonies. It is also useful to do "cytospins" of the colonies (which can be retrieved by plucking individual colonies with a pipette and suspending the cells in PBS for cytospins) for confirmation of colony type when you are first starting out with this method.

BFU-E can be stained with benzidine (which reacts with hemoglobin) for confirmation (note that you will not be able to continue to culture these plates if you do, so set up extra plates for continued culture). However, note that other cell types including granulocytes can also stain with benzidine [16, 17], so be aware of this if you do use this stain.

Troubleshooting Table for CFU Assay

Problem	Explanation	Potential Solutions
No colonies are visible	Too few cells have been plated	Increase the number of cells plated
	Methylcellulose mix is not supporting the colony formation	Check that your batch of methylcellulose is still viable. Use a new batch if uncertain.
Too many colonies are present/overlap with each other	Too many cells have been plated	Reduce the number of cells plated.
	The cells were not thoroughly mixed with the methylcellulose and hence the colonies are not well dispersed	Ensure thorough mixing of the cells and methylcellulose.

7.5 Radiation of Mice for In Vivo Assays

The major in vivo assays used in measuring HSC and progenitor cells require preconditioning of the mice prior to transplantation of the cell source. The amount of radiation normally used may depend on the radiation source and the sensitivity of the mouse strain (strains from different suppliers may even show differences in radiation sensitivity). The standard dose given to the mice ranges from 9 to 11 Gy of total-body radiation. Radiation is usually administered on the day of transplantation, but can be done the day prior to transplant if necessary.

The time required to radiate the mice depends heavily on the radiation source. Cesium sources, which are the most popular means of radiation for small animals, are very powerful (dose rate, approximately 1 Gy/minute), and it is highly recommended to administer the radiation at a split dose of even amounts (the total dose divided by two), given approximately 3 hours apart to minimize toxicity to the mice. Other radiation sources such as cobalt sources or linear particle accelerators are much more gentle (the dose rate can be adjusted to approximately 20 cGy/minute) and can be given in a single dose over the course of almost 1 hour (depending on the final dose required). The positioning of the mice and the number of mice that can be radiated at one time relies on the radiation source used.

Mice are susceptible to infection after radiation and transplantation, especially during the first 2 weeks after transplant, even when housed in sterile facilities. Antibiotics can be placed in the drinking water for the first 2 to 3 weeks after transplant to help prevent this from occurring.

Troubleshooting Table for Bone Marrow Transplantation

Problem	Explanation	Potential Solutions
Mice die before 3 weeks after transplantation	Too few cells have been transplanted	Increase the number of cells transplanted into the mice.
	The mice have received too much radiation	Lower the radiation dose.
	Mice may have succumbed to infection	Include antibiotics in their drinking water.
	Technical problems with the injections	Practice injections until you are confident they are successful.

7.6 Colony-Forming Unit-Spleen Assay

CFU-S are a population of in vivo radioprotective hematopoietic cells [6]. They are distinct from HSCs (being more mature than these very primitive cells), but are a relatively immature population of hematopoietic cells. After transplantation, these cells home to the spleen, where they give rise to colonies (hence the name). There are different classes of CFU-S, named for the day after transplantation in which they form macroscopic colonies [18, 19]. In general, the earlier forming CFU-S (such as CFU-S day 8) are more mature than the later forming CFU-S (e.g., CFU-S day 12). Examples of results of an assay are given in Figure 7.2.

Whole bone marrow cells are classically used in this assay; however, purified populations of HSC/progenitor cells can also be used.

7.6.1 Materials

7.6.1.1 Tools and plasticware

1. Syringe, 1 mL
2. Needle, 26G

7.6.1.2 Reagents, cells, and mice

3. Bone marrow cells (or other sources of hematopoietic cells such as enriched HSCs or progenitor cells)
4. Recipient mice (usually C57BL/6J)
5. PBS
6. Bouin's fixative (can be purchased from companies such as Sigma)
7. Neutral buffered formalin, 10%

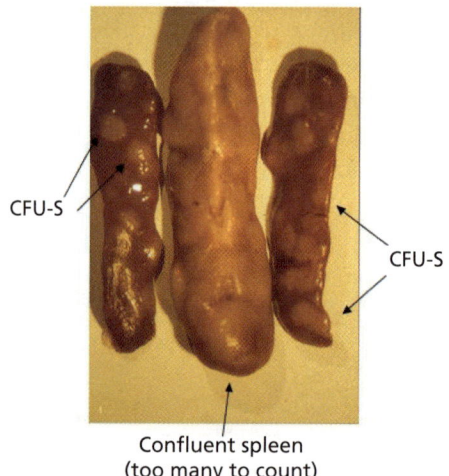

Figure 7.2 Examples of CFU-S visible on the surface of spleens. The middle spleen is confluent (too many colonies to count accurately), whereas the spleens on either side have distinct colonies that can be measured.

7.6.1.3 Equipment

8. Radiation source
9. Heat lamp
10. Mouse restrainer
11. Dissecting microscope

7.6.2 Methods

1. Radiate the recipient mice with a predetermined radiation dose.
2. Suspend the hematopoietic cells in 200 µL PBS per mouse to be injected. Allow for at least one mouse extra to account for the dead space of the needle.
3. Heat the mice under the heat lamp (this will allow the veins to be seen more easily for transplantation purposes).
4. Place the mouse in a mouse restrainer, hold tail with one hand (the hand you do not need to inject the cells with) and locate a good vein (either side of the top part of the tail).
5. Inject the mice intravenously with 200 µL cell suspension (for statistical purposes it is best to have four mice per group minimum).
6. Euthanize the mice 8 to 16 days after transplantation (the day depends upon which CFU-S population you wish to measure; day 12 is a popular time point to harvest).
7. Remove the spleens from the mice. Weigh the spleens using a sensitive balance so that you can accurately record the weights and monitor if there is any difference in spleen weights between different sources of cells.
8. Fix the spleens in Bouin's fixative (approximately 5 minutes).
9. Wash and place the fixed spleens in 10% neutral buffered formalin.
10. Count the CFU-S using a dissecting microscope (best to put them in PBS in a Petri dish under the microscope). Count all surface colonies on both sides of the spleens (make sure you do not count the same one twice if it is big enough to be seen on both sides of the spleen).

7.6.3 Data acquisition, anticipated results, and interpretation

Count the CFU-S and record numbers enumerated in each spleen. Excel spreadsheets can be used to determine the mean ±standard deviation or standard error of the mean for each group. Statistical analysis can be performed using Student's t-test comparing between the groups (if two groups) or using ANOVA if more than two groups.

The data can be presented as the number of CFU-S per number of cells transplanted; however, if there are significant differences between the numbers of cells per femur in the mice being assessed, it is more appropriate to present the data as the total number of CFU-S produced per femur. To do this, divide the number of CFU-S by the number of bone marrow cells transplanted and multiply this by the total number of bone marrow cells per femur for each respective mouse.

If the spleens are confluent (an indication of too many colonies; see Figure 7.2), the spleen weights can be compared between groups. Additional studies can be performed using lower cell doses to quantitate accurately the numbers of CFU-S in the samples.

The average number of day 12 CFU-S produced per 100,000 bone marrow cells from a wild-type C57BL/6 mouse is approximately 10 to 12. As for CFC assays, the strains of mice and even source of the mouse strains may influence the results obtained.

7.6.4 Discussion and commentary

It is better to prepare the cells for injection in PBS rather than PBS/2% FBS, because this minimizes bubbles when preparing to inject the mice. The cell dose to inject is a trial-and-error matter, depending upon the population of hematopoietic cells and mouse strain. In general, we find that $1 \cdot 10^5$ whole bone marrow cells or 500 LKS+ from C57BL/6J mice give measurable CFU-S. Other mouse strains and populations can be different. It is best to do a pilot study first, titrating different cell numbers. Some cell populations can contain so many CFU-S that the spleens become confluent (see Figure 7.2). In this instance, recording the weights is also very valuable, because differences can also be observed using spleen weights. If the numbers of CFU-S are required, the population can be further titrated in another experiment.

Tail vein injections can take a while to master. If resistance is felt when injecting, it is likely that the injection has not been successful (the needle is no longer in the vein, but has likely passed through it instead). If no resistance is felt, it is likely that the injection is successful.

Bouin's fixative is highly toxic and dangerous. It contains picric acid, which is extremely volatile and explosive if it dries out. Be extremely careful when using it, and discard it according to manufacturer directions. After the CFU-S have been enumerated, the spleens can be processed in paraffin and sectioned for staining with routine stains such as hematoxylin–eosin to determine whether the colonies are multipotential or lineage restricted.

Troubleshooting Table for CFU-S Assay

Problem	Explanation	Potential Solutions
Mice die before 3 weeks after transplantation	Too few cells have been transplanted	Increase the number of cells transplanted into the mice.
	The mice have received too much radiation	Lower the radiation dose.
	Mice may have succumbed to infection	Include antibiotics in their drinking water.
	Technical problems with the injections	Practice injections until you are confident they are successful.
The spleens are too confluent	Too many cells have been transplanted	Reduce the numbers of cells transplanted into the mice.
Mice have survived but very few colonies are visible on the spleen surface	Too few cells have been transplanted	Increase the number of cells transplanted into the mice.

7.7 Quantification of HSCs Using the Limiting Dilution Assay

There are a number of ways in which to measure HSC activity. One of the most widely used assays, the CRU assay, quantitates the number of HSCs in a given population of cells. This assay (initially reported by Szilvassy et al. [20, 21]) requires a minimum of three different cell doses of the sample, competed against a known reference cell population (originally compromised bone marrow that was obtained by serially transplanting the bone marrow; now a more widely used source is $2 \cdot 10^5$ congenic bone marrow cells). It is very useful in comparing two or more sources of HSCs—for example, when determining whether there are differences in the number of HSCs in mutant mice compared with their wild-type recipients.

This assay uses Poisson statistics to determine the number of HSCs in a given population, and is a limiting dilution assay. It relies on the number of mice that are negative for the test population (which is usually defined as being less than 1% multilineage repopulating donor cells); thus, one of the donor cell doses should be relatively low (we give an example of cell doses later). Furthermore, a minimum of eight (preferably 10) recipients per cell dose are required for the accuracy of this assay. A minimum of three cell doses (preferably four or more) are recommended for accurate analysis.

7.7.1 Buffers and materials

7.7.1.1 Tools and plasticware

1. Syringe, 1 mL
2. Needle, 26G

7.7.1.2 Reagents, cells, and mice

3. Test (donor) hematopoietic cell population
4. Congenic recipient mice
5. Competing bone marrow cells (cells from the recipient mice strain can be used.
6. PBS

7.7.1.3 Equipment

7. Radiation source
8. Heat lamp
9. Mouse restrainer

7.7.2 Methods

1. Lethally radiate the recipient mice
2. Prepare the hematopoietic cell populations to be injected into the recipient mice. If possible, allow for at least one extra mouse to account for the dead space of the needle. Allow a total of 200 μL cells in PBS per mouse to be injected. If using whole bone marrow, the suggested cell doses are as follows (for injection per mouse):
   - $1 \cdot 10^4$ donor cells + $2 \cdot 10^5$ competing cells
   - $5 \cdot 10^4$ donor cells + $2 \cdot 10^5$ competing cells
   - $2 \cdot 10^5$ donor cells + $2 \cdot 10^5$ competing cells
   - $1 \cdot 10^6$ donor cells + $2 \cdot 10^5$ competing cells
3. Inject 200 μL cells per mouse intravenously.
4. Wait for the appropriate time after transplantation before analyzing the cells by routine FACS methods. Commonly used times are 5 weeks (early engraftment), 3

months (short-term repopulating HSCs), and 6 months (long-term repopulating HSCs) [22].
5. Calculate the number of HSCs by Poisson statistics as described by Szilvassy et al. [21]. Alternatively, you can use the L-calc software that is available to download free from the StemCell Technologies website (www.stemcell.com). Note, however, that this is for PCs, not Macintosh computers.

7.7.3 Data acquisition, anticipated results, and interpretation

Analysis of long-term repopulating HSCs can be performed at 4 to 6 months (preferably 6 months) after transplantation via assessment of peripheral blood for hematopoietic lineage reconstitution by flow cytometry. Blood is hemolyzed to remove erythrocytes (which do not express CD45), and donor cell multilineage reconstitution is assessed. To detect a long-term repopulating HSC accurately, each mouse must have at least 1% donor-derived reconstitution in its myeloid (granulocytes and macrophages), B-lymphoid, and T-lymphoid populations. If a mouse has, for example, greater than or equal to 1% donor-derived B lymphocytes and T lymphocytes, but less than 1% donor-derived granulocytes and macrophages, it is considered to be negative for multilineage reconstitution. Note there are some complications that may arise in accurately interpreting data from CRU assays; we discussed them at length in our recent review [1].

After the raw data has been obtained for each mouse, the numbers of negative mice (<1% donor-derived multilineage repopulating cells) for each cell dose can be calculated. An example is given in Figure 7.3. The frequency of negative mice can then be plotted

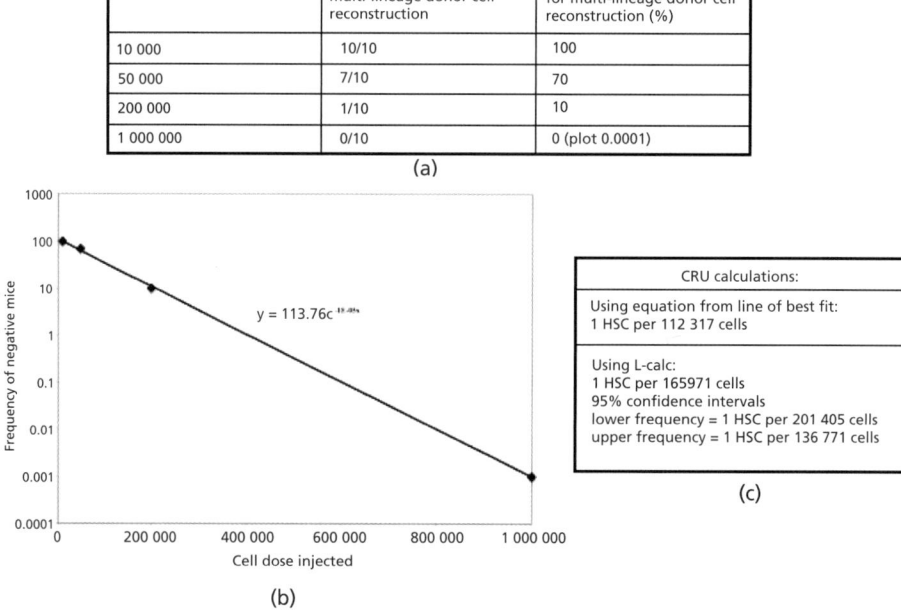

Figure 7.3 Calculation of the frequency of CRUs in a given sample. (a) Examples of numbers and frequencies of negative mice for each of four cell doses. (b) A logarithmic plot with line of best fit and its equation for the data. (c) Calculations of the CRU frequency based on the data shown in (a), comparing data obtained from the plot shown in (b) versus data obtained using L-calc software from StemCell Technologies.

on the y-axis (with a log scale) and the numbers of cells injected can be plotted on the x-axis. If using Excel, choose the scatterplot. Note that you cannot use the value zero in the logarithmic graphs, but you can adjust zero to a small fraction, such as 0.0001, for graphing purposes. A line of best fit can be obtained (choose "Add trend line" in the Chart toolbar, and select "Exponential"), and the equation for the line of best fit can be obtained (by double-clicking on the trend line and selecting "Display equation on chart" in the "Options" section). Based on Poisson statistics, which predicts that there is one HSC when 37% of mice are negative for multilineage reconstitution, $y = 37$. Using $y = 37$ in the equation for the line of best fit, the number of CRUs (x in the equation) can be assessed. The frequency of HSCs in a wild-type C57BL/6J mouse is approximately 1 per 100,000 cells (but this can vary according to mouse strain, source of mouse strain, and donor cell percentage defining multilineage reconstitution). The number of HSCs in a given sample (e.g., one femur) can also be calculated after the CRU frequency is known.

If using the L-calc software available from StemCell Technologies (which is free to download, but for PC users only), the numbers of positive mice are used to calculate the CRU. The L-calc software also generates the 95% confident intervals for any set of data, analyzes the statistical significance between groups, and is highly recommended for ease of use.

7.7.4 Discussion and commentary

The most widely used mouse models for transplantation are the congenic C57BL/6J and Ptprca mice, which differ only at the CD45 locus. CD45 is on all leukocytes, hence donor/host cells can be discriminated using antibodies for the different mouse strains, and a third color can be used to detect specific lineage cells. C57BL/6J mice are CD45.2+; Ptprca are CD45.1+. Progeny of C57BL/6J and Ptprca breeding pairs are CD45.1+/CD45.2+ and are good to use as the competing cells (you can also monitor endogenous recovery of the host mice if you use double-positive congenic competing cells).

If the mice are not on a congenic strain, there are two options: (1) backcross them at least 10 times onto a C57BL/6J background (this takes a lot of time and patience) or (2) use male donors into female recipients of the same strain and use female competing cells. This option is less sensitive, because quantitative polymerase chain reaction-based methods are used to detect the percentage of Y chromosomes in peripheral blood obtained from the female recipients. However, it is also an acceptable method [23].

It is best to mix the two populations together prior to injecting, so that a single injection of 200 μL gives the desired number of each population of cells per mouse (two separate injections is very messy and could lead to a lot of inaccuracies resulting from error in injecting and so forth). Other test HSC populations can be used, such as enriched HSCs and cultured HSCs, together with the same source of competing whole bone marrow cells.

The W^{41}/W^{41} mouse strain can be used as recipients instead of the congenic wild-type mice [24, 25]. These mice have significantly impaired numbers of HSCs as a result of partial impairment of the c-Kit receptor kinase activity in hematopoietic cells [26]. The test populations can be transplanted into sublethally radiated W^{41}/W^{41} mice without any competing marrow cells. Hence, smaller numbers of HSCs may be detected using this mouse model.

Survival of the mice is an important factor in the CRU assay, because the assay relies on the numbers of mice that show negative donor cell reconstitution (which is usually defined as less than 1% multilineage repopulating cells). If a mouse dies, it is difficult to determine why, especially because the competing bone marrow cells should contain sufficient HSCs and progenitors to keep the mouse alive. In this situation, the numbers of mice negative for reconstitution should be calculated from the number of surviving mice. However, if the number of surviving mice is very low, this introduces inaccuracies and the assay is best performed again with modifications to the protocol (see the troubleshooting table).

The number of repopulating units can also be assessed using this method, providing the competing cells are whole bone marrow cells [1, 27].

Note that the limiting dilution assay is not restricted to stem cell assays, but can be applied to any assays in which limiting dilutions are assessed. For example, it can be used to measure the frequency of a CFC in a population of unknown potential. In this instance, various cell doses are plated in CFC assays, the numbers of negative plates (i.e., those having no colonies) are determined for each cell dose, then the frequency of the CFC can be measured.

Troubleshooting Table for Limited Dilution Assay

Problem	Explanation	Potential Solutions
Mice die before 3 weeks after transplantation	Too few cells have been transplanted	Increase the number of cells (both test and competing) transplanted into the mice.
	The mice have received too much radiation	Lower the radiation dose.
	Mice may have succumbed to infection	Include antibiotics in their drinking water.
	Technical problems with the injections	Practice injections until you are confident they are successful.
Many mice die 3 weeks after transplantation	Too few cells have been transplanted	Increase the number of cells (both test and competing) transplanted into the mice.
	Mice may have succumbed to infection	Include antibiotics in their drinking water and assess the health status of the mice.
All mice have more than 1% multilineage reconstitution	Too many test cells have been transplanted for the lowest cell dose	Reduce the numbers of test cells transplanted into the mice.
All mice have fewer than 1% multilineage reconstitution	Too few test cells have been transplanted	Increase the number of test cells transplanted into the mice.

7.8 Summary Points

1. Competent skills in FACS analysis and sorting techniques are essential for HSC studies.
2. Intravenous injections are technically demanding skills and much practice is needed.
3. CFC assays require considerable practice to identify accurately the different colony types present.

4. Sufficient numbers of mice are required for accuracy in HSC quantification assays. Using fewer mice than recommended significantly compromises the integrity of the assay.
5. HSC transplant studies require a minimum of 4 months posttransplantation to achieve accurate results.
6. Different HSC phenotypes often represent different types of HSC populations and cannot be considered interchangeable.

References

[1] Purton, L. E., and D. T. Scadden, "Limiting Factors in Murine Hematopoietic Stem Cell Assays," *Cell Stem Cell*, Vol. 1, 2007, pp. 263–270.
[2] Dykstra, B., et al. "Long-Term Propagation of Distinct Hematopoietic Differentiation Programs in Vivo," *Cell Stem Cell*, Vol. 1, 2007, pp. 218–229.
[3] Jordan, C. T., and I. R. Lemischka, "Clonal and Systemic Analysis of Long-Term Hematopoiesis in the Mouse," *Genes Dev.*, Vol. 4, 1990, pp. 220–232.
[4] Yang, L., et al., "Identification of Lin(–)Sca1(+)kit(+)CD34(+)Flt3– Short-Term Hematopoietic Stem Cells Capable of Rapidly Reconstituting and Rescuing Myeloablated Transplant Recipients," *Blood*, Vol. 105, 2005, pp. 2717–2723.
[5] Adolfsson, J., et al. "Upregulation of Flt3 Expression Within the Bone Marrow Lin(–)Sca1(+)c-Kit(+) Stem Cell Compartment Is Accompanied by Loss of Self-Renewal Capacity," *Immunity*, Vol. 15, 2001, pp. 659–669.
[6] Till, J., and E. McCulloch, "A Direct Measurement of the Radiation Sensitivity of Normal Mouse Bone Marrow Cells," *Radiat. Res.*, Vol. 14, 1961, p. 213.
This study was the first to quantitate the in vivo clonogenic potential of "HSCs" (which were later recognized as more mature than HSCs) and pioneered HSC transplantation studies in the animal model.
[7] Spangrude, G. J., S. Heimfeld, and I. L. Weissman, "Purification and Characterization of Mouse Hematopoietic Stem Cells," *Science*, Vol. 241, 1988, pp. 58–62.
This is a pioneering study that described the first FACS-based method to isolate HSCs.
[8] Randall, T. D., and I. L. Weissman, "Phenotypic and Functional Changes Induced at the Clonal Level in Hematopoietic Stem Cells after 5-Fluorouracil Treatment," *Blood*, Vol. 89, 1997, pp. 3596–3606.
[9] Okada, S., et al., "In Vivo and In Vitro Cell Function of c-*kit*- and Sca-1-Positive Murine Hematopoietic Cells," *Blood*, Vol. 80, 1992, pp. 3044–3050.
[10] Ikuta, K., and I. L. Weissman, "Evidence That Hematopoietic Stem Cells Express Mouse c-Kit But Do Not Depend on Steel Factor for Their Generation," *Proc. Natl. Acad. Sci. USA*, Vol. 89, 1992, pp. 1502–1506.
[11] Osawa, M., et al., "Long-Term Lymphohematopoietic Reconstitution by a Single CD34-Low/Negative Hematopoietic Stem Cell," *Science*, Vol. 273, 1996, pp. 242–245.
[12] Goodell, M. A., et al., "Isolation and Functional Properties of Murine Hematopoietic Stem Cells That Are Replicating in Vivo," *J. Exp. Med.*, Vol. 183, 1996, pp. 1797–1806.
[13] Lin, K. K., and M. A. Goodell, "Purification of Hematopoietic Stem Cells Using the Side Population," *Methods Enzymol.*, Vol. 420, 2006, pp. 255–264.
[14] Kiel, M. J., et al., "SLAM Family Receptors Distinguish Hematopoietic Stem and Progenitor Cells and Reveal Endothelial Niches for Stem Cells," *Cell*, Vol. 121, 2005, pp. 1109–1121.
[15] Bradley, T. R., and D. Metcalf, "The Growth of Mouse Bone Marrow Cells in Vitro," *Austr. J. Exp. Biol. Med. Sci.*, Vol. 44, 1966, pp. 287–300.
This accomplishment is one of the most significant achievements in the HSC biology field. It pioneered the subsequent further development of methods to assay hematopoietic progenitor cells in vitro and led to the discovery of colony-stimulating factors.
[16] Kaplow, L. S., "Simplified Myeloperoxidase Stain Using Benzidine Dihydrochloride," *Blood*, Vol. 26, 1965, pp. 215–219.
[17] Kruszyna, R., R. P. Smith, and L. Ou, "Method for Measuring Increased Plasma Hemoglobin in the Presence of Erythrocytes," *Clin. Chem.*, Vol. 23, 1977, pp. 2156–2159.
[18] Ploemacher, R. E., and N. H. Brons, "Cells with Marrow and Spleen Repopulating Ability and Forming Spleen Colonies on Day 16, 12, and 8 Are Sequentially Ordered on the Basis of Increasing Rhodamine 123 Retention," *J. Cell Physiol.*, Vol. 136, 1988, pp. 531–536.
[19] Wolf, N. S., and G. V. Priestley, "Kinetics of Early and Late Spleen Colony Development," *Exp. Hematol.*, Vol. 14, 1986, pp. 676–682.
[20] Szilvassy, S. J., et al., "Isolation in a Single Step of a Highly Enriched Murine Hematopoietic Stem Cell Population with Competitive Long-Term Repopulating Ability," *Blood*, Vol. 74, 1989, pp. 930–939.

[21] Szilvassy, S. J., et al., "Quantitative Assay for Totipotent Reconstituting Hematopoietic Stem Cells by a Competitive Repopulation Strategy," *Proc. Natl. Acad. Sci. USA*, Vol. 87, 1990, pp. 8736–8740.
This assay, based on Poisson statistics, is a method that allows the numbers of HSCs in a given population to be calculated and compared with other sources of HSCs. It is routinely used in laboratories to quantitate the number of HSCs in a given sample.

[22] Purton, L. E., et al., "RARγ Is Critical for Maintaining a Balance between Hematopoietic Stem Cell Self-Renewal and Differentiation," *J. Exp. Med.*, Vol. 203, 2006, pp. 1283–1293.

[23] Walkley, C. R., et al., "Rb Regulates Interactions between Hematopoietic Stem Cells and Their Bone Marrow Microenvironment," *Cell*, Vol. 129, 2007, pp. 1081–1095.

[24] Trevisan, M., X. Q. Yan, and N. N. Iscove, "Cycle Initiation and Colony Formation in Culture by Murine Marrow Cells with Long-Term Reconstituting Potential in Vivo," *Blood*, Vol. 88, 1996, pp. 4149–4158.

[25] Miller, C. L., and C. J. Eaves, "Expansion in Vitro of Adult Murine Hematopoietic Stem Cells with Transplantable Lympho-Myeloid Reconstituting Ability," *Proc. Natl. Acad. Sci. USA*, Vol. 94, 1997, pp. 13648–13653.

[26] Nocka, K., et al., "Molecular Bases of Dominant Negative and Loss of Function Mutations at the Murine c-Kit/White Spotting Locus: W37, Wv, W41 and W," *EMBO J.*, Vol. 9, 1990, pp. 1805–1813.

[27] Harrison, D. E., "Competitive Repopulation: A New Assay for Long-Term Stem Cell Functional Capacity," *Blood*, Vol. 55, 1980, pp. 77–81.
This is another excellent method whereby the functional potential of HSCs can be quantitated in a competitive repopulating assay, and is also frequently used in laboratories. When combined with the CRU assay (which measures the quantity of HSCs), additional information about the quality of the HSCs in a given sample can be gained.

CHAPTER

8

Skeletal Stem Cells and the Hematopoietic Microenvironment: Biology and Assays

Benedetto Sacchetti and Paolo Bianco

Stem Cell Laboratory
Biomedical Science Park San Raffaele
Dipartimento di Medicina Sperimentale
Sapienza University of Rome
Rome, Italy

Abstract

Although the concept of mesenchymal stem cells is widely popular, formal proof of "stemness" for this class of postnatal progenitors rests with the formal demonstration of self-renewal in vivo. This in turn relies on the use of markers suited not only to isolate, but also to monitor in situ and in vivo, before explantation and after transplantation, the origin and fate of cultured mesenchymal progenitors. Self-renewal of postnatal skeletal progenitors found in the bone marrow stroma coincides, in vivo, with the establishment of human hematopoietic supporting stroma in a chimeric heterotopic ossicle generated by in vivo transplantation. Establishment of this stromal compartment also coincides with the transfer of the hematopoietic microenvironment to heterotopic sites.

Key Terms
Skeletal progenitors
mesenchymal stem cells
hematopoietic microenvironment
self-renewal
in vivo assays

8.1 Introduction

The pioneering work of Tavassoli and Crosby [1] established that heterotopic transplantation of boneless marrow fragments results in the generation of complete ossicles including hematopoietic tissues. The work of Friedenstein et al. (reviewed in [2–4]) later established that this function could be ascribed to nonhematopoietic stromal cells in mammalian bone marrow, and in particular to single cells capable of clonal growth. Analysis of the differentiation potency of the progeny of such clonogenic progenitors (colony forming unit-fibroblast [CFU-F]) through appropriate in vivo assays revealed that a single stromal cell could generate bone, cartilage, fibroblasts, and adipocytes (i.e., all skeletal tissues) in heterotopic ossicles, which would also accommodate host-derived hematopoiesis. From this data, the concept of stromal/osteogenic stem cells, later renamed *mesenchymal stem cells*, evolved. Important questions were left open by Friedenstein's work: (1) whether, besides multipotency, self-renewal of a subset of bone marrow stromal cells could be demonstrated, so that multipotent progenitors could be considered bona fide stem cells; and (2) which cell type in the varied cellular population found in the nonhematopoietic compartment of the bone marrow would be the in situ counterpart of the assayed multipotent (and possibly self-renewing) stromal progenitor. Intertwined with these two questions, and revived by a resurgent interest in the cells providing a niche for hematopoietic stem cells (HSCs), is the question of which cell types in the bone marrow environment are critical for establishing and maintaining cues permissive for homing, proliferation, self-renewal, differentiation, and maturation of hematopoietic progenitors (the hematopoietic microenvironment [HME])—a function reflected in the colonization of stromal cell-generated ossicles by hematopoietic cells in experimental systems.

Addressing these questions was made difficult by the lack of markers suited to bridge the gap between in vitro and in vivo observations. Although several markers are suited to enrich the bone marrow CFU-F prospectively [3, 5, 6], and most are extensively used to characterize mesenchymal stem cell populations in culture, few have been suited, and virtually none used, for coupling ex vivo observation with in vivo studies. Demonstration of self-renewal would imply for any kind of putative stem cells the reproduction of identical cells with identical phenotype and properties after transplantation of a phenotype and function-defined population of cells in vivo. Thus, demonstration of self-renewal of stromal progenitors in human bone marrow would imply identification of the same type of stromal cells (1) in human bone marrow prior to explantation and (2) in the chimeric bone marrow after in vivo transplantation.

The experimental approach leading to recognition of the ability of CD146+ stromal cells adventitial to bone marrow sinusoids to generate heterotopic ossicles, transfer the HME, and self-renew in vivo [6] is outlined here, along with a brief discussion of the applications and conceptual implications of these experiments.

8.2 Experimental Design

The fundamental experimental design rests on the use of a transplantation system in which the inherent capacity of test cells to generate histology-proved bone and bone marrow is probed in vivo. The transplant is made at a heterotopic site to exclude inductive influences from the host bone environment, and uses an osteoconductive carrier as necessary to provide a three-dimensional organization and a proper template for the newly deposited bone. The simplest readout is provided by the appearance of histology-proved tissues at defined time points. Based on this basic experimental framework, the isolation of phenotype-defined populations allows one to correlate the ability of stromal populations to form bone, or to establish heterotopic hematopoietic tissue or bone, to individual cell types that can in turn (1) be recognized in situ and (2) be probed for their clonogenic capacity and, thus, identity as CFU-Fs. In addition, the same fundamental approach, as applied to single clones generated by single CFU-Fs, allows for the analysis of multipotency through the detection of multiple tissues of donor origin, and of self-renewal in vivo through the detection of cells with phenotype and properties similar to those of the originally explanted cells.

8.3 Materials

8.3.1 Stromal cell isolation and culture

- Bone marrow stromal cell medium: α-modified minimum essential medium (αMEM; Invitrogen Life Technologies Corporation) supplemented with 20% fetal bovine serum (FBS; Invitrogen), 2 mM l-glutamate and 100 U/mL penicillin, 100 µg/mL streptomycin
- Ca^{2+}/Mg^{2+}-free phosphate-buffered saline (PBS; Invitrogen)
- Cell strainer, 40-µm pore size (Becton Dickinson Biosciences Discovery Labware)
- Sterile cloning cylinder (Sigma-Aldrich)

8.3.2 Isolation of CD45-CD146+ cells

- Magnetic activated cell sorting (MACS) blocking buffer: PBS (Invitrogen) without Ca^{2+}/Mg^{2+}; pH, 7.2; 1% BSA (Sigma-Aldrich) supplemented with 2 mM ethylenediaminetetraacetic acid (EDTA; Sigma-Aldrich)
- Anti-CD45, phycoerythrin (PE)-conjugated magnetic beads (Miltenyi Biotec)
- MiniMACS magnetic column separation unit (Miltenyi Biotec)
- Anti-CD146 (MUC-18, S-endo 1; P1H12 BD Biosciences)

8.3.3 In vivo transplantation

- Hydroxyapatite/tricalcium phosphate (HA/TCP) ceramic particles (Zimmer Corporation)
- Eight- to 15-week-old female nih/nu/xid/bg mice (Harlan-Sprague Dawley) (all animal procedures were approved by the relevant institutional committee)
- Human fibrinogen (Sigma-Aldrich) and human thrombin (Sigma-Aldrich)
- Antibodies for immunohistochemistry: human anti-CD146 NCL (Novocastra) and human antimitochondria MAB-1273 (Chemicon International)

8.4 Method

8.4.1 Bone marrow single-cell suspensions

Bone marrow aspirates are collected from the posterior iliac crest of patients with normal hematopoietic function after acquiring informed consent. The whole bone marrow aspirate, containing 100 U/mL sodium heparin, is mixed with Hank's balanced salt solution (HBSS; Invitrogen) without Ca^{2+}/Mg^{2+} (pH, 7.3) containing 30 mM HEPES (Sigma Aldrich), 100 U/mL penicillin, and 100 µg/mL streptomycin sulfate (Invitrogen) for 10 minutes at room temperature with gentle agitation. After washing, the cells suspensions are depleted of red cells by incubation in lysis buffer (10 mM Tris-NH_4Cl; pH, 7.3) for 10 minutes at room temperature with slow rotation. The cells are centrifuged at 1,200 rpm for 10 minutes at 4°C, and the pellet is resuspended in fresh Ca^{2+}/Mg^{2+}-free PBS (Invitrogen).

The marrow cell preparations are passed through 18G needles to break up cell aggregates. The resulting cell suspensions (bone marrow nuclear cells) are filtered through a 40-µm pore-size cell strainer (Becton Dickinson Biosciences Discovery Labware) to obtain a single-cell suspension. The total number of nucleated cells in cell suspension is determined using a hemocytometer.

8.4.2 Isolation of MCAM/CD146-expressing bone marrow osteoprogenitors

Cells are resuspended in HBSS/30 mM HEPES (Sigma), 100 U/mL penicillin, 100 mg/mL streptomycin, and 1% BSA (Sigma), and incubated on ice for 30 minutes. Cells are pelleted in HBSS/2 mM EDTA, 1% BSA, resuspended in 1 mL blocking buffer, and incubated with anti-CD45-conjugated magnetic beads (Miltenyi Biotec) for 20 minutes on ice. Cells are separated into CD45– and CD45+ fractions using a MiniMACS magnetic column separation unit per manufacturer instructions (Miltenyi). CD45 cells are incubated with PE-conjugated anti-CD146 antibody clone P1H12, and CD146+ and CD146– cells are separated using a FACS DIVAntageSE flow cytometer (BD Biosciences Labware).

Sorted cells are plated at densities of 1.6 (clonal density) to $1.6 \cdot 10^4$ cells/cm² in αMEM (Invitrogen), 20% FBS (Invitrogen), 2 mM l-glutamate, 100 U/mL penicillin, and 100 µg/mL streptomycin at 37°C. Nonadherent hematopoietic cells are removed after 1 day by washing twice with ca^{2t}/mg^{2t}-free PBS.

In colonies established at clonal density, individual colonies (>50 cells; Figure 8. 1) are counted after 14 days. Individual colonies are isolated using a cloning cylinder. The cylinder is attached to the dish so that each cylinder embraces an individual colony, and cells inside the cylinder are treated with one aliquot of 1× trypsin–EDTA for 5 minutes each at room temperature. The released cells are transferred to individual wells of six-well plates (Becton Dickinson Labware). Subsequent passages are performed before cells

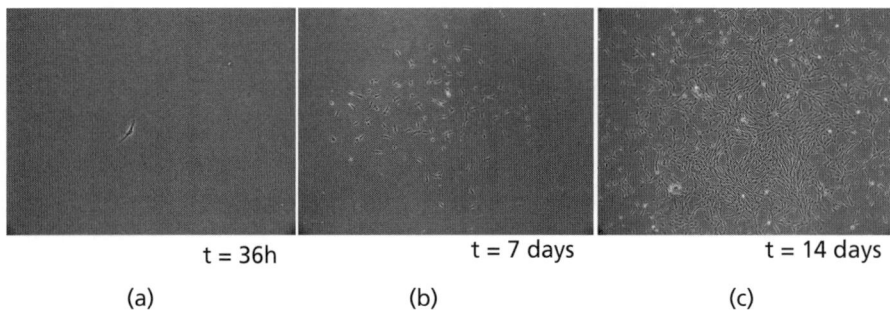

Figure 8.1 (a, b, c) Generation of a colony of stromal cells from a single CD146+ CFU-F. t, time.

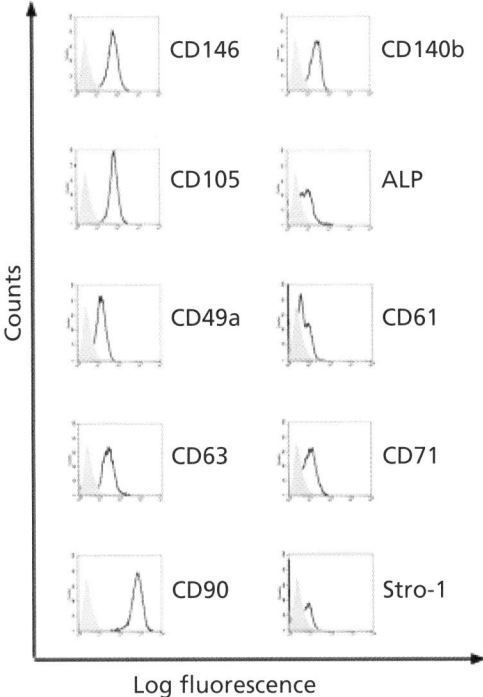

Figure 8.2 High and homogeneous expression of CD146 in a single clone of stromal cells generated by a CFU-F.

reach confluence, usually 5 to 10 days later. Samples are used for phenotype analysis in culture (Figure 8.2).

8.4.3 In vivo transplantation

The method for in vivo transplantation of CD146+ bone marrow osteoprogenitor is the same as previously designed and used for in vivo transplantation of total bone marrow stromal cell populations, as described in [7] and briefly summarized here. Further technical details can be found in [8] and [3].

Trypsin-released cells are centrifuged at 1,000 rpm for 5 minutes at 4°C and the cell pellet is resuspended in 1 mL fresh growth medium in 1.8-mL microtubes. A suspension of $2 \cdot 10^6$ adherent cells is mixed with 40 mg HA/TCP ceramic particles (Zimmer Corporation) and incubated at 37°C for 120 minutes with slow rotation (25 rpm).

The particles are collected after a brief centrifugation, and supernatant is discarded. Prior to transplantation, the vehicle with cells is incubated at 37°C for 5 minutes with 30 µL human fibrinogen (Sigma-Aldrich) and 30 µL human thrombin 100 U/mL (Sigma-Aldrich). The resulting constructs are implanted into subcutaneous pockets into the dorsal surface of 8- to 15-week-old female SCID beige mice (Harlan-Sprague Dawley).

Mid longitudinal skin incisions of about 1 cm in length are made on the dorsal surface of each mouse, and subcutaneous pockets are formed by blunt dissection. A single transplant is placed into each pocket with up to four transplants per animal (Figure 8.3). The incisions are closed with surgical staples.

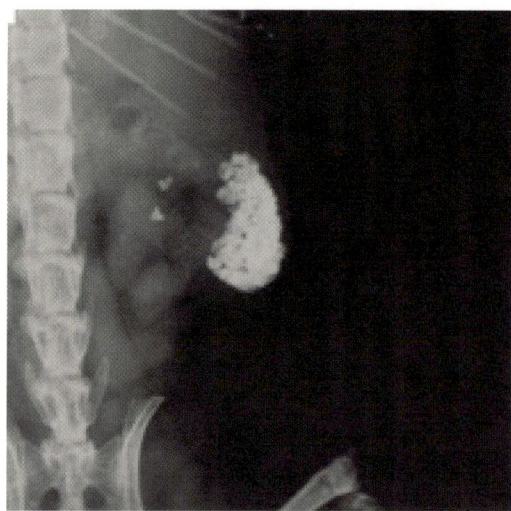

Figure 8.3 Radiograph of a mouse carrying a heterotopic transplant of CD146+ stromal cells.

8.4.4 Analysis of heterotopic ossicles

At 8 weeks posttransplantation, heterotopic ossicles are harvested and washed in pH 7.3 HBSS (Invitrogen) without Ca^{2+}/Mg^{2+} containing 30 mM HEPES (Sigma Aldrich), 100 U/ml penicillin, and 100 μg/mL streptomycin sulfate (Invitrogen) for 10 minutes at room temperature.

For histology, each transplant is fixed in 4% formaldehyde and decalcified in Ca^{2+}/Mg^{2+}-free PBS with 6% EDTA (0.2M; pH, 7.0) prior to embedding in paraffin. Bone and hematopoietic tissues are assessed histologically, and individual cell types are analyzed immunohistochemically (Figure 8.4). Donor origin of stromal cells is demonstrated by detection of human mitochondria-specific antigens. CD146-expressing cells are demonstrated by immunolocalization of human CD146.

For cell analysis, the harvested transplants are digested twice with 100 U/mL *Clostridium histolyticum* type II collagenase (Invitrogen) supplemented with 3 mM CaCl in PBS for 40 minutes at 37°C with gentle agitation. A total of $5 \cdot 10^5$ vital cells harvested from the two digestions are used to analyze human CD146+ cells using a FACScalibur flow cytometer (BD Biosciences) and CellQuest software (BD Biosciences), or other cells of interest based on relevant markers.

8.5 Anticipated Results

Single CD146+ cells will generate clonal colonies of stromal cells, noted for a high and homogeneous expression of CD146, and simultaneous expression of multiple putative markers of mesenchymal stem cells. Cell strains derived by passaging and expansion of either a single colony or multiple colonies will retain the phenotype through culture. Upon in vivo transplantation, these cells will generate bone and establish the HME in the heterotopic ossicle. Immunohistochemical analysis will demonstrate the presence of human bone and human stromal cells interspersed in the hematopoietic tissues and residing over the abluminal surface of sinusoids. These cells will express human CD146.

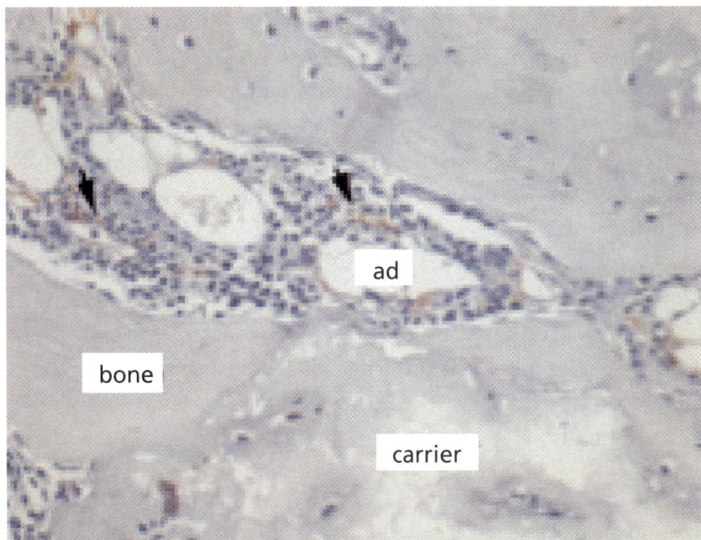

Figure 8.4 Histology of a transplant, demonstrating heterotopic bone and bone marrow including adipocytes (ad) and hematopoietic cells. A compartment of CD146+ stromal cells, residing over sinusoids, has been reconstituted.

Upon digestion of the harvested ossicles, it will be possible to sort human cells, or human CD146+ cells, and to show the presence of secondary CFUFs.

Success in generating heterotopic ossicles including host hematopoiesis is highly dependent, first of all, on the nature of the cell population used. Cell populations capable of generating heterotopic osteoblasts and bone are not necessarily able to establish the HME at the same time. This is the case, for example, for periosteum-derived or trabecular bone-derived cell populations. Apparently, this correlates with a low representation of CD146-expressing cells in the cell strains. Second, success in generating the heterotopic HME is dependent on culture conditions used. Among these, lot selection of serum batches is critical, as is the use of growth factor complements. For example, addition of fibroblast growth factor 2 (FGF-2) retains, and perhaps extends, the osteogenic capacity of a stromal cell strain, but tends to abrogate its ability to establish heterotopic CD146-expressing stromal cells and HME. Third, the carrier used must be at least partially resorbable. In this respect, materials including tricaclium phosphate are to be chosen, and each particular material needs to be tested for composition, crystal size, and physical aggregation (particle size). Nonresorbable materials cannot be used. Analysis of the HME can be adjusted to specific experimental needs.

8.6 Discussion and Commentary

The identification of cells that generate heterotopic ossicles, within the heterogeneous population of cells in the nonhematopoietic fraction of human bone marrow, has remained elusive for a long time. This property, previously ascribed to the clonogenic subset of bone marrow stromal cells, can now be ascribed to CD146+ cells, which in turn can be identified histologically as the CD146+ adventitial reticular cells in the intact bone marrow, and functionally as the CFU-F in bone marrow cell suspensions. These cells can generate, in vivo and within the heterotopic ossicles, bone and bone marrow adipocytes, and at the same time CD146+ adventitial reticular cells, and CFUF that can be passaged secondarily. This represents evidence for the ability of CD146+ cells to self-renew, suggesting that they represent bona fide stem cells. The original Friedenstein and Owen hypothesis [2] that multipotent skeletogenic progenitors in the bone marrow could represent a second type of stem cell in the bone marrow seems validated by these results. It must be noted that self-renewal of putative stem cell populations needs to probed by relevant in vivo assays, which postulate the definition of a minimum phenotype whereby the reconstitution of the originally explanted cell population can be assessed in vivo. It is also important to note that the rate and extent of cell proliferation in vitro does not represent proof of self-renewal in any case, contrary to statements in the literature, particularly in the field of mesenchymal stem cells.

This data also suggests that the ability to transfer the HME to heterotopic sites is ascribed to the same cell type that exhibits the capacity to generate bone and to self-renew. It is important to note that the ability to form bone and the ability to transfer the HME, while coupled, can be dissociated from one another, and are dissociated from one another in cell populations that can establish bone and osteoblasts, but not the HME, at the heterotopic transplantation site. For example, osteoblastlike cells derived in culture from trabecular bone surfaces, although capable of establishing heterotopic osteoblasts and bone, do not establish a heterotopic HME. Further developments of this type of experimental approach would lend themselves to a more detailed definition of the specific role of individual nonhematopoietic cell types in hematopoietic cell support [9, 10]. Interestingly, the ability to transfer the HME coincides with the ability of stromal progenitors to reestablish stromal progenitors in the transplant-generated tissues in vivo, linking self-renewal of stromal progenitors to a hematopoiesis-supporting function.

Troubleshooting Table

Problem	Explanation	Potential Solutions
Inconsistent clonogenic efficiency, cell expansion	Commercial serum lots are not equivalent	Serum should be lot selected.
Poor yield of stromal cells from relatively large volumes of bone marrow	Dilution of marrow with peripheral blood, which negatively influences growth of bone marrow stem cells	Relatively small volumes of bone marrow tissue should be used (typically, 0.5 mL).
Poor expansion of individual clones	Clonal heterogeneity	Increase the number of isolated clones.

8.7 Application Notes

In vivo transplantation assays for assessment of the osteogenic capacity of stromal progenitors have been in use for decades, and multiple versions thereof, besides the one described in detail here, exist. The value of these system is multifold. First, they represent the golden standard for claiming true osteogenic potency of any test cell population. A formal comparison of the ability of given cell strains to generate heterotopic ossicles, and to generate Oil red O stainable adipocytelike cells, or mineral deposits in vitro, demonstrates that no in vitro assays of adipo-, osteo-, or chondrogenic differentiation predicts, or substitutes for, in vivo assays. Many cell strains that are incapable of generating bone, cartilage, or fat in vivo are indeed capable of "differentiation" as artificially assessed in vitro. In this respect, this type of assays represents a must during the early steps of translational work aiming at bone regeneration using stem cells. In this particular context, the use of these assays can also be reverted to the assay of the osteoconductive competence of test materials in the presence of a validated osteogenic cell strain. Critical in both instances is the use of culture conditions that rigorously exclude bone morphogenic proteins, because these factors can reprogram cell types that are not natively osteogenic to an osteogenic function, without implying an osteogenic nature or commitment.

Second, these assays allow for the assessment of the ability of individual cell strains to establish the HME. This property does not coincide with the ability of individual cell strains to establish osteoblasts and bone in vivo. The ability to form bone and to establish the HME can even be dissociated from one another experimentally in a single, clonal, or nonclonal cell strain by ex vivo manipulation. For example, prolonged exposure of cells competent to establish the HME to FGF-2 abrogates this ability while leaving their osteogenic capacity unscathed. The ability of stromal progenitors to establish the HME appears to coincide, to a large extent, with the ability of a specific, early subset of stromal cells, defined by the expression of MCAM/CD146, to guide the organization of a bone marrow-specific type of local vasculature. Conceivably, although the role of stromal cells in this particular process seems critical, there may be other determinants that remain to be established. For this, this type of assay seems indispensable, at least as long as the use of human cells rather than murine models is envisioned. From a more application-specific point of view, the relevance of stromal progenitors to the support of hematopoietic function is linked to their current or conceivable use in multiple clinical settings, many of which are related to bone marrow transplantation procedures. In this area, the HME aspect of the in vivo transplantation assay provides a starting point for addressing relevant biological questions in preclinical studies.

Third, the use of these assays with phenotype-defined cell populations seems a reasonable way to go to dissect precisely the relative contribution of specific cell subsets to the important function of hematopoietic support.

Fourth, these systems lend themselves well either to the use of transgenic murine cell strains or to ex vivo manipulation of human cell strains (transfer and silencing of individual genes prior to in vivo transplantation). Murine cells transplanted with nonosteoconductive carriers (such as collagen-based carriers) can generate heterotopic ossicles. In sharp contrast, an osteoconductive material (i.e., a material based on a mineral phase) is necessary for human osteoprogenitors to generate bone in vivo.

8.8 Summary Points

1. In vivo transplantation assays represent the crucial assays to probe genuine skeletogenic potential of known or putative osteoprogenitors.
2. These assays can be used to generate heterotopic, chimeric hematopoietic tissue in which the hematopoiesis-supporting stroma is of donor origin and the hematopoietic cells are of host origin. These assays can thus be used to probe the functional interaction between bone cells and hematopoiesis, and between osteoprogenitors and hematopoiesis.
3. These assays can be used to probe the ability of phenotype-enriched cell populations to self-renew.

Acknowledgments

This work was supported by grants from MIUR, Telethon, and AIRC of Italy to P. B.

References

[1] Tavassoli, M., and W. H. Crosby, "Transplantation of Marrow to Extramedullary Sites," *Science*, Vol. 161, 1968, pp. 54–56.
[2] Friedenstein, A. J., "Bone Marrow Osteogenic Stem Cells." In D. V. Cohn, F. H. Glorieux, and T. J. Martin (eds.), *Calcium Regulation and Bone Metabolism*, Cambridge, U.K.: Elsevier, 1990, pp. 353–361.
[3] Bianco, P., et al., "Post-natal Skeletal Stem Cells," *Methods Enzymol.*, Vol. 419, 2006, pp. 117–149.
[4] Bianco, P., P. G.. Robey, and P. J. Simmons, "Mesenchymal Stem Cells: Revisiting History, Concepts, and Assays," *Cell Stem Cell*, Vol. 2, 2008, pp. 313–319.
[5] Gronthos, S., et al., "The STRO-1+ Fraction of Adult Human Bone Marrow Contains the Osteogenic Precursors." *Blood*, Vol. 84, 1994, pp. 4164–4173.
[6] Sacchetti, B., et al., "Self-Renewing Osteoprogenitors in Bone Marrow Sinusoids Can Organize a Hematopoietic Microenvironment," *Cell*, Vol. 131, 2007, pp. 324–336.
[7] Krebsbach, P. H., et al., "Bone Formation in Vivo: Comparison of Osteogenesis by Transplanted Mouse and Human Marrow Stromal Fibroblasts," *Transplantation*, Vol. 63, 1997, pp. 1059–1069.
[8] Kuznetsov, S. A., et al., "Postnatal Skeletal Stem Cells: Methods for Isolation and Analysis from Postnatal Murine and Human Bone Marrow." In J. Celis, et al. (eds.), *Cell Biology: A Laboratory Handbook*, New York: Academic Press, 2005, pp. 79–86.
[9] Calvi, L. M., et al., "Osteoblastic Cells Regulate the Haematopoietic Stem Cell Niche," *Nature*, Vol. 425, 2003, pp. 841–846.
[10] Kuznetsov, S. A., et al., "The Interplay of Osteogenesis and Hematopoiesis: Expression of a Constitutively Active PTH/PTHrP Receptor in Osteogenic Cells Perturbs the Establishment of Hematopoiesis in Bone and of Skeletal Stem Cells in the Bone Marrow," *J Cell. Biol.*, Vol. 167, 2004, pp. 1113–1122.

CHAPTER 9

Targeting the Stem Cell Niche In Vivo

Gregor B. Adams

Eli and Edythe Broad Center for Regenerative Medicine and Stem Cell Research
Keck School of Medicine
University of Southern California
Los Angeles, CA 90033

Abstract

The specialized microenvironment or niche where stem cells reside provides regulatory input governing stem cell function. Reasoning that the success of stem cell-based therapies relies on the ability of the stem cells both to engraft and self-renew sufficiently in their niche, one potential approach to augment these therapies is to target the stem cell niche. Using the hematopoietic stem cell (HSC) niche as a model system, we have demonstrated that the osteoblast is a key component of the HSC niche and that daily treatment with parathyroid hormone (a clinically approved method for increasing osteoblast function) resulted in therapeutic benefit in clinically relevant models of stem cell therapy. These results suggest that the niche may be a pharmacological target for altering stem cell function in settings of regenerative medicine.

Key Terms

Hematopoietic stem cell
stem cell niche
bone marrow
osteoblast
parathyroid hormone
stem cell mobilization

9.1 Introduction

Hematopoietic stem cells (HSCs) are an effective cell-based therapy because of their unique ability both to self-renew and to give rise to all cell lineages of the hematopoietic system for the life of the individual organism. Therefore, a single treatment targeted at the HSCs can achieve lifelong therapeutic benefit. This has been realized since the first reports were published more than 40 years ago of patients being given infusions of blood or bone marrow to treat various diseases [1]. However, the method by which HSCs are used as a therapy has not changed during this time—that is, the cells are simply infused into the peripheral circulation and allowed to home and engraft in the bone marrow. Therapeutic approaches to enhance the engraftment and function of the HSCs in the bone marrow niche have been limited.

One approach to increase the engraftment of HSCs is to understand and manipulate the mechanisms involved in the expansion of stem cells in their niche. Following the identification of the localization of the HSCs, it was hypothesized that adult HSCs reside within the context of a complex microenvironment of different cell types and extracellular matrix molecules that dictate stem cell self-renewal and progeny production in vivo [2]. These regions were termed the stem cell *niches*. One proposed role of the stem cell niche is to prevent the stem cell from becoming accessible to the differentiating influences of the surrounding microenvironment. Within the adult bone marrow, HSCs have been shown to reside in proximity to the endosteal surface of bone and blood vessels [3–6]. Our previous work used a transgenic mouse model in which a constitutively active form of the parathyroid hormone/parathyroid hormone-related peptide (PTH/PTHrP) receptor was expressed specifically in cells of the osteoblastic lineage. This led to a specific expansion of the HSC pool mediated through activation of the Notch pathway. We further demonstrated that these effects could be recapitulated through administration of exogenous PTH to a wild-type mouse [7]. Therefore, the components of this niche may provide targets for therapies aimed at altering stem cell fate.

Other methods for targeting the stem cell niche to achieve therapeutic benefit may also exist. These include the extracellular matrix molecule hyaluronic acid, a single-chain, large-molecular weight polysaccharide that is known to promote cell interaction through its known receptor CD44. Administration of hyaluronic acid results in a marked improvement in the recovery from bone marrow injury models using myelotoxic chemotherapy [8]. Recent studies have also demonstrated that the sympathetic nervous system is involved in the bone marrow HSC niche by stimulation of the osteoblastic cells [9]. This led to treatment approaches showing that stimulation of the sympathetic nervous system with an $\alpha 2$ adrenergic agonist, when used in conjunction with a mobilizing agent such as granulocyte–colony-stimulating factor, led to enhanced stem cell mobilization [10]. In addition, studies demonstrating the role of the Tie-2 receptor on HSCs identified that its ligand Ang-1 can improve survival of mice after lethal doses of myelotoxic drugs [11].

In this chapter we describe the specific methods for the manipulation of the osteoblastic cell that results in expansion or protection of the HSCs. However, it should be noted that simply targeting cells of the osteoblastic lineage may not be sufficient to achieve expansion of the HSCs in the bone marrow. A recent report has suggested that treatment of mice with strontium, which increases numbers of osteoblasts and indicators of bone formation, does not actually increase the number of HSCs in vivo [12].

However, our method provides a proof-of-principle that targeting the adult niche is a viable therapeutic option for therapies dependent upon HSCs. This also highlights the question of whether targeting the stem cell niche is a reasonable means of modifying stem cell responses in other tissues.

9.2 Experimental Design

The observation that the osteoblasts are a key component of the HSC niche and that activation of those cells leads to an expansion of the stem cell population offers a possibility for a novel stem cell therapy: targeting the microenvironmental niche rather than direct targeting of the stem cell itself. Using this approach we demonstrated that stimulation with PTH can result in expansion of resident HSCs, expansion of exogenously delivered HSCs, or protection of HSCs from myelotoxic injury [13] (Figure 9.1). In addition, because our studies used recombinantPTH, which is a drug currently approved for use in humans in the setting of osteoporosis, the potential for translating our studies into a clinical setting is therefore readily testable.

Using this method we are testing the hypothesis that treatment with PTH results in a significant expansion of the HSC population. As outlined later, the primary outcome measurement is the increase in the HSC population. This can be measured by both a phenotypic method or a functional method (but preferably both). In these experiments we typically have a control-treated group (saline-only group) plus the treatment group, although the treatment group may vary according to dose of PTH and duration of treatment. The number of subjects in each group depends on the variability of the measurement of HSC frequency, but typically requires at least five mice per group.

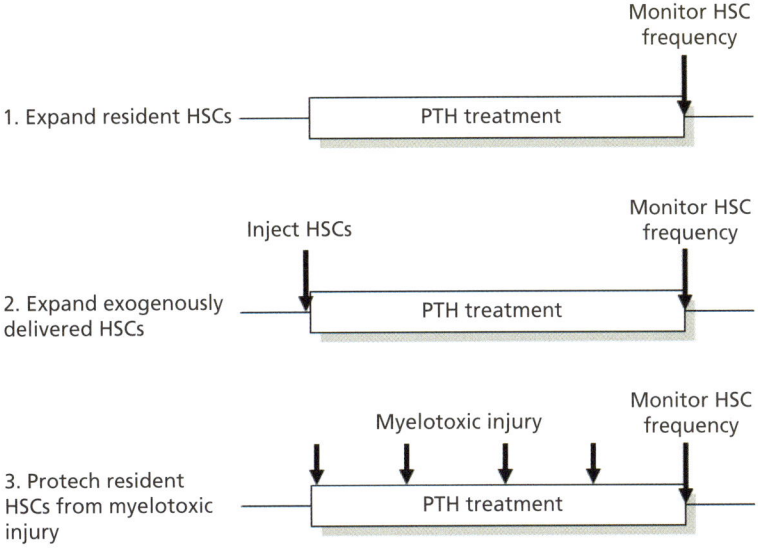

Figure 9.1 Diagrammatic representation of the options for PTH treatment to enhance stem cell-based therapies. Targeting of the stem cell niche can be performed (1) prior to collection of the HSCs to expand resident HSCs, (2) after transplantation of HSCs to enhance the engraftment of the cells or (3) during settings of myelotoxic injury to protect resident HSCs.

9.3 Materials

9.3.1 PTH treatment

- Rat PTH (1-34) (Bachem Bioscience)
- Sterile saline
- Syringe, 1 mL, with attached needle

PTH should be reconstituted at a concentration of 1 mg/mL, aliquoted into 20-μL aliquots and stored at –20°C.

9.3.2 Obtaining bone marrow mononuclear cells

- Scissors and forceps for dissection of bones
- Alcohol to sterilize tools and mice
- Syringe with attached needle
- Phosphate-buffered saline to flush out the mononuclear cells (MNCs) from bone

9.3.3 Immunophenotypic enumeration of HSC number

- Biotinylated "lineage" antibodies, including anti-CD3, CD4, CD8, B220, CD11b, Gr-1, and Ter-119
- Fluorescence-conjugated anti-Sca-1, anti-c-Kit, and anti-Flk-2 antibodies (all antibodies from BD Biosciences)
- Phosphate-buffered saline

Other phenotypic methods from marking HSCs can be similarly used, including side population cell analysis or signaling lymphocytic activation molecule (SLAM) family markers [6].

9.3.4 Functional enumeration of HSC number

- C57Bl/6 or B6.SJL mice (obtained and used in accordance with appropriate guidelines)
- Radiation source
- Fluorescence-conjugated anti-CD45.1 and anti-CD45.2 antibodies (BD Biosciences) to assess engraftment from different cell populations
- Fluorescence-conjugated anti-CD11b, B220, CD3, and so forth, antibodies to test for multilineage engraftment
- Ethylenediaminetetraacetic acid-containing Microtainer tubes (Becton Dickinson) to collect blood to monitor engraftment

9.4 Methods

9.4.1 Treatment of mice with PTH

1. Weigh mice.
2. Dilute stock of PTH to a dose of 80 μg/kg/day in sterile saline (final volume, 0.2 mL).
3. Inject mice intraperitoneally.

4. Repeat daily for 4 weeks.

Control mice receive a daily injection of 0.2 mL sterile saline for the same time period.

Analysis of the HSC content of the bone marrow is accomplished by two independent means: immunophenotype (lin$^-$Sca-1$^+$c-Kit$^+$Flk-2$^-$) [14] and function as measured by competitive repopulation assay of radiated mice [15, 16].

9.4.2 Immunophenotypic enumeration of HSC number

1. Sacrifice mouse, dissect bones, and obtain bone marrow MNCs by using a syringe and needle to flush the bones.
2. Stain cells with lineage cocktail, as well as anti-Sca-1, c-Kit, and Flk-2 antibodies according to standard methods.

9.4.3 Functional enumeration of HSC number

1. Sacrifice mouse, dissect bones, and obtain bone marrow MNCs by using a syringe and needle to flush the bones.
2. Prepare serial dilutions of MNCs and transplant with standard number of competitor cells into lethally radiated secondary hosts.
3. At regular time intervals, collect peripheral blood and monitor engraftment of the cells through analysis of the CD45.1 and CD45.2 alleles, and also multilineage engraftment (as referenced earlier).

9.5 Anticipated Results

As discussed earlier, the primary endpoint for these studies is the enumeration of the frequency of the HSC population. Therefore, both the immunophenotypic and functional enumeration methods will result in quantitative analysis of HSC number. From these studies it is anticipated that you will be able to observe an increase in the frequency of the HSC population. Although the measured frequency may differ between the methods, it is anticipated that an increase in the range of two- to threefold will be observed by both methods. It should, however, be observed that PTH treatment does not result in an alteration of mature cell counts or progenitor frequency, because this treatment affect should be restricted to the HSC subpopulation of cells.

As a result of the quantitative nature of the measurement of the effect, standard statistical analyses can be used for the analysis of the results obtained between the control and treated groups. As mentioned previously, though, the numbers of subjects may need to be increased as a result of the inherent variability in using murine models of hematopoiesis.

The exact influence on the HSC may depend somewhat on which setting the PTH is being used. As discussed earlier, targeting the HSC niche can be used to expand resident stem cells, expand exogenously delivered (transplanted) stem cells, or protect HSCs during conditions of myelotoxic stress. Our previous data has shown that although expansion of resident stem cells under relatively homeostatic conditions results in a twofold increase in stem cells, treatment with PTH under conditions of severe myelotoxic stress results in a much larger increase [13]. In addition, the quantitative enumeration may not accurately reflect key functional differences in the animal as a whole. Our previous data demonstrated that treatment with PTH after bone marrow transplant resulted in a twofold increase in the expansion of the HSCs [13]. However, when this same treatment protocol was used in setting of limiting cell number, we observed a much more impressive increase in the survival of the animals from approximately 30% in control-treated groups to 100% survival in PTH-treated groups [7]. Therefore, secondary endpoints should be used to evaluate the full affect of the treatment.

9.6 Discussion and Commentary

There are likely multiple sites within the bone marrow where HSCs reside and are regulated. The region about which we have the most information in terms of molecular regulation is the endosteal region. Defining that the osteoblast is a component of the stem cell niche has permitted targeting of osteoblast function to affect stem cell function. This was achieved by pharmacological manipulation through targeting of the osteoblast with PTH. As mentioned previously, therapeutic targeting of the niche is not restricted to using PTH; however, this drug is currently used clinically for the treatment of osteoporosis, making it readily translatable into the clinical setting [17]. As more components of the stem cell niche are elucidated, it could be envisioned that these, too, could potentially be targeted with clinically approved drugs leading to improvements in HSC-based therapies.

Our method is designed to outline the therapeutic targeting of a cellular component of the stem cell niche. The observed results were a marked improvement in HSC engraftment and thus animal survival after transplantation that supports the general strategy of manipulating the microenvironment to alter stem cell fate. Therefore, defining the HSC niche components is of biological interest and has practical utility in designing therapies to enhance stem cell number or function. When we have achieved this, more novel therapies can be developed that target the stem cells in various therapeutic and disease settings. It is envisioned that these approaches used in the hematopoietic system would then serve as a model for the treatment of various stem cell disorders through the manipulation of the stem cell microenvironment. Defining and manipulating niche constituents provides insight into the complex interactive system that governs physiological stem cell control.

Troubleshooting Table

Problem	Explanation	Potential Solutions
No increase in HSC frequency	Dose of PTH is not optimal	Adjust dose of PTH (either increase or decrease).
	Duration of treatment is not optimal	Either increase or decrease length of treatment, or increase frequency from once per day to two or three times per day.
	No PTH activity is left in stock solutions	Make new stock solutions of PTH.
HSC frequency is very variable	Mice have infection	Monitor mice daily for infection and remove from study if infection is found.

9.7 Application Notes

The protocol for targeting the HSC niche outlined in this chapter represents a proof-of-principle method that targeting of the niche can result in therapeutic benefit in stem cell-based therapies. One benefit to the use of PTH in these studies is that it is a clinically approved drug in the treatment of osteoporosis. Therefore, translation of the use of this drug in the setting of clinical stem cell therapies has been rapid [17]. It is conceivable that other factors known to increase the activity of the osteoblasts may have similar therapeutic benefit. In addition, as other components of the HSC niche are identified, it is similarly conceivable that pharmacological targeting of these components may have similar therapeutic benefit. This method provides a guide for the preclinical testing of these potential treatments for stem cell therapies.

9.8 Summary Points

1. The hematopoietic stem cell niche is a complex microenvironment consisting of many different cellular and extracellular components.
2. The role of the niche is to promote self-renewal of the stem cells to enable the cells to repopulate the hematopoietic system.
3. Cells of the osteoblastic lineage have been identified to be a key component of the bone marrow HSC niche.
4. The activity of osteoblastic cells can be enhanced through pharmacological treatment with PTH.
5. PTH treatment can expand resident stem cells, promote expansion of transplanted stem cells, or protect resident stem cells from myelotoxic insult.
6. Targeting of the niche cells could have therapeutic potential.
7. Targeting of the HSC niche with PTH serves as a model system for other stem cell niche-based therapies.

References

[1] Thomas, E. D., "Bone Marrow Transplantation from Bench to Bedside," *Ann. N. Y. Acad. Sci.*, Vol. 770, 1995, pp. 34–41.
[2] Schofield, R., "The Relationship between the Spleen Colony-Forming Cell and the Haematopoietic Stem Cell," *Blood Cells*, Vol. 4, 1978, pp. 7–25.
[3] Lord, B. I., N. G. Testa, and J. H. Hendry, "The Relative Spatial Distributions of CFUs and CFUc in the Normal Mouse Femur," *Blood*, Vol. 46, 1975, pp. 65–72.
[4] Gong, J. K., "Endosteal Marrow: A Rich Source of Hematopoietic Stem Cells," *Science*, Vol. 199, 1978, pp. 1443–1445.
[5] Nilsson, S. K., H. M. Johnston, and J. A. Coverdale, "Spatial Localization of Transplanted Hemopoietic Stem Cells: Inferences for the Localization of Stem Cell Niches," *Blood*, Vol. 97, 2001, pp. 2293–2299.
[6] Kiel, M. J., et al., "SLAM Family Receptors Distinguish Hematopoietic Stem and Progenitor Cells and Reveal Endothelial Niches for Stem Cells," *Cell*, Vol. 121, 2005, pp. 1109–1121.
[7] Calvi, L. M., et al., "Osteoblastic Cells Regulate the Haematopoietic Stem Cell Niche," *Nature*, Vol. 425, 2003, pp. 841–846.
This article was one of the first reports to identify that cells of the osteoblastic lineage are key components of the adult bone marrow HSC niche in vivo.
[8] Matrosova, V. Y., et al., "Hyaluronic Acid Facilitates the Recovery of Hematopoiesis following 5-Fluorouracil Administration," *Stem Cells*, Vol. 22, 2004, pp. 544–555.
[9] Takeda, S., et al., "Leptin Regulates Bone Formation via the Sympathetic Nervous System," *Cell*, Vol. 111, 2002, pp. 305–317.

[10] Katayama, Y., et al., "Signals from the Sympathetic Nervous System Regulate Hematopoietic Stem Cell Egress from Bone Marrow," *Cell*, Vol. 124, 2006, pp. 407–421.
This article demonstrates that modulating the sympathetic nervous system can be used to enhance stem cell mobilization using standard regimens. This highlights the interaction between the nervous system, bone, and the HSC niche.

[11] Arai, F., et al., "Tie2/Angiopoietin-1 Signaling Regulates Hematopoietic Stem Cell Quiescence in the Bone Marrow Niche," *Cell*, Vol. 118, 2004, pp. 149–161.

[12] Lymperi, S., et al., "Strontium Can Increase Some Osteoblasts without Increasing Hematopoietic Stem Cells," *Blood*, Vol. 111, 2008, pp. 1173–1181.
This article identifies that strontium treatment increases osteoblast cell number in vivo, but this treatment has no effect on the HSC population.

[13] Adams, G. B., et al., "Therapeutic Targeting of a Stem Cell Niche," *Nat. Biotechnol.*, Vol. 25, 2007, pp. 238–243.

[14] Christensen, J. L., and I. L. Weissman, "Flk-2 Is a Marker in Hematopoietic Stem Cell Differentiation: A Simple Method to Isolate Long-Term Stem Cells," *Proc. Natl. Acad. Sci. USA*, Vol. 98, 2001, pp. 14541–14546.

[15] Harrison, D. E., "Competitive Repopulation: A New Assay for Long-Term Stem Cell Functional Capacity," *Blood*, Vol. 55, 1980, pp. 77–81.

[16] Harrison, D. E., et al., "Primitive Hemopoietic Stem Cells: Direct Assay of Most Productive Populations by Competitive Repopulation with Simple Binomial, Correlation and Covariance Calculations," *Exp. Hematol.*, Vol. 21, 1993, pp. 206–219.

[17] Ballen, K. K., et al., "Phase I Trial of Parathyroid Hormone to Facilitate Stem Cell Mobilization," *Biol. Blood Marrow Transplant.*, Vol. 13, 2007, pp. 838–843.

CHAPTER

10

Parabiosis in Aging Research and Regenerative Medicine

Michael J. Conboy and Irina M. Conboy

Department of Bioengineering
University of California Berkeley
Berkeley, CA 94720

Abstract

The surgical technique of parabiosis may very well be much older than scientific publications. However, in 1864, Paul Bert published what is regarded as the first widely read report of parabiosis in his "Sur la Greffe Animale." Largely focused on the nature of tissue grafts and rejection, this work also describes "greffe par approche," the surgical joining of two rats to make artificially, as Bert described, a siamese twin. Since then, parabiosis (or joining two separate animals through blood circulation) has been used in many evolutionary distinct species with diverse scientific goals, ranging from understanding immune response to studies of aging and carcinogenesis, to stem cell research, understanding obesity, and so forth This chapter is focused on experimental parabiosis with detailed protocol of this technique and on the past, current, and future implementations of this technique.

Key Terms

Parabiosis
transfusion
life support
extracorporeal
artificial organ
transplantation
aging
stem cell
niche

10.1 Introduction

10.1.1 What is parabiosis?

Our Greek friends would (proudly) explain that *para* means "next to" or adjacent, *bios* means "life," and the *-is* at the end refers to the condition of something. Parabiosis is the condition of more than one living organism joined to another, with blood and other circulatory fluids being exchanged among the parabionts. Parabiosis can happen "naturally"—typically, in utero or in an egg mass in which embryos breach their respective egg sacs or amnions to touch. Not yet having developed self versus non-self mechanisms, the two or more embryos grow together and develop to give a conjoined twin, triplet, and so on. In mammalian gestation, the placentas might also grow together to give the same shared circulation, and this also has been referred to as *parabiosis in utero*. Although such arrangements are certainly uncommon, sometimes the babies are born or hatch to live, at least for some time. Conjoined identical twins, politically incorrectly referred to in humans as *siamese twins*, could even-more-politically incorrectly be thought of as *parabionts*; in this case, the cleaved egg gives rise to two embryos that never completely separate. The formation of an animal chimera, in which some parts of one type of animal are grafted, fused, or joined to another, often during early development, shares some similarity in many ways to parabiosis, and has been used to answer some similar questions. Chimeras between chick/quail, for example, have been invaluable for developmental studies. A practical distinction would be that whole animals are joined in parabiosis whereas only parts, cells, or tissues are shared in a chimera—typically, a singular animal.

10.1.2 Animal species

There appears to be no biological limit to the type of animal that may be "parabiosed," as there are reports in hydra [1], insects (houseflies [2], the silkworm *cecropia* [3]), Amphibia, and Mammalia. For example, Wallace [4] studied the growth of a genetic mutant frog strain in which every cell lacked nucleoli—the structure in the nucleus where ribosomal RNAs are processed. These mutant animals died quickly after hatching from lack of feeding and respiration, but they could be kept alive through the metamorphosis stage by parabiosis with a wild-type partner. By this approach, the developmental defects from lack of the nucleolus could be better studied. Although this review focuses on parabiosis in mammals, in principal most of the discussion would apply to any animal parabiosis. Experimental parabiosis in mammals has been successful so far only with inbred or genetically very similar partners.

10.1.3 Physiology of joining

By and large, most studies use the technique to achieve a shared circulation between the partner animals via the capillary beds that regrow at the join, called the *anastomosis*. In addition, there is the oft-ignored lymph flow and more passive fluid exchange under the skin and, with technique variations, through the peritoneal wall. This is in many ways similar to a "cross-circulation" (e.g., connection of major arteries and veins, as might be achieved by a cross-transfusion), but there are a few fundamental differences: The kinetics of cross-circulation through the skin are much slower (days to a week) to achieve, the rate of exchange once established is relatively slow (about 10 blood volumes per day in rodents), and the immunological status of skin is fundamentally different from the endothelial blood system, as is expounded upon later in the discussion of parabiotic disease. For what is still an excellent review of the physiology of parabiosis, refer to Finerty [5]. The key points to consider for experimental parabiosis, and whether to use parabiosis, are the time course of anastomosis, the exchange kinetics of the parabiotic state, and the time course after separation, if the animals are to be separated. All studies to date capitalized on these points and weighted them favorably against the technical challenges of the technique.

10.1.4 History of parabiosis and the range of its biomedical applications

In 1864, Paul Bert [6] published the first widely read report of parabiosis in his "Sur la Greffe Animale," which describes the surgical joining of two rats to make artificially, as he described, a siamese twin. It would make a valuable project for an undergraduate student to translate Bert's paper from the original French to at least English for the less cultured among us, and post this on the Internet. (Online translation websites are inaccurate. Babelfish, for example, consistently translates "le greffe" into "county official"—far more humorous than helpful.)

The early 20th century saw a number of publications using the technique, most published in German (again, we see a valuable translation project for a student). Sauerbruch and Heyde [7] introduced joining the peritonea (celio-anastomosis), with the goal of increasing abdominal cross-circulation and perhaps better "tolerizing" the animals to each other. A problem that arose during those early experiments was that the individuals of the pair might rotate and twist around the join, constricting the skin into necrosis. Bunster and Meyer [8] addressed the problem by ligating the animals at the shoulder (scapula). Recent investigators ligated the animals at the elbows and or knees for the same purpose [9].

Quite the variety of biomedical fields turned to parabiosis to answer questions. Falls and Kirschbaum [10] examined tumor growth and remission. One partner had a "remissed" tumor; the other was implanted with a fresh tumor and the tumor regressed from the shared circulation, suggesting an immune component. Kamrin [11] looked at dental caries in pairs of rats in which one partner was fed glucose daily. The results that only the glucose-fed partner got caries ruled out that dental caries were from the blood sugars in a high-sugar diet, because both partners of a pair shared similar blood glucose levels. Thus, caries were likely from the oral sugars given to one partner of the pair. Parameswaran et al. [12] looked at the body weight changes in pairs when one of the pair is stimulated to feed. The feeding partner gets fat, not surprisingly, but the other partner gets thin! They proposed a humoral mechanism of satiety that does not rely on insulin or glucagon—conclusions that were confirmed much later by Harris and Martin [13], who suggest leptin as the circulating factor [14]. In muscle studies, Hall et al. [15] prolonged the life of dystrophic mice through parabiosis to wild-type partners and argued that the wild-type partner was feeding the weakling through the parabiotic union. Montgomery [16] parabiosed healthy and dystrophic mice, and also crossed their inner sciatic nerves per Matzke and Kamrin [17] to determine whether the primary defect in a particular type of dystrophy was innervation or the muscle fibers themselves.

Parabiosis was a key technique for investigations of the immune system, which interestingly is an intertwined story with investigations into the nature of radiation sickness. Hasek and Hraba [18], in 1955, determined that self-tolerance happens during embryogenesis and via the blood by parabiosing chick embryos through the extraembryonic blood supply—in the egg, of course—and showed that even after separation, the partners were immunotolerant to each other. Zaiman et al. [19], in 1954, investigated the development of immunity by immunizing one partner of parabiotic pairs and then disconnecting the pair at different time points to determine when immunity took hold and for how long it lasted. A series of investigations highlighted by Barnes and Furth [20], Binhammer et al. [21], Warren et al. [22], and Carroll and Kimeldorf [23] showed that parabiosis allows a lethally radiated partner to survive a dose that would destroy the endothelial digestive tract, resulting in a gross imbalance of fluids, and later cause anemia. Survival was dependent on the ability of the healthy partner to maintain fluid and electrolyte homeostasis, and to feed the other through the die-off and regeneration of the digestive epithelium, and later through the die-off and repopulation of the hematopoietic system. These studies, following the observation that the new blood system in the radiated partner was seeded by cells migrating from the shielded partner, helped ground the stem cell theory of hematopoiesis. For an extensive review, see Nisbet [24]. Recent investigations into stem cell identity and regenerative properties have exploited parabiosis in their studies, in combination with robustly identifiable genetic differences between partners (e.g., green fluorescent protein) to identify the cross-engrafting cells. Currently, the general conclusion would be that, aside from the circulating blood cells, few other cells cross-engraft, and that the only stem cells to cross-engraft to a significant extent are of the hematopoietic system. Even then, engraftment becomes substantial only if the partner's own system is depleted, such as by radiation. Engraftment and/or transdifferentiation into other cell types, such as neurons or muscle, is normally rarely seen (muscle [25], brain [26], heart [27], ovary [28], fat [29], endothelium [30]). However, if the local population of stem cells is depleted, then contribution from the partner may be observed. Whether this contribution is tissue-specific stem cells, transdifferentiating hematopoietic stem cells, or from fusion of differentiated, infiltrating leukocytes is still debated (for an honest review, see Vieyra et al. [31]).

10.1.5 Parabiosis in aging studies

One view of aging is that it is systemic; all the tissues and organs age together because they share a common circulation and are interdependent. Another view is that aging is the result of a decline and eventual failure in tissue maintenance and regeneration. Young individuals regenerate and maintain their tissues well whereas the elderly do not. Both views may very well be correct. Two lines of investigations have suggested that a youthful circulatory milieu can have a restorative effect on tissues. The first is that if old tissues are transplanted into a young host, they often survive and do well, but young tissues in an old host fare poorly, adopting the aged characteristics of the host. These heterochronic transplant studies indicate that the host environment dictates the phenotypic age of a tissue—specifically, how well it engrafts and grows—and implicates local or systemic cues [32]. The second line of investigation again used heterochronic parabiosis and here the results were generally consistent with the age of the circulation governing the age of the tissue. Fifty years ago, it was proposed that if aging is systemic, then an old animal might be rejuvenated by the circulatory factors or system of a young animal. This experiment was first attempted by McCay et al. [33] using parabiosis instead. The results of these experiments suffered from a limited number of joined animals, but suggested that in the old animal some tissues (specifically, collagen, bones) appeared more youthlike whereas those of the young partner were unchanged or slightly older. The few surviving pairs did not live on average longer than nonparabiosed rats, although one pair did live notably long. In 1972, Ludwig and Elashoff [34] published the results of a more rigorous test of heterochronic parabiosis and longevity, with more controls and enough pairs in each cohort to get statistically meaningful data. Two- to 3-month-old rats were joined with 1-year-old partners. The results were that the older partners of the heterochronic pairs lived, on average, 4 to 5 months longer. Here it should be described that a rat (or mouse) is generally considered youthful from the onset of maturity at about 2 months until fertility drops at around 1 year. At 1 year, one can already detect a decline in function of various parameters. After that, the performance of many tissues and organs declines dramatically so that, by 1.5 to 2 years, the animal is clearly decrepit and mortality is high. In the Ludwig experiment, the old animals shared circulation with a young animal for as long as 2 years and, during most of this time, the young partner was certainly not young anymore. These experiments, although limited in number, do suggest that a young circulation may have some effect on longevity, or at least beg the question to be investigated further.

Recently we revisited the effect of heterochronic parabiosis on the aging phenotype using a regeneration model in muscle. Here we scored the age of the tissue not in its basal maintenance state, but during and after a bout of injury-induced regeneration. In this model, the old muscle tissue regenerated as well as the young when it was exposed to the young–old shared circulation, and this rejuvenation was of the old tissue and regenerative "old" stem cells, not by invading cells from the young partner. The young muscle regeneration suffered only slightly from exposure to the old circulation. We also noted a significant improvement in the basal stem cell proliferation in the liver of old partners, with a decrease in that of the young, even though the livers were not specifically injured or forced to regenerate (although it was argued that the whole surgical procedure might stimulate or stress the liver). These experiments suggest that regardless of the age of the circulatory factors affecting life span, at least the age of the circulation affects the age of many tissues in the body, and their regenerative response [35]. Investigations are currently underway to identify those circulatory factors that are responsible for the rejuvenating effect.

So the question remains that if a younger circulation or milieu can effect the basal phenotype and even more so the regeneration of various organs and tissues, can these changes have a significant effect on the overall life span and health of the individual? If the factors in the young that support young regeneration and those in the old that drive aging are identified, will modulating them be expected to extend functional life span, or is there more to aging than just the age of the circulation or regenerative ability? We propose, and describe here, that the aging researchers address these specific questions by repeating the work of Ludlow with the following twist: Instead of allowing the young partners to age along with the old after parabiosis, and thus diminish any positive influence over time, the young partners should be replaced at regular intervals to ensure that the old partner always shares a truly young circulation. In addition to overall life span, various parameters of the aging phenotype in different organ systems should be measured along the way to determine whether any improvements are seen over time.

10.2 Experimental Design for Aging Studies

The general design would be to join an experimental group of animal pairs, with the old partner initially just entering "old age" at about 1 year of age, and the young partner at 2 to 3 months (a young adult). The control group would be isogenic pairs of old animals both initially at 1 year of age. Because reproductive fecundity drops at around 8 months of age, the young partner may be considered young for an additional 6 months after joining. Every 6 months, the young partner would therefore be replaced with a new 2-month-old partner. For the control pairs, the replacement partner should be the same age as the old partner (e.g., the first replacement will be with a 1.5-year-old; the second, with a 2-year-old; and so on). Pairs would also be compared with age-matched individuals from the same colony. Retired breeders may be preferred because they are readily available and can be matched to their progeny. We suggest an initial target of 60 pairs of each group, control and experimental, to be joined to hedge against mortality from parabiotic disease and to ensure sufficient data for mortality curves. Ludlow obtained significant data with 20 surviving pairs in each cohort.

A number of parameters should be measured, preferably noninvasively or with minimal invasion (obviously, one would not want to jeopardize the health of the parabiotic pairs): weight, heart rate, blood profile (glucose, insulin, peripheral blood count, lipid profile), hair regrowth or some assay on a hair plug (may combine with skin biopsy), teeth, blood and/or urine glucose, and skin biopsy.

There is a 6-month cycle of joining and rejoining animal pairs, so the time requirements each 6 months would be as follows. Two groups of 60 pairs equals 120 person-hours just for surgery. Postoperative care for the first week is relatively quick: examination and medication, with a few percent of pairs requiring additional surgery, so a reasonable average would be 0.5 hour per pair for the first week, for an additional 60 hours. Care for the following 2 weeks until anastomoses is established and the risk of parabiotic disease passes involves daily examination, medication if needed (rarely), and surgery to separate those pairs that appear to be rejecting (typically from 20% to 50%). This will average another hour per pair, or 120 hours. This time requirement would be repeated every 6 months as partners are replaced. From this point onward until the next parabiosis surgery, the work would consist of a brief daily examination of the pairs for viability, and monthly examination and data collection of age-related parameters. This should take 1 hour per pair per month—120 hours total, plus another 60 hours for the individual animal controls. Summing up, the first 6-month segment of work equals 480 person-hours or 60 person-days (of the traditional 8 hours). It would be expected that all the pairs could be joined during the first 6 months, and then the surviving pairs rejoined every 6 months afterward in an ongoing process. During this time, data would be collected and analyzed. The hands-on animal time will, of course, decrease as the pairs age and die, increasing the time for data analysis and reporting.

10.3 Materials

1. Animals to be paired, from a highly inbred or isogenic strain, preferably related to each other by birth. Expect 50% survival past week 2, so order extra animals.
2. Shaving device. A quality electric "mustache and beard" trimmer will work almost as well as a veterinary shaver on small rodents. The use of Nair or a similar depilatory product is also helpful if the animal can be rinsed with warm water afterward.
3. Betadine or other surgical scrub
4. Sterile swabs and pads, small for wiping the animals and larger for making the sterile field
5. Two sets (for one in use, one in the sterilizer) of small surgical instruments: blunt forceps, sharp forceps, scissors, scalpel, 7- or 9-mm wound clips and stapler (Clay Adams Autoclip is excellent), wound clip remover, small suture tool. A small hemostat or two is also handy.
6. Bead heat sterilizer. Wash and place surgical instruments in the sterilizer as directed between animals and as needed.
7. Sterile saline solution in 15-mL conical tubes
8. Ophthalmic ointment
9. Rubbing alcohol, 70%
10. An isoflurane/oxygen anesthesia apparatus for small animals, with some kind of nosepiece for two (or more) animals. Alternatively, an injectable solution of xylazine/ketamine or Avertin (tribromoethanol/amylene hydrate). One injection typically will anesthetize an animal for 40 minutes, so the novice might prepare to inject a second smaller dose should the animals begin to awaken during the procedure. The animals may also be shaved on one day and then joined the next day. We found isoflurane, although cumbersome, gives an easier controlled dose, a safer long dose, and quicker recovery than the injectables.
11. Small heating pad unless the procedure room is very warm (>25°C)
12. Bright spotlight to see well. Note that a few hundred watts of spotlight can make the surgery area uncomfortably warm and even kill a small animal. The new compact fluorescent bulbs run much cooler than incandescent and so the temperature of the surgery area can be modulated by the choice of bulb with no loss of light. If your hands are too hot at the surgery site then the animal will be too hot also, and too cool is better than too hot.
13. Suture material: 4-0 nylon or braided silk, curved cutting needle for closing the skin, 2-0 to 4-0 nylon monofilament, curved tapered needle for joining the inner limbs, 6-0 absorbable or silk, curved tapered needle for ligating peritoneal membranes
14. Antibiotics preparation, broad spectrum such as Baytril
15. An analgesic preparation: for moderate pain and for long-lasting pain, such as Buprenex
16. Small cages (the standard size for one to five animals), one per pair of animals

10.4 Methods

10.4.1 Parabiosis protocol

Before embarking on this procedure, secure all necessary approvals from your institute's animal use committee and animal care facility. Meet and plan with your facility's veterinary staff. This is not a discreet procedure; parabiotic pairs are obvious and can attract a lot of attention in a facility and so make sure you have prepared all involved. Last, although the techniques are rather crude, unless you have a lot of experience in surgery, it would be worth the effort to get training from someone familiar with these procedures. Practice on euthanized animals until you feel confident with the procedure, before working with live experimental animals.

This procedure is written for approximately 30g adult mice, so scale up or down as needed for other animals. If one joins the pair at the inner limbs, then the skin need only be joined from limb to limb, but if the limbs are not to be joined, then a longer stretch of skin must be joined to keep the animals from rotating around and constricting the flap of skin; in such a case, join from ear to rump. Joining internally at the peritoneal wall is optional in either case and may reduce the incidence of parabiotic disease or may be redundant when limbs are joined. An experienced surgeon can set up a pair in about 30 minutes, but expect twice that for a novice.

10.4.2 Experimental method

1. Mice are anesthetized to full muscle relaxation.
2. Because the procedure can take an hour for a novice, the eyes are dabbed with ophthalmic ointment [Figure 10.1(a)].
3. Mice are shaved completely on the side to be joined and rubbed down with rubbing alcohol to clean and remove loose fur. Use Nair or similar product as directed if the animal can be rinsed in warm water [Figure 10.1(b)]. Shave well, because it will make subsequent steps easier and reduce the chance of infection.

Figure 10.1 Steps of the parabiosis procedure. Animals are oriented with the head pointing up or to the right. The animal models shown were euthanized for this demonstration, and we suggest practicing on euthanized animals before performing experiments. (a) After the animals are anesthetized to complete relaxation, dab the eyes with ophthalmic ointment to protect them from drying. (b) A cosmetic depilatory may be used in place of or in addition to shaving. Fur can be difficult to wet, so wipe with rubbing alcohol first, then water, then the depilatory. Wash off the depilatory well. (c) Visualize where the skin should be joined before cutting. (d) Mark the incision line, in this optional case, planning access to the elbow and knee joints. Other options might include an incision from behind the ear to just before the tail. (e) A sterile or aseptic wrap may be useful for keeping fur, excrement, and so forth, out of the surgical site. (f) Apply surgical scrub as directed. (g) Lift the skin and cut along the line, then spread free the skin flaps with a blunt instrument. (h) Approximate the ventral skin edges and apply staples from the middle outward. (i) Place staples from one-half to one staple-width apart, as far anterior and posterior as practical, leaving tight areas for later suture. (j–l) (Optional) Ligate the elbows and knees, passing the suture through the flesh around the joint but not through the cartilage joint itself, preferably using a tapered needle and monofilament suture. Tie the knot outside of contact between the snug limbs. (m) (Optional) If the peritoneal walls will be ligated, carefully pull out and cut an approximately 1-cm incision in each abdomen. (n) Pass suture through all four edges of the peritoneal walls, spiraling from one end to another. Make sure that suture is not crossed or trapped inside the spiral. Absorbable suture material is required; 5-0 suture is shown for clarity, but thinner material works well also for mice, and a tapered, curved needle is much preferred over a cutting needle. (o) After the spiral is complete, snug up the suture to close the peritoneal openings together, pass the needle back through the join to the starting end of suture, and tie off. (p) Staple the dorsal skin flaps as in (h) and (i). (q) Close any remaining openings in the skin with suture as indicated by the white arrow. Here, a cutting needle with 4-0 or larger suture is preferred. (r) A joined pair.

10.4 Methods

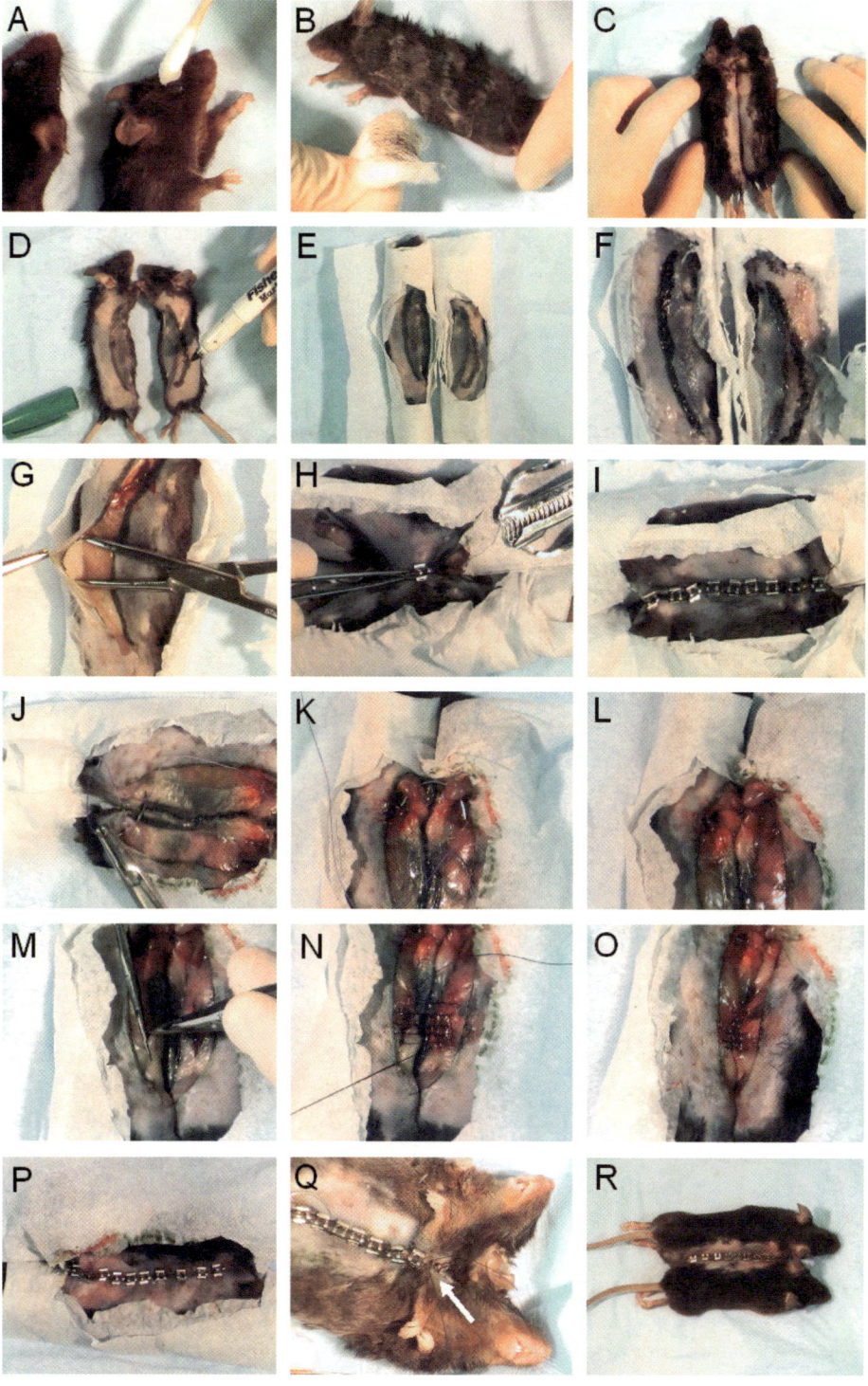

4. Wrap each animal lightly in a sterile material like gauze, and expose only the shaved area by cutting through the gauze [Figure 10.1(e)].
5. Swab the side with Betadine or other surgical scrub [Figure 10.1(f)].
6. On the first mouse, a skin incision is made extending in a slight curve up from the side of the elbow across the side of the body and down to the side of the knee [Figure 10.1(d)]. The elbow and knee joints must be accessible, but more cutting than that just means more sutures later. If the joints will not be ligated, the longest practical incision should extend in a straight line from just behind the ear to the flank of the rump—the contact line if two animals were pressed side by side [Figure 10.1(c)].
7. Free the skin from the subcutaneous fascia using a moist swab or blunt forceps in difficult areas [Figure 10.1(g)].
8. Lightly irrigate the wound with saline and keep tissues moist throughout the procedure.
9. Make a mirror-image incision on the second mouse as just described.
10. Place the animals on their backs, incisions next to each other, approximate the skin from one animal to the other, and staple together using 7- or 9-mm wound clips [Figure 10.1(h)]. Work from the middle outward. Space the clips from one-half to one clip length apart [Figure 10.1(i)].
11. Carefully flip the animals over so that dorsal is up.
12. If the inner limbs will be joined, join them with the 4-0 monofilament. Visualize the joined, "lock-step" joints before suturing and make sure the suture passes through the flesh and the joint, and that the ends are accessible to tie off [Figure 10.1(k)]. Try to keep the knot away from the bend of the joint. Tie several square or self-locking knots in the nylon and snug the knots tight, but do not constrict the joints [Figure 10.1(l)].
13. If the peritonea will be joined, carefully make approximately 1-cm mirror-image incisions to the abdominal walls of each partner in the area below the ribs but above the thigh. To avoid damaging internal tissue, pinch and pull the peritoneal wall away from the abdomen with the forceps and cut with the scissors [Figure 10.1(m)].
14. Visualize the joined peritoneal walls and a spiral suture closing the four edges to only one line: dorsal and ventral edges of one animal joined to the dorsal and ventral edges of the other animal. The goal is not to make a tube between the peritoneal cavities, but to join the edges so that fluids may still ooze past, but intestine may not. Start by passing the needle into an end of the dorsal edge of one partner and out the ventral edge, into the ventral edge of the other partner and out the dorsal edge. Pull the peritoneal tissue out from the abdomen with the forceps while pushing the needle through the tissue to avoid puncturing internal organs. Repeat passing the needle as noted while progressing along the edges a few millimeters at a time until the spiral is complete [Figure 10.1(n)]. Gently pull on the edges of the suture, using the forceps to snug the windings of suture and close the openings. Pass the needle once more through the edges back to the starting free end of suture and tie off [Figure 10.1(o)].
15. On the dorsal side, close the skin with wound clips, again working from the middle outward [Figure 10.1(p)].
16. Close the hard-to-reach areas of skin with 4-0 cutting sutures [Figure 10.1(q)].
17. After closure, wipe off excess surgical scrub with a gauze pad and a minimum of rubbing alcohol, avoiding the joined skin, and check the integrity of the join [Figure 10.1(r)].

10.4.3 Postoperative care

1. Each mouse is injected subcutaneously with warm Baytril antibiotic solution (as directed, 5 µg/g), diluted in saline to give a volume of approximately 1% of the animal's weight.
2. Hydrate each animal if needed intraperitoneally with warm saline.
3. Place the pair on a warm, but not hot, heating pad or under an incubation lamp if the room is cool, or in a clean cage if the room is warm. Mice should awaken within minutes of removal from isoflurane inhalation, longer from the injectable anesthetics.
4. Administer Buprenex or equivalent as directed for pain, but only after the animal has completely awakened from anesthesia.
5. House the animals at one joined pair per small cage. Although the pair will likely not eat or drink much the first day, they may have trouble accessing food and water until they learn to work together. Place wetted food and/or hydrating gel on the bottom of the cage for the first few days.
6. Observe the pair at least daily for signs of infection, distress, or wound opening, and administer Baytril antibiotic subcutaneously for the next 5 days at 2.5 µg/g per mouse.

10.4.4 Removing the staples

The pair should achieve a stable join in approximately 1 week, longer if infection is present. Because parabiotic disease typically manifests itself at about 1 to 2 weeks, removing the staples at about 2 weeks allows one to examine the animals thoroughly.

1. Anesthetize the mice as described earlier.
2. Clean the joined area as best as possible and blot dry.
3. Observe for signs of separation and consider restapling or suturing the area, or signs of parabiotic disease and consider separating the pair.
4. Undo the staples, and cut and remove any remaining stitches.
5. Smear a thin layer of antibiotic ointment around the joined area.
6. Allow the pair to recover and return to their cage.

10.4.5 Separating a pair

It may be desirable to separate a joined pair, either as part of the experiment or because one partner is sick, or worse.

1. Set up for surgery as described earlier.
2. Anesthetize the mice as described earlier.
3. Clean the joined area as best as possible, reshaving if needed, and swab the skin between the animals with scrub.
4. If still present, undo staples, and cut and remove any remaining stitches.
5. Recall if the peritoneal tissues are joined, and cut the skin to separate the animals. Cut the dorsal-side skin then the ventral, and not both together.
6. Cut and remove sutures at the elbow or knee if they were joined.
7. Carefully cut through the peritoneal join if it had been ligated, and close that opening on each animal with 5-0 or 6-0 Vicryl or silk using a tapered needle as noted previously.

8. Clean up the edges of skin on each animal, removing scarred or stretched tissue so that the ends approximate easily but there is not such extra loose skin that it might drag on the ground.
9. Flush with saline if needed and close the skin using wound clips and suture.
10. Hydrate, administer antibiotic and analgesic, and observe as noted earlier.

10.5   Troubleshooting Parabiotic Disease

10.5.1   "Parabiotic intoxication"

The most obvious and immediate problem encountered in experiments using parabiosis is the mortality that arises approximately 1 to 2 weeks after the partners are joined, coinciding with the formation of anastomosis and sharing of circulation. Originally termed *parabiotic intoxication*, this referred (in the language of a century ago) to the toxicity or poisoning of one or both partners from the shared blood. Today, this is more commonly referred to as *parabiotic disease*. For those considering using the technique in their studies, note that the incidence of mortality from parabiotic disease is typically several tens of percent, and that is with highly inbred strains of mice or rats. Pairings between different strains of animals are almost certain to react, a few anecdotal examples aside. Separation of the diseased partners or surviving partner is no guarantee of survival, although it increases the odds. To our knowledge, immunosuppression therapy has not been investigated for parabiosis. Of course, with the current developments in cloning, one may be considering parabiosing cloned animals, to each other or to the "original," in which case parabiotic disease should not be an issue, although this is yet untested.

The history of investigation regarding the cause of this disease is enlightening and itself has offered a great deal of knowledge to our understanding of graft-versus-host compatibility and tissue rejection in grafts and transplants. Early descriptions and hypotheses for this disease were published in German around the beginning of the 20th century. Again, the translation and posting of these works would make a valuable project for the student. The most obvious sign of parabiotic disease was that one partner becomes shriveled, pale, and anemic whereas the other is almost swollen with blood, red, plethoric. Because the blood was affected and an immunoreaction was involved, the most common explanation of the disease was rejection of the partner as foreign tissue, although differences in blood pressure or other physiology was also proposed to explain the pale/red asymmetry in the partners.

Finerty and Panos [36] reviewed the disease and noted that the more closely related (genealogy) the partners, the less likely the disease, again suggesting immunoincompatibility. Chute and Sommers [37] observed what looked similar to blood type incompatibility. They reported that the pale partner was found to suffer immunoreaction and necrosis in the marrow whereas the red partner suffered blood clotting and inflammation in the internal organs, particularly the spleen, inflamed lymph nodes, and general swelling. It was proposed that, because of the location of new and old erythrocytes, the blood from the white partner went to the other, was attacked by antibodies, and then got "caught" on the red side, unable to cross back over the anastomosis. Why blood would not also get caught on the pale partner's side of the anastomosis was not clear.

Hall and Hall [38] induced shock in one partner by severing the spinal cord, which resulted in, among other things, hypotension at the capillaries. This was proposed to be the cause of the previously mentioned symptoms. However, this work did not address the root cause of "shock" in parabiotic animals, because separated animals may also later develop parabiotic disease. That later heterologous grafts can exacerbate parabiotic disease in separated animals supported the idea of a developing immunoincompatibility [39]. Andresen et al. [40] joined rabbits at the ears, which must offer an ample joining surface but with very slow transfer of fluids, and then examined cross-transplants of musculofascial tissue. The graft-versus-host reactions were diminished and the grafts better tolerated, but what was interesting was the site of the parabiotic union. Even in cases with obvious inflammation and "rejection" at the union site, the scar (collagen) itself was not attacked and served to maintain the union, typically until the reaction subsided to a more "neutral" tolerance.

10.5.2 Suggestions for the side effects associated with parabiotic disease

Given that the skin is especially immunoreactive and the gut more immunotolerant, we propose the crude and untested theory that ligating inner tissues and/or sharing peritoneal or subvisceral fluids may help avoid developing or may diminish the reactions that lead to parabiotic disease. Or perhaps, if the shock/hypertension theories of the disease have merit, joining the peritoneum allows fluids accumulating in one partner to drain back to the hypertense partner. We have not seen an attempt to mitigate parabiotic disease through the use of immunosuppressing drugs, and suggest that this might be a worthwhile investigation. Toward the alternative theory for the disease, if it is caused by an imbalance in circulation, then by comparing the rates of blood exchange from one partner with the other would strengthen this correlation. For example, if a dye injected into one partner's tail vein appears sooner in the other partner than vice versa, this would support an alternative theory for the disease. If true, such disparate pairs would show higher incidence of parabiotic disease than pairs with equal primary circulation exchange.

10.6 Discussion and Commentary

The idea of parabiosis has not only survived the test of time, but has yet another entirely novel and important ramification in the age of bioengineering, tissue engineering, and artificial organogenesis—namely, it would be very tempting to manufacture an extracorporeal organ or even a set of organs as an alternative to conventional organ transplantation. Such an extracorporeal organ system could be connected to the physiological circulation, and in this regard would emulate prototypical parabiosis as described here. Although design and manufacture of such a parabiotic extension of a living organism is definitely challenging, it would solve many of the current problems inherently associated with tissue and organ transplantation.

Organ transplantation has been used for decades for treating the terminal malfunction of vital organs, and pioneering work in this field added years of productive life to many people and was recognized by several Nobel Prizes, starting with 1912 Nobel Prize to Alexis Carrel for the innovative technique to connect blood vessels and organs

[41, 42]. Although more than a million people live with transplanted livers, kidneys, lungs, and hearts, the side effects associated with allogeneic or xenogeneic organ transplants are many and include tissue rejection as well as ischemic injury and a shortage of suitable donor organs. Even with constant immunosuppression there is progressive deterioration of allogeneic tissue, which severely limits the life span of transplanted organs [41, 43].

In addition, in some cases, the reason for organ failure is an autoimmune disease mounted against a tissue, be these cells of host or donor origin, such as against pancreatic β cells in type 1 diabetes mellitus [44, 45]. The same is true with respect to multiple sclerosis, in which an autoimmune response against the person's own myelin proteins results in demyelination, progressive dysfunction of the central nervous system, and, ultimately, paralysis [45, 46]. Therefore, even if sources of pancreatic β cells and oligodendrocytes were abundantly available (which is not the case), the transplanted cells or tissues would suffer the same elimination by the host immune system as the host's own endogenous cells.

With the advent of stem cell science and technology, significant progress has been achieved in developing specific protocols that allow the directed differentiation of embryonic stem cells into pancreatic β-like cells [47, 48], oligodendrocytes [49], dopaminergic neurons [50–52], cardiomyocytes [53], and many other cell types that are of great therapeutic value for combating tissue degenerative disorders. Moreover, functional integration of these cells into organ systems was successfully demonstrated in animal models of human diseases. Although using fetal or embryonic human stem cells and/or cloning parts of human beings has ethical concerns, the idea of induced pluripotency (e.g., directed dedifferentiation of somatic cells into embryoniclike stem cells), followed by the directed differentiation of these induced pluripotent stem (iPS) cells into the tissue of interest solves these ethical issues and potentially provides for syngeneic transplantable cells and tissues [54, 55].

Another alternative to organ replacement that is free of human leukocyte antigen-based tissue rejection and does not require the destruction of human embryo is artificial organ design. Extracorporeal replacement of organ function was first achieved in 1943 with the clinical use of dialysis to substitute for renal function [56]. Since then, technologies have evolved for high-volume hemofiltration or extracorporeal blood purification, with the capacity for removal of not only toxins and metabolic by-products, but also microorganisms, endotoxins, and inflammatory mediators. These artificial systems are able to provide support for multiorgan dysfunction and, in the future, have the promise of restoring circulatory homeostasis [56, 57]. In this regard, extracorporeal membrane oxygenation or gas exchange systems are used for artificial lung and heart support, pioneered by the first heart–lung bypass surgery in 1953 [58, 59]. Extracorporeal liver function can be, to some degree, obtained with the help of the molecular adsorbents recirculating system, which is capable of removing albumin-bound and water-soluble toxins [60, 61]. Such a mechanical extracorporeal liver support system provides an alternative to liver transplantation, which was first performed more than 50 years ago, and is an alternative to the first use of liver cells for liver function replacement, which was first accomplished in 1963 [56]. An alternative promising method for combating liver failure is hepatic engineering, during which exogenous cells are expanded and organized into a functional tissue with the help of three-dimensional biopolymers [62, 63]. With respect to the endocrine system, and specifically the idea of an extracorporeal pancreas, such artificial support could be potentially accomplished with the help of an acellular system (e.g., an insulin pump guided by a glucose sensor), and the first steps in this direction are already being taken [64]. Alternatively, pancreatic β cells could be produced (from embryonic or a person's iPS cells, for example), and transplanted into a protective membrane that is impervious to the host's immune cells, but allows fluid and nutrient exchange [65]. Finally, an entirely synthetic organ could be recreated based on a physiological template—for example, a person's own heart—using the recently described process of decellularization [66]. Using this method, the macro- and microarchitecture of the organ is maintained with exact precision, while cells are lysed and removed by perfusion. Subsequently, new tissue-specific progenitor cells may colonize the vacant extracellular matrix of the organ shell with the hope of ultimately forming a new functional organ [66].

All these techniques are currently being developed for clinical applications and all are amenable to the idea of an artificial, multiorgan parabiosis-based support system. In such a system, mechanical, cellular, or hybrid (synthetic and biological) devices that replace the function of vital organs would be connected to a person's systemic milieu through an engineered microvasculature. With respect to establishing such anastomosis between physiological and artificial circulation, synthetic vascular channels could be successfully organized with the help of endothelial progenitor cells guided by three-dimensional polymeric porous scaffolds [67, 68]. However, blood exchange between physiological and artificial organs results in platelet degranulation, coagulation, and activation of the complement system, all of which are highly undesirable and limit the functional life of an organ. Thus, novel biomaterials for extracorporeal fluidic channels are needed to enable viable blood exchange between the physiological and artificial organ systems.

In summary, parabiosis was broadly used for more than a 100 years and helped answer a range of biomedical questions. The experimental technique of parabiosis and its applications described here would likely evolve into "parabiotic engineering," enabling an ideal multiorgan transplant that is free of side effects associated with immune rejection, withstands autoimmune responses, and is accessible for maintenance, repair, and modifications with relative ease. In addition, based on the heterochronic parabiosis results and current models of stem cell aging, methods of purification of blood and lymph fluids could be further modified for removal of age-specific inhibitory molecules that negatively influence tissue repair. This would greatly help to combat degenerative disorders that commonly accompany aging and might even increase the productive life span. Although seemingly futuristic, these ideas are supported by the development of state-of-the-art artificial organs that currently undergo miniaturization [69], and by the rapid evolution of stem cell engineering and tissue engineering, and by understanding the molecular mechanisms of aging and the advent of smart biomaterials [68, 70].

Acknowledgments

We thank Laura Gigliello, BS, LATG, and Penelope Collins, DVM, of the Palo Alto VA Veterinary Medical Unit for the improvements to this protocol since publication [35]. We include the following: We acknowledge funding of Irina Conboy by the National Institutes of Health (R01 AG 027252) and the California Institute for Regenerative Medicine New Faculity Award.

References

[1] Tardemt, P., "Experiments about Sex Determination in *Hydra attenuata Pall*," *Dev. Biol.*, Vol. 17, 1968, pp. 483–511.
[2] Sharma, R. N., "A Technique for Establishing Parabiosis between Houseflies (*Musca domestica L.*)," *Experientia*, Vol. 29, 1973, pp. 1179–1180.
[3] Williams, C. M., "Physiology of Insect Diapause: II. Interaction between the Pupal Brain and Prothoracic Glands in the Metamorphosis of the Giant Silkworm, *Platysamia cecropia*," *Biol. Bull.*, Vol. 93, 1947, pp. 89–98.
[4] Wallace, H., "Prolonged Life of Anucleolate *Xenopus* Tadpoles in Parabiosis," *J. Embryol. Exp. Morphol.*, Vol. 10, 1962, pp. 212–223.
[5] Finerty, J. C., "Parabiosis in Physiological Studies," *Physiol. Rev.*, Vol. 32, 1952, pp. 277–302.
[6] Bert, P., "Experiences et Considerations Sur la Greffe Animale," *J. Anat. Physiol.*, Vol. 1, 1864, pp. 69–87.
[7] Sauerbruch, F., and M. Heyde, "Uber Parabiose Kunstleichvereinigter Warmbluter," *Munchener Med. Wochenschrift*, Vol. 55, 1908, pp. 153.
[8] Bunster, E., and R. K. Meyer, "An Improved Method of Parabiosis," *Anat. Rec.*, Vol. 57, 1933, pp. 339–343.
[9] Wright, D. E., et al., "Physiological Migration of Hematopoietic Stem and Progenitor Cells," *Science*, Vol. 294, 2001, pp. 1933–1936.
[10] Falls, N. G., and A. Kirschbaum, "Passive Immunization of Mice in Parabiosis against a Transplanted Lymphosarcoma," *Cancer Res*, Vol. 13, 1953, pp. 741–743.
[11] Kamrin, B. B., "Local and Systemic Cariogenic Effects of Refined Dextrose Solution Fed to One Animal in Parabiosis," *J. Dent. Res.*, Vol. 33, 1954, pp. 824–829.
[12] Parameswaran, S. V., et al., "Involvement of a Humoral Factor in Regulation of Body Weight in Parabiotic Rats," *Am. J. Physiol.*, Vol. 232, 1977, pp. R150–R157.
[13] Harris, R. B., and R. J. Martin, "Specific Depletion of Body Fat in Parabiotic Partners of Tube-Fed Obese Rats," *Am. J. Physiol.*, Vol. 247, 1984, pp. R380–R386.
[14] Harris, R. B., R. J. Martin, and R. C. Bruch, "Dissociation between Food Intake, Diet Composition, and Metabolism in Parabiotic Partners of Obese Rats," *Am. J. Physiol.*, Vol. 268, 1995, pp. R874–R883.
[15] Hall, C. E., O. Hall, and A. H. Nevis, "Prolongation of Survival by Parabiosis in Strain 129 Dystrophic Mice," *Am. J. Physiol.*, Vol. 196, 1959, pp. 110–112.
[16] Montgomery, A., "Parabiotic Reinnervation in Normal and Dystrophic Mice. Part 1: Muscle Weight and Physiological Studies," *J. Neurol. Sci.*, Vol. 26, 1975, pp. 401–423.
[17] Matzke, H. A., and B. B. Kamrin, "Regeneration of Resected and Crossed Sciatic Nerves in Parabiotic Rats," *Science*, Vol. 118, 1953, pp. 623–624.
[18] Hasek, M., and T. Hraba, "Immunological Effects of Experimental Embryonal Parabiosis," *Nature*, Vol. 175, 1955, pp. 764–765.
[19] Zaiman, H., et al., "Studies on the Nature of Immunity to *Trichinella spiralis* in Parabiotic Rats. IV: The Immune Response in Uninfected Parabiotic Rats Surgically Separated from their Mates 2, 3, 4, or 5 Days after the Latter Received an Immunizing Infection," *Am. J. Hyg.*, Vol. 59, 1954, pp. 39–51.
[20] Barnes, W. A., and O. B. Furth, "Studies on the indirect effect of roentgen rays in single and parabiotic mice", *AJR Am. J. Roentgenol.*, Vol. 49, 1943, pp. 662.
[21] Binhammer, R. T., M. Schneider, and J. C. Finerty, "Time as a Factor in Postirradiation Protection by Parabiosis," *Am. J. Physiol.*, Vol. 175, 1953, pp. 440–442.
[22] Warren, S., R. N. Chute, and E. M. Farrington, "Protection of the Hematopoietic System by Parabiosis," *Lab. Invest.*, Vol. 9, 1960, pp. 191–198.
[23] Carroll, H. W., and D. J. Kimeldorf, "Protection through Parabiosis against the Lethal Effects of Exposure to Large Doses of X-rays," *Science*, Vol. 156, 1967, pp. 954–955.
[24] Nisbet, N. W., "Parabiosis in Immunobiology," *Transplant Rev.*, Vol. 15, 1973, pp. 123–161.
[25] Wagers, A. J., et al., "Little Evidence for Developmental Plasticity of Adult Hematopoietic Stem Cells," *Science*, Vol. 297, 2002, pp. 2256–2259.
[26] Massengale, M., et al., "Hematopoietic Cells Maintain Hematopoietic Fates upon Entering the Brain," *J. Exp. Med.*, Vol. 201, 2005, pp. 1579–1589.
[27] Balsam, L. B., et al., "Haematopoietic Stem Cells Adopt Mature Haematopoietic Fates in Ischaemic Myocardium," *Nature*, Vol. 428, 2004, pp. 668–673.
[28] Eggan, K., et al., "Ovulated Oocytes in Adult Mice Derive from Non-circulating Germ Cells," *Nature*, Vol. 441, 2006, pp. 1109–1114.
[29] Koh, Y. J., et al., "Bone Marrow-Derived Circulating Progenitor Cells Fail to Transdifferentiate into Adipocytes in Adult Adipose Tissues in Mice," *J. Clin. Invest.*, Vol. 117, 2007, pp. 3684–3695.
[30] Purhonen, S., et al., "Bone Marrow-Derived Circulating Endothelial Precursors Do Not Contribute to Vascular Endothelium and Are Not Needed for Tumor Growth," *Proc. Natl. Acad. Sci. USA*, Vol. 105, 2008, pp. 6620–6625.
[31] Vieyra, D. S., K. A. Jackson, and M. A. Goodell, "Plasticity and Tissue Regenerative Potential of Bone Marrow-Derived Cells," *Stem Cell Rev.*, Vol. 1, 2005, pp. 65–69.
[32] Carlson, B. M., and J. A. Faulkner, "Muscle Transplantation between Young and Old Rats: Age of Host Determines Recovery," *Am. J. Physiol.*, Vol. 256, 1989, pp. C1262–C1266.

[33] McCay, C. M., et al., "Parabiosis between Old and Young Rats," *Gerontologia*, Vol. 1, 1957, pp. 7–17.
[34] Ludwig, F. C., and R. M. Elashoff, "Mortality in Syngeneic Rat Parabionts of Different Chronological Age," *Trans. N. Y. Acad. Sci.*, Vol. 34, 1972, pp. 582–587.
[35] Conboy, I. M., et al., "Rejuvenation of Aged Progenitor Cells by Exposure to a Young Systemic Environment," *Nature*, Vol. 433, 2005, pp. 760–764.
[36] Finerty, J. C., and T. C. Panos, "Parabiosis Intoxication," *Proc. Soc. Exp. Biol. Med.*, Vol. 76, 1951, pp. 833–835.
[37] Chute, R. N., and S. C. Sommers, "Hemolytic Disease and Polycythemia in Parabiosis Intoxication," *Blood*, Vol. 7, 1952, pp. 1005–1016.
[38] Hall, C. E., and O. Hall, "On the Nature of Parabiosis Intoxication: Shock as the Precipitating Cause," *J. Exp. Med.*, Vol. 103, 1956, pp. 263–272.
[39] Nakic, B., and V. Silobrcic, "Tolerance of Skin Homografts Related to Fatal Disease in Separated Rat Parabionts," *Nature*, Vol. 182, 1958, pp. 264–265.
[40] Andresen, R. H., et al., "Postparabiotic Tissue Reactions of Rabbits to Musculofascial Cross-transplants," *J. Exp. Med.*, Vol. 105, 1957, pp. 85–92.
[41] Sayegh, M. H., and C. B. Carpenter, "Transplantation 50 Years Later: Progress, Challenges, and Promises," *N. Engl. J. Med.*, Vol. 351, 2004, pp. 2761–2766.
[42] Cascalho, M., B. M. Ogle, and J. L. Platt, "The Future of Organ Transplantation," *Ann. Transplant.*, Vol. 11, 2006, pp. 44–47.
[43] Rowinski, W., "Future of transplantation medicine," *Ann. Transplant.*, Vol. 12, 2007, pp. 5–10.
[44] Leibiger, I. B., B. Leibiger, and P. O. Berggren, "Insulin Signaling in the Pancreatic Beta Cell," *Annu. Rev. Nutr.*, Vol. 28, 2008, pp. 233–251.
[45] Yanaba, K., et al., "B-Lymphocyte Contributions to Human Autoimmune Disease," *Immunol. Rev.*, Vol. 223, 2008, pp. 284–299.
[46] Oksenberg, J. R., et al., "The Genetics of Multiple Sclerosis: SNPs to Pathways to Pathogenesis," *Nat. Rev. Genet.*, Vol. 9, 2008, pp. 516–526.
[47] Jiang, J., et al., "Generation of Insulin-Producing Islet-like Clusters from Human Embryonic Stem Cells," *Stem Cells*, Vol. 25, 2007, pp. 1940–1953.
[48] Stanley, E. G., and A. G. Elefanty, "Building Better Beta Cells," *Cell Stem Cell*, Vol. 2, 2008, pp. 300–301.
[49] Faulkner, J., and H. S. Keirstead, "Human Embryonic Stem Cell-Derived Oligodendrocyte Progenitors for the Treatment of Spinal Cord Injury," *Transplant. Immunol.*, Vol. 15, 2005, pp. 131–142.
[50] Cohen, M. A., P. Itsykson, and B. E. Reubinoff, "Neural Differentiation of Human ES Cells," *Curr. Protoc. Cell Biol.*, Volume 36, 2007, pp. 23.7.1–23.7.20.
[51] Vazin, T., et al., "Assessment of Stromal-Derived Inducing Activity in the Generation of Dopaminergic Neurons from Human Embryonic Stem Cells," *Stem Cells*, Vol. 26, 2008, pp. 1517–1525.
[52] Cho, M. S., et al., "Highly Efficient and Large-Scale Generation of Functional Dopamine Neurons from Human Embryonic Stem Cells," *Proc. Natl. Acad. Sci. USA*, Vol. 105, 2008, pp. 3392–3397.
[53] Xu, X. Q., et al., "Chemically Defined Medium Supporting Cardiomyocyte Differentiation of Human Embryonic Stem Cells," *Differentiation*, 2008. Volume 76, Issue 9, 2008, pp. 958–970.
[54] Takahashi, K., et al., "Induction of Pluripotent Stem Cells from Adult Human Fibroblasts by Defined Factors," *Cell*, Vol. 131, 2007, pp. 861–872.
[55] Park, I. H., et al., "Reprogramming of Human Somatic Cells to Pluripotency with Defined Factors," *Nature*, Vol. 451, 2008, pp. 141–146.
[56] Malchesky, P. S., "Artificial Organs and Vanishing Boundaries," *Artif. Organs*, Vol. 25, 2001, pp. 75–88.
[57] Cruz, D., et al., "The Future of Extracorporeal Support," *Crit. Care Med.*, Vol. 36, 2008, pp. S243–S252.
[58] Hill, J. D., "John H. Gibbon, Jr. Part I: The Development of the First Successful Heart–Lung Machine," *Ann. Thorac. Surg.*, Vol. 34, 1982, pp. 337–341.
[59] Cooper, D. S., et al., "Cardiac Extracorporeal Life Support: State of the Art in 2007," *Cardiol. Young*, Vol. 17, 2007, pp. 104–115.
[60] Krisper, P., and R. E. Stauber, "Technology Insight: Artificial Extracorporeal Liver Support: How Does Prometheus Compare with MARS?," *Nat. Clin. Pract. Nephrol.*, Vol. 3, 2007, pp. 267–276.
[61] Mitzner, S. R., et al., "Improvement of Hepatorenal Syndrome with Extracorporeal Albumin Dialysis MARS: Results of a Prospective, Randomized, Controlled Clinical Trial," *Liver Transplant.*, Vol. 6, 2000, pp. 277–286.
[62] Nahmias, Y., F. Berthiaume, and M. L. Yarmush, "Integration of Technologies for Hepatic Tissue Engineering," *Adv. Biochem. Eng. Biotechnol.*, Vol. 103, 2007, pp. 309–329.
[63] Fiegel, H. C., et al., "Hepatic Tissue Engineering: From Transplantation to Customized Cell-Based Liver Directed Therapies from the Laboratory," *J. Cell Mol. Med.*, Vol. 12, 2008, pp. 56–66.
[64] Weinzimer, S. A., and W. V. Tamborlane, "Sensor-Augmented Pump Therapy in Type 1 Diabetes," *Curr. Opin. Endocrinol. Diabetes Obes.*, Vol. 15, 2008, pp. 118–122.
[65] Best, M., et al., "Embryonic Stem Cells to Beta-Cells by Understanding Pancreas Development," *Mol. Cell Endocrinol.*, Vol. 288, 2008, pp. 86–94.

[66] Ott, H. C., et al., "Perfusion-Decellularized Matrix: Using Nature's Platform to Engineer a Bioartificial Heart," *Nat. Med.*, Vol. 14, 2008, pp. 213–221.

[67] Hoganson, D. M., H. I. Pryor, II, and J. P. Vacanti, "Tissue Engineering and Organ Structure: A Vascularized Approach to Liver and Lung," *Pediatr. Res.*, Vol. 63, 2008, pp. 520–526.

[68] Kohane, D. S., and R. Langer, "Polymeric Biomaterials in Tissue Engineering," *Pediatr. Res.*, Vol. 63, 2008, pp. 487–491.

[69] Ronco, C., and L. Fecondini, "The Vicenza Wearable Artificial Kidney for Peritoneal Dialysis (ViWAK PD)," *Blood Purif.*, Vol. 25, 2007, pp. 383–388.

[70] Karp, J. M., and R. Langer, "Development and Therapeutic Applications of Advanced Biomaterials," *Curr. Opin. Biotechnol.*, Vol. 18, 2007, pp. 454–459.

CHAPTER 11

Utilization of the Mixed Lymphocyte Reaction Assay to Determine Stem Cell Immunogenicity and Suppression

Kevin R. McIntosh

Cognate BioServices, Inc.
Baltimore, MD 21227

Abstract

Allogeneic transplantation of stem cells provides a cost-effective approach for their clinical utilization. Because of multiple methodologies used for the production and utilization of stem cells, a method to assess the immunogenicity of stem cells prior to and after preclinical studies in animals would be extremely beneficial. The use of the mixed lymphocyte reaction (MLR) assay is described for this purpose. The MLR assay is a technique in which responder cells containing T lymphocytes are mixed with allogeneic stimulator cells, and T-cell proliferation is measured as an index of reactivity. Variations of this assay are described in which stem cells are used as stimulators to determine immunogenicity, stem cells are added to MLR cultures to determine suppression, and T cells obtained from animals treated with stem cells are cultured with cells from the stem cell donor to determine whether the animals were primed to the stem cell allograft.

Key Terms

Mixed lymphocyte reaction
stem cell immunogenicity
stem cell suppression
alloreactivity
T-cell priming
immune rejection
universal donor

11.1 Introduction

The utilization of stem cells for tissue regeneration and repair is fast becoming a reality. One of the primary considerations for clinical utilization of these cells is economic: How can stem cell therapies be affordable in view of the fact that the production of clinical-grade cell products is extremely expensive? One way of overcoming this hurdle is to produce large amounts of stem cells from one donor that could be used in multiple patients. Establishment of a cell bank from early-passage cells could be expanded as needed to produce clinical lots of stem cells that could be shipped to clinics for administration to patients. Production and testing of a donor lot for clinical release would be considerably less expensive than production and testing cell lots specific for each patient. Other advantages of this "universal donor" strategy include availability and donor cell characteristics. A universal product would be available for administration to a patient immediately whereas patient-specific cells would require tissue procurement, stem cell expansion, and release testing, all of which could take a month or longer. In some cases, autologous stem cells may not be available (e.g., neural stem cells derived from fetal tissue). There are also several advantages inherent in using stem cells derived from other individuals. First, the disease or genetic defect responsible for damaging the patient's tissues would be expected to be missing in an unrelated donor population. Second, universal donor populations could be screened for potency in performing the functions they are meant to treat. For example, stem cell populations from multiple donors could be prescreened for osteogenic differentiation and the best of these could be selected for bone regeneration therapies.

A major problem with the universal donor cell strategy is that stem cells derived from an unrelated donor (allogeneic stem cells) should be rejected by the patient's immune system after they are transplanted. However, this may not be the case. Several types of stem cells have been shown to be poorly immunogenic by in vitro studies, suggesting that they can be transplanted to allogeneic recipients without immune rejection. These primarily include mesenchymal stem cells (MSCs) derived from bone marrow [1–4], adipose tissue [5, 6], placenta [7], umbilical cord matrix [8], and amniotic fluid [9]. Other types of stem cells may be immune privileged as well, including embryonic stem cells [10] and neural progenitor cells [11]. MSCs are typically characterized by low levels of major histocompatability (MHC) class I antigens and negligible expression of MHC class II antigens and costimulatory molecules CD40, CD80, and CD86 [3, 4]. Moreover, many stem cells have been shown to suppress alloreactive immune responses actively [1–4, 5–9], which probably contributes to the lack of a T-cell response that is observed in these cells in vitro. Suppression has been attributed to soluble factors elaborated by stem cells, including transforming growth factor a plus human growth factor [1], indoleamine 2,3-dioxygenase (IDO) [12], prostaglandin E2 [13], human leukocyte antigen (HLA)-G [8, 14], heme oxygenase 1 [15], and nitric oxide [16]. Although it has been demonstrated that MSCs maintain their suppressive effects in vivo [2, 15,17–19] and persist in allogeneic and xenogeneic hosts [20–22], contradictory studies have shown that these cells lose their suppressive properties in vivo [23–25] and are rejected after transplantation to immunocompetent recipients [26, 27]. The reason for the divergent outcomes in these experiments may be attributed to the species origin of the MSCs, how the cells were propagated in expansion medium, and how they were used in animals (dosage, route of delivery, scaffold type, and so on). Propagation of MSCs in medium containing fetal bovine serum (FBS), for example, has been shown to sensitize animals to FBS proteins after injection [28]. Investigators interested in using allogeneic stem cells for tissue repair or replacement will want to evaluate the immunological properties of stem cell populations produced by their specific methodology and used in their specific animal model.

The purpose of this chapter is to describe an immunological tool, the mixed lymphocyte reaction (MLR) assay, that can be used to assess the immunological properties of the unique population of stem cells produced by the investigator (immunogenicity and suppression assays) as well as determine whether these cells induce a cellular immune response after their utilization in animals (T-cell priming assay). The application of these assays will usually occur in a linear fashion, during which the investigator will first characterize the stem cells for immunogenicity and suppression by in vitro experiments, followed by studies to determine whether the cells are immunogenic in vivo. The immunogenicity and suppression MLR assays have been described in a number of publications [1–10]; the use of the MLR to measure T-cell priming in animals that have received a transplant of allogeneic stem cells has been described in rats [29], pigs [30], and baboons [21].

The MLR involves the culture of two populations of cells: one responder population containing T lymphocytes and one stimulator population. The two populations are derived from different individuals, making them allogeneic to each other (i.e., they express different MHC antigens on their cell surfaces). MHC antigens are powerful signals of self, and the immune system is geared toward recognizing deviations from self. If the stimulator population expresses different MHC antigens from the responder T cells, alloreactive T cells specific for these antigens will initiate a rejection response that is characterized by T-cell proliferation that can be measured by uptake of ^{3}H-thymidine and expressed as counts per minute (cpm). Proliferation can also be measured by colorimetric and chemiluminescent assays offered by many companies. Although they are not described here, the MLR setup can also be used to obtain additional information such as cytokine profiles (by measuring different cytokines in MLR supernatants), expression of activation markers on T cells (by flow cytometry), and induction of immunological tolerance (by restimulating T cells in secondary MLR cultures) [3, 4].

The MLR assay is a screening tool that can provide information useful in decision making. If a stem cell population induces a powerful response when cultured with allogeneic T cells in an immunogenicity assay, the investigator will want to think twice about proceeding with this population in animal experiments. If the stem cells do not induce a T-cell response in vitro, or they induce a small response, there is no guarantee that this population will be nonimmunogenic in vivo, but at least the investigator has some positive information to move forward in performing animal experiments. Likewise, the T-cell priming assay will measure whether a T-cell response was induced in an animal treated with allogeneic stem cells, but it will not tell you whether the stem cell graft survived. Thus, additional assays should be performed to gauge stem cell engraftment, such as functional readouts of tissue repair, histological assessments of immune cell infiltration, and assays of stem cell survival at the site of implantation. Given these limitations, the MLR assay continues to be the method of choice for screening stem cell immunogenicity because of its simplicity and obvious parallels to in vivo transplantation.

11.2 Experimental Design

Basic experimental designs utilizing the MLR assay will be described for determining stem cell immunogenicity, suppression by stem cells, and T-cell priming to allogeneic stem cell transplantation in vivo. The designs are suitable for human or animal experiments.

11.2.1 Immunogenicity assay

This assay determines whether a stem cell population can elicit a proliferative response from allogeneic T cells. A positive response indicates that the stem cells are immunogenic.

11.2.1.1 Basic features

Immunogenicity of a stem cell population is determined by culturing responder cells with three different stimulator cell populations: (1) autologous or syngeneic cells to obtain a background response, (2) allogeneic cells to obtain a positive control response, and (3) the test stem cell population. The stimulator cells must be mitotically inactivated by radiation or chemical treatment to prevent their division in the MLR cultures. The assay is set up in 96-well flat-bottom microtiter plates using tissue culture medium that contains homologous serum matched to the cells used in the assay to minimize background proliferation of T cells. After incubation at 37°C in a humidified atmosphere of 5% CO_2 for 4 to 6 days, the cultures are pulsed with ^{3}H-thymidine for 18 hours and the cells are harvested on filter mats for scintillation counting to determine the amount of incorporated isotope. The amount of radioactivity incorporated is proportional to the degree of proliferation by responder T cells in the wells. The response to syngeneic/autologous cells provides a baseline response with which the response against the test cells are compared. If the response to the stem cell population is significantly higher than the response to the syngeneic/autologous control cells, the stem cell population is considered immunogenic.

11.2.1.2 Responder cells

For human or large-animal experiments that can utilize cells of peripheral blood mononuclear cell (PBMC) origin, unfractionated PBMCs ($4 \cdot 10^5$ cells/well) or T cells purified from PBMCs ($2 \cdot 10^5$ cells/well) can be used as responder cells in the MLR. For rodent experiments, responder cells can be derived from lymphoid organs (lymph nodes, spleen) as unfractionated cells, or T cells can be purified from these organs. The decision to use unfractionated cells or purified T cells will depend on the investigator's resources (including time constraints) as well as the rationale for using one population over the other (see Section 11.6, Discussion and Commentary). Our laboratory performs human immunogenicity assays routinely.

Multiple responder donors should be utilized if the relationship (HLA disparity) between the responder donor and stem cell donor is not known to avoid misinterpretation of negative results. Although unlikely, it is possible that the lack of response to the stem cell population may be the result of HLA similarity between responder and stimulator populations and not a result of a nonimmunogenic profile of the stem cell population. The use of multiple responder donors diminishes this possibility. We normally use at least two different responder populations in this situation.

11.2.1.3 Stimulator cells

There are three different stimulator populations that are utilized in the immunogenicity MLR assay: autologous cells (baseline response), allogeneic cells (positive control), and the stem cell test population. The autologous cells must be matched to the responder population to give an accurate baseline response with which the other responses will be compared. Allogeneic positive control cells should be from the stem cell donor, but because this may not be possible, any allogeneic donor will suffice. This control will establish that the assay is functioning properly and, if the cells are from the stem cell donor, it will establish that the responder and stimulator donors are suitably mismatched, validating interpretation of the stem cell results. Stem cells and control cells should be titrated in the MLR, starting at the highest number of stem cells that can be cultured per microtiter well at confluence. For MSCs that have a large cell diameter, confluence occurs at 20,000 to 25,000 cells/microtiter well. For smaller stem cells, such as neural stem cells, the number to attain confluence will be higher and should be determined by the investigator. Serial dilution of this cell number to give two or three lower stimulator cell concentrations in the assay will establish whether T-cell proliferation is influenced by stem cell number and should give a dose–response effect.

All stimulator populations must be mitotically inactivated prior to cell culture. This ensures that any cell proliferation detected in the cultures is the result of responder T cells. The stimulator cells can be radiated or they can be treated with mitomycin C. We prefer radiation of cells because of high cell losses incurred from mitomycin C treatment. In either case, the investigator should determine whether the treatment is sufficient to inhibit cell proliferation. For cell populations containing T cells, this can be done by stimulating the cells with a T-cell mitogen, such as concanavalin A (Con A) or phytohemagglutinin (PHA).

11.2.1.4 Plate setup

A typical configuration for an immunogenicity assay is depicted in Figure 11.1. The setup is shown for testing the immunogenicity of human stem cells derived from two donors using one responder lot (purified T cells from Resp$_A$ plated at $2 \cdot 10^5$ cells/well). This setup should be replicated on a second plate using a different responder lot (not shown). Three different stimulator populations are utilized: autologous (Auto) PBMCs, allogeneic (Allo) PBMCs (donor B), and stem cells (donors C and D). These populations, radiated (x) before use, are shown seeded at 1,000, 5,000, and 25,000 cells/well. Each treatment is performed in quadruplicate wells. Note that additional controls are incorporated to evaluate background responses by responder and radiated stem cell populations cultured alone. Radiated autologous and allogeneic PBMC stimulator populations cultured alone can also be included, but we have found that proliferation produced by these cells is consistently negligible.

11.2.1.5 Small animals

Responder and stimulator cells derived from rats and mice are obtained from mechanically dissociated lymphoid organs such as lymph nodes and spleen because of the inability to derive sufficient numbers of cells from peripheral blood. In rats, we have found that using lymph node cells as responders and spleen cells as stimulators works well; in

Immunogenicity Assay

	1	2	3	4	5	6	7	8	9	10	11	12	
	\multicolumn{12}{c}{**Number of Irradiated Stimulator Cells Per Well**}	
	\multicolumn{3}{c}{1,000}	\multicolumn{3}{c}{5,000}	\multicolumn{3}{c}{25,000}				
Resp$_A$ T Cells+ xAuto PBMC$_A$	145	255	165	230	165	280	145	250	245	195	260	145	A
Resp$_A$ T Cells+ xAllo PBMC$_B$	1200	1000	950	1500	9500	15000	12000	10000	45000	50000	40000	55000	B
Resp$_A$ T Cells+ xStem Cells$_C$	120	135	160	145	95	100	80	75	45	25	40	35	C
Resp$_A$ T Cells+ xStem Cells$_D$	145	255	165	235	1165	1280	945	1250	2245	3195	2260	2145	D
xStem Cells$_C$ Cultured Alone	45	50	50	75	150	100	75	60	25	50	40	55	E
xStem Cells$_D$ Cultured Alone	20	35	60	45	95	100	80	75	45	25	40	35	F
2×10^5 Cells/Well													G
Resp$_A$ T Cells+ Cultured Alone	200	250	300	150									H

Figure 11.1 Typical plate setup for the immunogenicity assay. Responder T cells from one donor (A) are shown cultured with autologous PBMCs (baseline control), allogeneic PBMCs from donor B (positive control), and stem cells from donors C and D. The number of radiated stimulator cells has been varied from 1,000 to 25,000 cells/well. Control cultures of stem cells or T cells cultured alone are shown in the lower half of the plate. Sample count-per-minute values are shown for each well.

mice, spleen cells can be used as both responder and stimulator cells. In our laboratory, freshly prepared rodent cells are best used for MLR assays as opposed to cryopreserved cells, because of low recovery and viability of thawed cells.

11.2.2 Suppression assay

The purpose of this assay is to determine whether a stem cell population can suppress alloreactive T-cell proliferation in MLR cultures.

11.2.2.1 Basic features

The suppression assay is performed by setting up MLR assays in either the one-way or two-way configuration. If performed with the immunogenicity assay, it will be most efficient to set up one-way MLR cultures, because the cells are already available in this format. The assay can also be performed as a two-way MLR in which unfractionated PBMCs from two different donors are cocultured to generate a response. Because neither population is radiated, they respond against each other. This is the easiest system to set up because T-cell purification and radiation treatments are not required. Using either the one-way or two-way MLR indicator system, stem cells are titrated into the wells in various numbers, starting at confluence (approximately 25,000 cells/well for MSCs) and titrating down to a number of cells that would not be expected to mediate significant suppression (approximately 1,000 cells/well). Cell culture, ^{3}H-thymidine pulse, and cell harvest are performed as described for the immunogenicity assay. The determination of suppression is made by comparing the MLR responses of cultures containing stem cells with control MLR cultures containing no stem cells.

11.2.2.2 Plate setup

A typical configuration for a suppressor assay is depicted in Figure 11.2. The setup is shown for testing the suppression by one stem cell lot on two different MLR combinations (i.e., two different responder populations cultured with one stimulator population). Assessing suppression on two different MLR combinations addresses issues of reproducibility and magnitude of suppression in different systems. The MLR cultures are incubated alone to provide baseline responses, or stem cells are added at the numbers shown in Figure 11.2. Each treatment is performed in quadruplicate wells with the exception of the MLR cultured alone, which is shown performed in 12 wells.

11.2.3 T-cell priming assay

The purpose of this assay is to determine whether an allogeneic stem cell treatment induced a T-cell response in a recipient animal. This assay will often be performed in conjunction with an experiment in which the goal is to determine whether stem cells can perform a certain function in vivo (e.g., mitigating tissue damage from stroke [29] or myocardial infarction [30]).

11.2.3.1 Basic features

The premise for this assay is that T cells derived from an animal treated with vehicle (or untreated) will give a certain baseline response to allogeneic donor cells in the MLR assay. If a similar animal is treated with stem cells from that allogeneic donor and becomes sensitized to the donor cells, T lymphocytes obtained from that animal should produce an enhanced proliferative response of higher magnitude and faster kinetics

Suppression Assay

Number of Stem Cells Added Per Well

	1,000				5,000				25,000				
MLR$_1$ – No Stem Cells	45,000	60,000	75,000	40,000	55,000	65,000	60,000	45,000	55,000	50,000	45,000	65,000	A
MLR$_1$ + xStem Cells$_c$	40,000	50,000	55,000	60,000	20,000	30,000	35,000	25,000	5,000	2,500	3,000	4,000	B
													C
MLR$_2$ – No Stem Cells	25,000	30,000	45,000	30,000	25,000	35,000	40,000	25,000	35,000	30,000	25,000	20,000	D
MLR$_2$ + xStem Cells$_c$	12,500	15,000	10,000	7,500	2,000	3,000	3,500	2,500	1,500	1,200	900	1,700	E
													F
													G
													H
	1	2	3	4	5	6	7	8	9	10	11	12	

Figure 11.2 Typical plate setup for the suppression assay. Two different MLR cultures are shown (MLR$_1$ and MLR$_2$) cultured with and without stem cells. The number of stem cells added to the MLR has been varied from 1,000 to 25,000 cells/well. Sample count-per-minute values are shown for each well.

relative to the baseline response. In experiments in which rats or mice are used, control animals treated with vehicle (or untreated) are required to produce a baseline response. If large animals are used, prebleeds performed prior to stem cell treatment can be used to establish baseline responses.

11.2.3.2 Responder cells

Lymphocytes to be used as responder cells are harvested from treated animals at designated time points determined by the investigator. In rat and mouse models, the animals will need to be sacrificed at these time points to procure responder cells from lymphoid tissues. We have used the time points of 4 and 8 weeks after stem cell treatment as the harvest intervals in our experiments. In our experience, freshly harvested cells produce the best responses in MLR assays; cryopreserved cells perform poorly. Lymphoid organs shipped overnight in cold phosphate-buffered saline have produced adequate responses when processed upon receipt. For large-animal studies, multiple bleedings at 2- to 4-week intervals can be obtained. For example, a baseline bleeding can be done several weeks before treatment, followed by posttreatment bleeds at 2 weeks, 4 weeks, 8 weeks, and 12 weeks. In this situation, peripheral blood can be collected at each time point and PBMCs can be purified and cryopreserved until needed. PBMCs from all the bleeds can then be thawed and run in one MLR assay.

11.2.3.3 Stimulator cells

Cell populations to be used as stimulator cells can be spleen or lymph node cells (rats/mice) or PBMCs (large animals) derived from donors of the stem cells. The use of stem cells as stimulators in the MLR is not recommended, because stem cell populations tend to be immunosuppressive. In rodent studies that have used inbred strains of animals as stem cell donors and recipients, lymph nodes or spleens can be obtained from any animal of the donor strain because they are all genetically identical. However, in large-animal studies that typically use outbred species, stimulator PBMCs must be obtained from the same animals from which the stem cells were derived. These same rules apply to the procurement of syngeneic/autologous cells to be used as controls in the MLR assay. For this reason, it will be necessary to obtain one large bleed or multiple smaller bleeds from stem cell donors in large-animal studies.

11.2.3.4 Specificity controls

In some studies, the investigator may wish to determine whether an effect on the MLR is antigen specific (i.e., if the antidonor response is higher or lower than baseline). An investigator will need to determine if the result is an antigen-specific response against the cells or whether a general up- or downregulation of the immune response was the result of something else. For example, a scaffold used to deliver the cells may have inflammatory properties that could have generalized consequences on the immune system [31]. To control for specificity, third-party stimulator cells can be used in the MLR assay. These cells do not share MHC antigens with the donor stem cells; thus, a modulated response to donor cells that is not replicated in the response to third-party cells would demonstrate that the donor response is antigen specific. Choice of a third-party cell donor is dictated by MHC typing, which can be determined by the investigator or is available through the published literature.

11.2.3.5 Mitogenic controls

To gauge the overall health of responder T cells from individual animals, the proliferative response to a T-cell mitogen (Con A or PHA) is used. If the responder populations derived from individual rats have similar numbers of healthy T cells, their proliferative responses to mitogen should be similar. This control is most important if lymphoid organs are shipped prior to processing or if they are processed by multiple individuals. Low responses by individual animals could indicate that problems occurred during organ procurement or shipping.

11.2.3.6 Plate setup

A typical configuration for a T-cell priming assay is shown in Figure 11.3. The setup is shown for testing four rats treated with vehicle (baseline control) and four rats treated with allogeneic stem cells. Note that this setup is for demonstration purposes and that typical experiments have more treatment groups and more rats per group. Also note that a second plate, identical to the one shown in Figure 11.3, is set up for harvest at a second time point to assess kinetics of the MLR response. Plates are usually harvested at days 3 and 7. Specificity and mitogen controls are not shown. Responder lymph node cells from each rat are cultured in medium alone, with syngeneic spleen cells, or with allogeneic spleen cells in quadruplicate cultures. The rationale for two control groups is that we have observed that responder cells often produce a larger response when cultured with autologous/syngeneic stimulators than in medium alone. Whether this is the result of a property of the syngeneic cells, cell density effects, the serum used to culture stem cells, or a possible autoimmune response is not currently clear, so it is worthwhile to collect these data.

T-Cell Priming Assay

Responder Population	No Stim				Syn Spleen				Allo Spleen				
Rat #1 – Vehicle	150	170	140	155	130	145	170	220	22,500	20,000	25,000	30,000	A
Rat #2 – Vehicle	130	150	155	180	150	130	185	170	20,500	26,500	32,500	22,500	B
Rat #3 – Vehicle	180	250	175	150	250	300	350	275	19,500	20,500	13,000	15,500	C
Rat #4 – Vehicle	150	190	250	225	310	350	345	400	21,000	16,500	23,000	17,000	D
Rat #5 – Allo SC	170	250	190	200	350	400	420	375	32,500	30,000	28,500	30,750	E
Rat #6 – Allo SC	250	220	280	225	430	375	350	450	40,500	43,000	49,500	47,000	F
Rat #7 – Allo SC	150	200	250	220	200	250	250	275	42,050	52,500	50,000	45,000	G
Rat #8 – Allo SC	200	350	275	250	300	350	400	325	37,250	35,500	34,500	37,000	H
	1	2	3	4	5	6	7	8	9	10	11	12	

Figure 11.3 Typical plate setup for the T-cell priming assay. Responder lymph node cells from four control rats treated with vehicle and four rats treated with allogeneic (Allo) stem cells are shown cultured alone, with syngeneic (Syn) spleen cells, and with allogeneic spleen cells (SC). Sample count-per-minute values are shown for each well. No Stim, no stimulator cells.

11.3 Materials

Materials and equipment required to perform basic MLR assays are listed here. Commonly available equipment and general supplies can be obtained from major companies (VWR, Fisher Scientific). Specialized reagents and equipment for MLR assays are supplied with sources listed here and in Section 11.4, Methods.

- In a biological safety cabinet (BSC), assemble the equipment required to perform tissue culture. These include a 1- to 2-L beaker containing bleach for liquid waste disposal; P-20, P-200, and P-1000 Pipetman; a repeat pipetter; and a multispeed pipet-aid.
- In or adjacent to the BSC, assemble the materials required to perform tissue culture. These include a spray bottle containing 70% ethanol; Kimwipes or nonscratching, lint-free wipes; 5-, 15-, and 50-mL polypropylene centrifuge tubes; pipet tips for Pipetman P-20, P-200, and P-1000; pipet tips for the repeat pipetter; 96-well flat-bottom, low-evaporation tissue culture plates; and 2-, 5-, and 10-mL pipets.
- To count cells, assemble the following: a 1.5-mL flip-top Eppendorf tube, trypan blue (0.4%) (Gibco), hemacytometer with coverslip, binocular light microscope, and tally cell counter.
- We have used a cesium 137 source gamma radiator (Isomedix Inc.; Gammator B) and an X-ray machine (Faxitron X-Ray) for inactivating stimulator cells. If none is available, use mitomycin C (Sigma) as described in Section 11.4, Methods.
- Con A or PHA (Sigma) is used for stimulation of lymphocytes
- A refrigerated centrifuge set at 10°C is best for washing cells.
- Hepa-filtered CO_2 incubators are best for cell culture.
- An inverted light microscope is useful for monitoring cell cultures (e.g., assessing contamination, colony formation as an indication of T-cell activation).
- Cell cultures are pulsed with ^{3}H-thymidine (Amersham Biosciences); Code TRA120, 5 Ci/mmol, 1 mCi/mL, in aqueous sterilized solution. A repeat pipetter (designated for radioactivity) facilitates this procedure.
- For harvesting cells from 96 well plates, we use a Skatron Micro96 Cell Harvester (Molecular Devices Corporation). The cells are harvested on filter mats, placed in plastic bags with scintillation fluid, sealed with a plate sealer, and loaded into a cassette (all reagents and equipment from Perkin Elmer). The cassette is placed into a Microbeta Trilux Scintillation and Luminescence Counter (Wallac-Perkin Elmer) for counting.

11.4 Methods

11.4.1 General considerations

Methods are described for the general set up of MLR assays. Methods associated with extrinsic protocols (PBMC and T-cell purification, dissociation of lymphoid tissues, cryopreservation, and so forth) will need to be fleshed out by the investigator. *Current Protocols in Immunology* (John Wiley & Sons) is a good reference text for these protocols. All procedures, except as indicated, must be performed in a BSC using sterile technique.

11.4.2 Safety

- Tissue and blood products from humans and animals are potentially infectious and must be treated according to Occupational Safety and Health Administration (OSHA) regulations and universal precautions for preventing transmission of blood-borne pathogens. Add approximately 100 mL bleach to a 1- to 2-L beaker and place it at the rear of the working surface of the BSC. All fluids that contact tissue and blood products can be disposed of in this beaker prior to pouring the contents in the sink. Plasticware that contacts tissue and blood products should be rinsed with bleach prior to disposal in a biohazard container.
- Radioactivity must be handled according to the rules and regulations stipulated by the laboratory in which these materials are used.
- Chemical, radioactive, and biohazardous wastes must be disposed according to laboratory regulations.

11.4.3 Media preparation

Remove 15.5 mL medium from a 500-mL bottle of Iscove's Modified Dulbecco's Medium containing 25 mM HEPES and l-glutamine, and discard. Add 5 mL each of 100× non-essential amino acids, 100× sodium pyruvate, and 100× antibiotic/antimycotic. Add 0.5 mL 1,000× 2-mercaptoethanol (medium and medium supplements from Gibco). Supplemented media are stored at 4°C in the dark. Media are stable under these conditions for 1 month.

Culture medium is produced by adding 5 mL of the appropriate serum to 95 mL supplemented Iscove's Modified Dulbecco's Medium (final 5% serum concentration). Homologous serum can be produced by the investigator from whole blood or purchased from a reputable supplier. We have purchased human AB serum that was screened for MLR assays from Sigma, animal sera from Pel-Freez, and FBS from HyClone and Atlas Biologicals. Culture medium is stable for 2 weeks when stored at 4°C in the dark.

11.4.4 Prepare responder cell populations

11.4.4.1 Small-animal studies (rat/mouse)

Using aseptic technique, remove cervical and mesenteric lymph nodes and spleen. Pool lymph nodes but keep separate from spleen during processing. Process lymph nodes/spleen into a single cell suspension by grinding tissue in cell strainers (Falcon, Sigma). Transfer cells to a 15-mL centrifuge tube, wash twice, and determine viable cell count by diluting the cells in 0.4% trypan blue in an Eppendorf tube. Count live and dead cells on a hemacytometer. Cell viability more than 70% is optimal. If the viability is less than 50%, remove dead cells by centrifugation over a density gradient formulated for rodent cells (Cedarlane Laboratories). "Pellet" cells by centrifugation and resuspend in culture medium at a concentration of $4 \cdot 10^6$ viable cells/mL. Cells should be used fresh.

11.4.4.2 Human and large-animal studies

Obtain peripheral blood from responder donor and purify PBMCs by centrifugation over Ficoll-Hypaque density gradient (Cambrex/Lonza, Cedarlane). Determine the percentage of viable cells by diluting cells in 0.4% trypan blue in an Eppendorf tube, and count live and dead cells on a hemacytometer. Cell viability should be more than 90% for PBMCs isolated over Ficoll-Hypaque density gradients. Pellet cells by centrifugation and resuspend in culture medium at a concentration of $4 \cdot 10^6$ viable cells/mL. Cells can be used fresh or cryopreserved for future studies.

If purified T cells are desired as responder cells, use negative selection techniques to remove non-T cells. We use magnetic beads coated with antimouse immunoglobulin G antibodies (Invitrogen-Dynal) to remove non-T cells that we have treated with mouse monoclonal antibodies (anti-CD14, CD19, CD56, and MHC class II; antibodies from BD Biosciences Pharmingen). The T-cell population should be at least 85% pure by flow cytometry as assessed using fluorescence-tagged anti-CD3 monoclonal antibodies (BD Biosciences). If cells are to be used fresh, resuspend at $2 \cdot 10^6$ cells/mL in culture medium.

11.4.5 Prepare stimulator cell populations

Methods used for the preparation of responder cells can be used for the preparation of stimulator populations. Stimulator cells must be mitotically inactivated prior to cell culture. Cells should be radiated with approximately 5,000 rads by X-ray or gamma radiation. If this is not possible, cells can be treated with mitomycin C [10 μg/mL for 1–2 hours at 37°C (Sigma)] followed by extensive washing to remove the chemical. Mitomycin C is toxic and care must be exercised in using this chemical as well as in disposing of it. Expect high cell losses as a result of toxicity and extensive cell washing.

Preliminary experiments should be performed to determine that the inactivation protocol was successful. We have tested our inactivation protocols using lymphoid populations stimulated with the T-cell mitogens PHA and Con A (10 μg/mL, Sigma).

Stimulator cells should be resuspended in culture medium at densities appropriate for the protocol used. Radiated PBMCs can be cryopreserved for future studies.

11.4.6 Performance of immunogenicity assays

See Figure 11.1 for the experimental setup of the MLR performed in flat-bottom 96-well microtiter plates. Unfractionated responder cells are cultured at $4 \cdot 10^5$ cells/well; if purified T cells are used as responders, they are cultured at $2 \cdot 10^5$ cells/well. Responder cells should be suspended in complete culture medium containing 5% homologous serum at 10× higher density so that they can be added at 100 μL/well.

Radiated stimulator cells are cultured at various numbers per well. Cells should be serially diluted in 5 mL polypropylene tubes at 10× higher density so that they can be added at 100 μL/well. Final volumes in all wells should be 250 μL/well. The remaining volume is made up with complete culture medium.

11.4.7 Performance of suppression assays

See Figure 11.2 for the experimental setup of the MLR performed in flat-bottom 96-well microtiter plates. Add 100 μL of each responder cell ($4 \cdot 10^6$ cells/mL) and radiated allogeneic stimulator cells ($2 \cdot 10^6$ cells/mL) to each well to set up the MLR.

Radiated stem cells (5,000 rads) are serially diluted in 5 mL polypropylene tubes at 20× higher density so that they can be added at 50 μL/well. Final volumes in all wells should be 250 μL/well. The remaining volume in wells containing control MLR cultures (no stem cells added) is made up with complete culture medium.

11.4.8 Performance of T-cell priming assays

See Figure 11.3 for the experimental setup of the MLR performed in flat-bottom 96-well microtiter plates. Unfractionated responder cells are cultured at $4 \cdot 10^5$ cells/well; if purified T cells are used, they are cultured at $2 \cdot 10^5$ cells/well (100 µL/well). Radiated stimulator cells are cultured at $2 \cdot 10^5$ cells/well (100 µL/well). Final volumes in all wells should be 250 µL/well. The remaining volume is made up with complete culture medium.

Mitogenic controls should be set up on a separate plate. Responder cells are cultured with medium or mitogen. We use Con A at 10 µg/mL. The plate is pulsed with ^{3}H-thymidine on day 2 and harvested on day 3.

11.4.9 MLR plate culture, pulsing with ^{3}H-thymidine, cell harvest, and scintillation counting: applicable to all three MLR assays

Place the MLR plate in an incubator providing a humidified atmosphere of 5% CO_2 at 37°C. Pulse the plate with ^{3}H-thymidine on the fourth through sixth day of culture (optimum culture period should be determined in preliminary experiments). All the following procedures are to be performed in a designated radioactive area. Dilute stock ^{3}H-thymidine (1.0 mCi/mL, located in designated radioactive refrigerator) 1:50 with culture medium to obtain a concentration of 20 µCi/mL. Determine volume to be prepared by multiplying the number of wells by 50 µL and add 0.5 mL to account for overage. Add 50 µL diluted ^{3}H-thymidine (1.0 µCi) to each well containing cells.

Label pulsed plates with radiation stickers and place them in the CO_2 incubator (5% CO_2, 37°C) designated for radioactive materials. Incubate plates for approximately 18 hours (a range of 12–24 hours is acceptable). Harvest cells from the plates on filters for scintillation counting. We use a Skatron plate harvester that harvests all 96 wells onto a filter mat. The filter mat is placed in a plastic bag containing scintillation fluid and is heat sealed. To count ^{3}H-thymidine incorporated in the cells, we use a Microbeta scintillation counter that counts each of the 96-well culture deposits on the filter mat.

11.5 Data Acquisition, Anticipated Results, Interpretation, and Statistical Guidelines

11.5.1 Immunogenicity assay

Sample data are presented in Figure 11.1 in accordance with the experimental design. Data are expressed as counts per minute. The means and standard deviations of quadruplicate cultures are shown in Table 11.1. Data transfer from the scintillation counter into an Excel spreadsheet will facilitate these calculations.

The summarized data from Table 11.1 are shown in typical graphical form in Figure 11.4. The upper panel bar graph shows T-cell proliferative responses to autologous stimulators, allogeneic stimulators, and to both stem cell populations at various stimulator cell numbers. The lower panel bar graph does not show the response to allogeneic cells to enhance visualization of the responses to the autologous and stem cell populations.

The T-cell response to autologous stimulators serves as the baseline response to which all other responses are compared. The two-tailed Student's t-test is used to assess signifi-

Table 11.1 Summary of Immunogenicity Data

Group	1,000 Cells/Well	5,000 Cells/Well	25,000 Cells/Well
$Resp_A$ T Cells + xAuto $Stim_A$ (baseline response)	199 ± 52	210 ± 65	211 ± 52
$Resp_A$ T Cells + xAllo $Stim_B$	$1,162 \pm 250*$	$11,625 \pm 2496*$	$47,500 \pm 6455*$
$Resp_A$ T Cells + xStem $Cells_C$	140 ± 17	$88 \pm 12*$	$36 \pm 9*$
$Resp_A$ T Cells + xStem $Cells_D$	200 ± 53	$1,160 \pm 151*$	$2,461 \pm 492*$
xStem $Cells_C$ cultured alone	55 ± 14	96 ± 39	43 ± 13
xStem $Cells_D$ cultured alone	40 ± 17	88 ± 12	36 ± 9
$Resp_A$ T cells cultured alone, $2 \cdot 10^5$ cells/well	225 ± 65		

$*P < 0.05$.

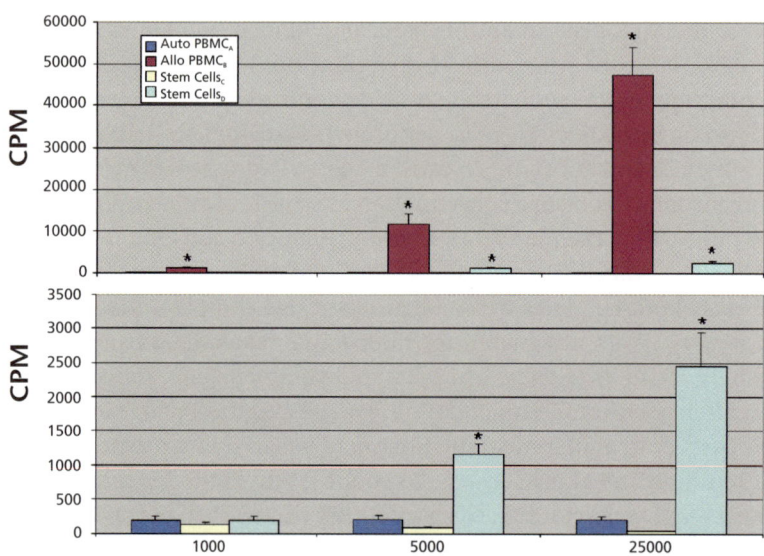

Figure 11.4 Graphical representation of immunogenicity assay data. The data from Figure 11.1 has been summarized and represented in this graph. The top panel shows count-per-minute (cpm) data from all groups (mean ±standard deviation); the bottom panel shows data from all groups less the positive control group, allowing expansion of the count-per-minute scale to enhance visualization of the differences between the baseline and stem cell treatment groups (mean ±standard deviation).

cance of difference between populations. Significant differences are held at $P < 0.05$. In the example shown, significant differences were found between the baseline response and the response to allogeneic stimulator cells (all three cell doses), and to stem cells derived from donor D at the 5,000 and 25,000 cell doses. The stem cell population from donor C is not immunogenic.

With regard to anticipated responses, T cells cultured alone should give a similar response to the baseline response (not significantly different). T cells cultured with allogeneic stimulator cells should give a vigorous response, significantly higher than baseline (usually by thousands of counts per minute). If the control allogeneic stimulator population does not induce a significant response above the baseline response, the MLR assay is not valid. T cells cultured with allogeneic MSCs that have been passaged repeatedly will generally give low responses, similar to baseline [1–9]. Responses to other types of stem cells may vary.

11.5.2 Suppression assay

Sample data are presented in Figure 11.2 in accordance with the experimental design, which assessed suppression by one stem cell population on two different MLR cultures. The means and standard deviations of control MLR cultures (12 wells) and those cultured with stem cells (quadruplicate cultures) are shown in Table 11.2. The summarized data from Table 11.2 are shown in two graphic formats in Figure 11.5.

Table 11.2 Summary of Suppression Data

Group	No Stem Cells Added (Baseline Response)	1,000 Stem Cells/ Well	5,000 Stem Cells/ Well	25,000 Stem Cells/ Well
MLR_1	55,000 ± 10,445	51,250 ± 8,539 (7%)	27,500 ± 6,455* (50%)	3,625 ± 1,109* (93%)
MLR_2	30,417 ± 7,217	11,250 ± 3,227* (63%)	2,750 ± 645* (91%)	1,325 ± 350* (96%)

*Significantly different from baseline response ($P < 0.05$).

( ), percent suppression relative to baseline response.

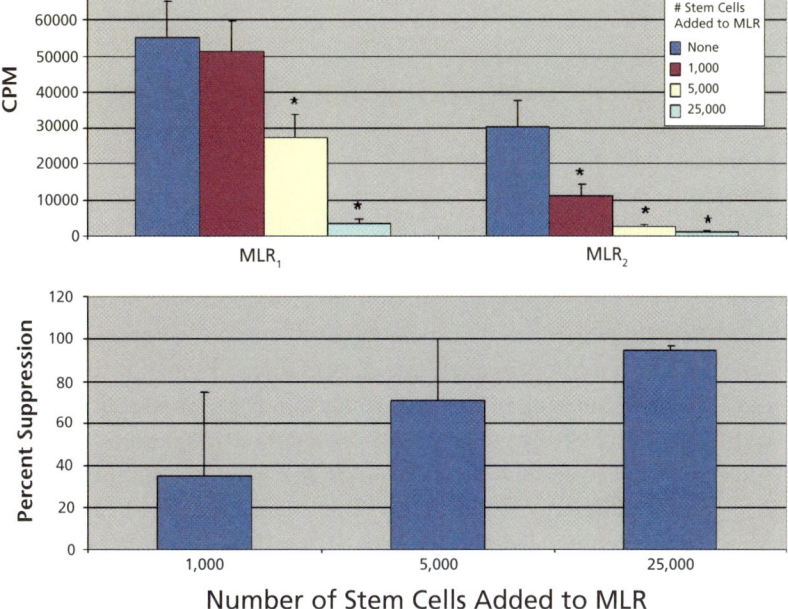

Figure 11.5 Graphical representation of suppression assay data. The data from Figure 11.2 has been summarized and represented in this graph. The top panel shows count-per-minute data from all groups (mean ±standard deviation); the bottom panel shows percent suppression data (1 − [stem cell + MLR cpm ÷ MLR cpm]), mean ±standard deviation).

The upper bar graph shows control MLR responses and responses to which various numbers of stem cell control have been added. The MLR response (no cells added) serves as the baseline response to which all other responses are compared. The two-tailed Student's *t*-test can be used to assess whether a putative suppressor cell population significantly enhances or suppresses this response. This format is most suitable for displaying stem cell inhibition on each MLR culture. The lower bar graph displays the data as percent suppression of the control MLR response. This format is most suitable for summarizing results of one stem cell population tested on multiple MLR cultures.

With regard to anticipated responses, the investigator should ensure that the MLR baseline response is optimized and vigorous. MLR responses are typically more than 20,000 cpm for rat and human cultures; lower numbers can be expected for mouse cultures.

The amount of suppression of MLR cultures by stem cells is variable. For MSCs, a range of 30% to 70% maximum suppression is typical, depending on species, MSC passage number, and so forth. Greater degrees of suppression at stem cell numbers higher than confluence may be the result of cell crowding effects and should be regarded with caution.

11.5.3 T-cell priming assay

Sample data are presented in Figure 11.3 in accordance with the experimental design, which assessed T-cell responses from four rats in each of two groups injected with vehicle or allogeneic stem cells. In the example shown, the animals are sacrificed at one time point after stem cell treatment, and their lymph nodes are removed and processed as responder cells. Spleen cells obtained from the recipient strain (syngeneic) and from the stem cell donor strain (allogeneic) are used as stimulator cells. The plate setup shown is replicated for harvest at two time points: day 3 and day 7. Sample data derived from the day 7 culture is shown.

The means and standard deviations of quadruplicate cultures are shown in Table 11.3 for the day 3 and day 7 time points. Raw data are expressed as counts per minute ±standard deviation of quadruplicate wells. The last two columns show processed data for graphic representation in which the response to syngeneic cells has been subtracted from the response to allogeneic cells.

Summarized data from Table 11.3 is shown graphically in Figure 11.6. The vehicle control group's response to stimulation with allogeneic donor cells serves as the baseline response with which the allogeneic stem cell group is compared.

The bar graph (upper panel) summarizes *averaged* data (mean Δcpm ±standard error of the mean) from each of the two groups of rats to stimulation with allogeneic donor cells at the day 3 and day 7 MLR assay time points. Background responses to syngeneic spleen cells have been subtracted to arrive at the Δcpm responses shown in Figure 11.6. A significant difference between the vehicle- and stem cell-treated groups in the day 7 MLR assay is denoted by an asterisk ($P < 0.05$, two-tailed Student's *t*-test).

The lower panel shows *individual* rat responses at day 7. A threshold response has been calculated for the vehicle control group equal to the group mean plus two standard deviations (30,688 cpm). The threshold response, indicated on the graph by a dotted line, represents the value under which 97.8% of the control group would be expected to fall (empirical rule). Any response exceeding the threshold response has only a 2.2%

11.5 Data Acquisition, Anticipated Results, Interpretation, and Statistical Guidelines

Table 11.3 Summary of T-Cell Priming Data

Group	Medium (cpm)		Syngeneic Spleen Cells (cpm)		Allogeneic Spleen Cells (cpm)		Allogeneic Spleen Cells (Δcpm)	
	Day 3	Day 7	Day 3	Day 7	Day 3	Day 7	Day 3	Day 7
Rat #1 – vehicle	89 ± 15	196 ± 31	110 ± 22	166 ± 39	550 ± 87	24,375 ± 4,270	440	24,209
Rat #2 – vehicle	76 ± 11	154 ± 21	125 ± 25	159 ± 24	640 ± 68	26,750 ± 4,193	515	26,591
Rat #3 – vehicle	60 ± 10	189 ± 43	103 ± 30	294 ± 43	700 ± 92	17,125 ± 3,497	597	16,831
Rat #4 – vehicle	93 ± 27	204 ± 43	142 ± 27	351 ± 37	680 ± 56	19,375 ± 3,146	538	19,024
Group mean response ±standard error	80 ± 7	186 ± 11	120 ± 9	243 ± 48	643 ± 33	21,906 ± 2,214	523 ± 32	21,664 ± 2,256
Rat #5 – Allo SC	100 ± 17	203 ± 34	96 ± 39	386 ± 30	750 ± 110	30,438 ± 1,663	654	30,052
Rat #6 – Allo SC	95 ± 20	244 ± 28	88 ± 12	401 ± 47	780 ± 95	45,000 ± 4,021	692	44,599
Rat #7 – Allo SC	70 ± 8	205 ± 42	62 ± 14	244 ± 31	840 ± 78	47,388 ± 4,731	778	47,144
Rat #8 – Allo SC	86 ± 12	269 ± 63	55 ± 11	344 ± 43	910 ± 135	36,063 ± 1,297	855	35,719
Group mean response ±standard error	88 ± 7	230 ± 16	75 ± 10	344 ± 35	820 ± 35	39,722 ± 3,939	745 ± 45	39,379 ± 3,957

Allo, allogeneic; SC, spleen cell.

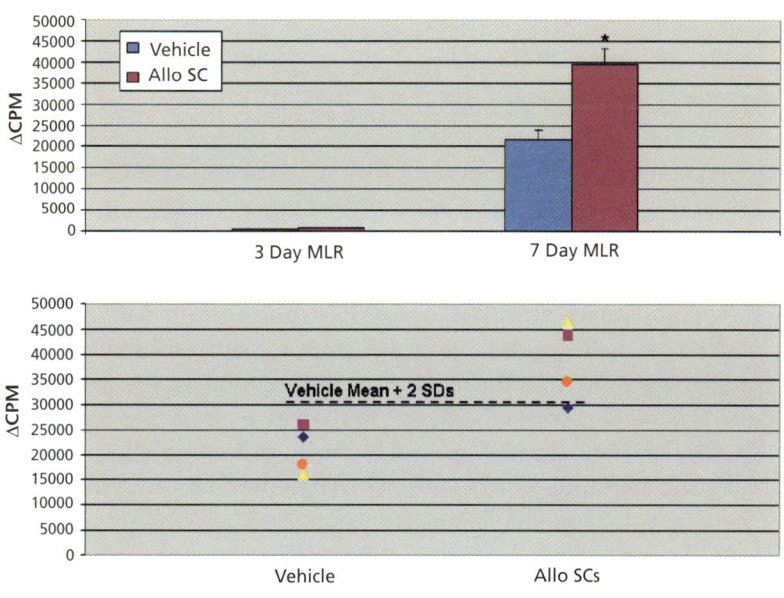

Figure 11.6 Graphical representation of T-cell priming assay data. The data from Figure 11.3 has been summarized and represented in this graph. The top panel shows Δcpm data (allogeneic spleen cpm minus syngeneic spleen cpm) from vehicle control and stem cell groups (mean ±standard error) from day 3 and day 7 MLR assays. The bottom panel shows individual rat data from vehicle and allogeneic (Allo) stem cell (SC) groups at the day 7 MLR time point relative to the vehicle mean plus two standard deviations, which defines the upper limit of the vehicle response with 97.8% confidence. In this example, three of four rats treated with allogeneic stem cells exceeded this threshold, indicating that these rats were primed by allogeneic stem cell treatment.

probability of falling in the vehicle response range. In the example given, three of the four rats treated with stem cells exceed the threshold response, placing them significantly outside the vehicle response range. This type of data presentation is useful when significant variation exists between individual responses within the treatment group, preventing significance between group means.

With regard to anticipated responses, the vehicle control baseline response should be higher at day 7 than at day 3. If a response cannot be demonstrated in the control group at day 7, the assay is invalid.

If animals treated with allogeneic stem cells were primed to donor alloantigens, they should produce an MLR response that is significantly greater in magnitude than the baseline response. In the example, allogeneic stem cells induced a significant T-cell response in the recipient rats.

In a well-primed recipient, T-cell proliferation may exhibit accelerated kinetics, showing a higher response at day 3 than day 7. Although we have not found this in animals treated with unmanipulated MSCs, which do not induce T-cell priming, we have found enhanced kinetics in goats treated with MSCs transduced with green fluorescent protein [32].

Responder T cells harvested from recipient animals should be tested for responsiveness by a mitogenic stimulus to ensure that the population of cells has not been unintentionally compromised during cell processing. The overall T-cell response to stimulation with PHA or Con A should not be significantly different between groups.

11.6 Discussion and Commentary

11.6.1 General considerations

The MLR assay should be optimized by the investigator prior to performing the study of interest. Although human MLR assays are fairly robust over a range of conditions, animal MLRs tend to produce responses of lower magnitude and thus require more preliminary investigation for optimization. When working with allogeneic strain combinations in rats or mice, the investigator should choose inbred strains that exhibit major mismatches at the MHC class I and class II loci to obtain a good response when cells from both donors are mixed in the MLR. Animal strain MHC genotypes can often be obtained from literature developed by companies that sell research animals. Performing MLR assays in larger animals may require preliminary studies to determine the magnitude of MLR responses between breeds of animals or between individuals of outbred species. The optimization protocol can include analysis of responder-to-stimulator cell ratio, number of responder cells per well, serum screening for serum used in culture medium, and culture duration. The optimal culture period typically varies between 5 to 7 days and is dependent on the degree of disparity between donors of responder and stimulator cells, species, and the use of fresh versus frozen cells.

The serum used in culture medium should be homologous to the cells used in the MLR assay. For example, rat serum should be used in rat MLRs, goat serum in goat MLRs, and so forth. The use of matched serum will result in low background responses by T cells cultured in medium or with syngeneic/autologous stimulator cells. Unfortunately, many serum lots will not support a good MLR response to positive control cells, and the use of FBS may be necessary to generate a response. FBS contains a rich source of growth factors and will increase background responses significantly, but at least a response can be elicited. We have resorted to using FBS in cases when responder cells were obtained in less than optimal condition (e.g., after overnight shipping).

Results obtained from MLR assays can be expressed as Δcpm (treatment counts per minute minus background counts per minute) and as a stimulation index (treatment counts per minute divided by background counts per minute). Δcpm values should always be provided, because stimulation index alone can be misleading: A stimulation index of 10 appears like a vigorous response was induced to a stimulator population, but the interpretation changes dramatically if the treatment response was 500 cpm and the background response was 50 cpm (Δcpm = 450).

11.6.2 Immunogenicity assay

The investigator has a choice of whether to use unfractionated cells or purified T cells as responder cells in the MLR. Unfractionated cells may replicate the in vivo scenario more accurately because the entire complement of immune cells is present in this population (including macrophages), allowing indirect presentation of alloantigens to T cells. By contrast, using purified T cells as responders tests the ability of the stem cell population to behave as an antigen presenting cell, requiring both the presentation of alloantigens on MHC molecules and the expression of costimulatory molecules. When MSCs were cultured with unfractionated cells, they elicited a low but discernible response, likely as a result of their expression of MHC class I antigens that were presented by antigen presenting cells within the responder population [4]. When cultured with purified T cells, no response was observed, because MSCs lack costimulatory molecules [3, 4] and possibly the cellular machinery for antigen processing. From a purely technical point of view, purified T cells produce a cleaner response with lower backgrounds to syngeneic/autologous control stimulator populations and higher responses to allogeneic positive control cells.

How does the investigator interpret the MLR data in terms of rejection or survival of the stem cell population after transplantation in vivo? Although there are no hard-and-fast rules, there are commonsense guidelines. A stem cell population that generates a T-cell proliferative response that is not significantly different from the baseline response is considered nonimmunogenic and would not be expected to generate a T-cell response in an immunocompetent recipient. Conversely, a stem cell population that generates a vigorous response similar to the positive control would be expected to be immunogenic and rejected after transplantation. Interpretation of the gray area in between both of these scenarios seemingly depends on the magnitude of the MLR response and where it lies on the continuum between the baseline response and the positive control. Unfortunately, there are no data on which a count-per-minute threshold can be calculated to predict a rejection response.

This does not prevent investigators from fine-tuning their stem cell population for allogeneic use. For example, a stem population that induces a significant T-cell response in the immunogenicity assay should not be used as a therapeutic treatment in an animal model. However, the population may be rendered nonimmunogenic by removal of contaminating antigen presenting cells by specific antibodies and magnetic beads or by simply passaging the cells further [6]. The modified population can be reevaluated by the immunogenicity assay to determine whether the depletion protocol was successful.

11.6.3 Suppression assay

A solid MLR response is essential for assessing immunosuppression by stem cells. We have noticed that poor responses can be enhanced by the addition of MSCs whereas strong responses are suppressed. A possible explanation for this finding may be that stem cell suppression is activated by cytokines produced in the MLR. For example, interferon γ has been reported to induce MSCs to produce IDO, which suppresses T-cell proliferation [33].

A major pitfall of the suppression assay is distinguishing stem cell suppression effects from cell crowding effects. To diminish the effect of cell crowding, we limit the upper number of stem cells added per well to the number that results in cell confluence (approximately 25,000 cells/well for MSCs). In one suppression study, we included nonsuppressive cells similar in size to MSCs (human splenic fibroblasts; CRL-7433, American Type Culture Collection) to determine the cell number threshold that induced artifactual inhibitory effects on the MLR response [6]. Once determined, results derived at this threshold or higher were eliminated. Unfortunately, the use of such a control is arbitrary, because one can never be sure that a cell population is nonsuppressive, only relatively nonsuppressive when compared with other cells.

When comparing multiple stem cell populations for suppression, it may be useful to determine the "suppression titer" of each stem cell population by determining the minimal number of stem cells capable of significantly suppressing the MLR response. If suppression titer is expressed as the ratio of suppressor cells to responder cells, a range of 1:10 (20,000 suppressor cells:200,000 responder T cells) and more would signify significant suppression. Ratios approaching 1:1 suggest that suppression is weak or may be artifactual (e.g., as a result of cell crowding).

11.6.4 T-cell priming assay

Immunologic studies of sensitization are often performed in conjunction with a study set up to investigate stem cell function (e.g., the ability of MSCs to mediate spinal fusion or mitigate the effects of stroke). The number of experimental groups and the number of animals per group are dictated by the functional model and the requirements to obtain good immunological data. Rodent models, in which individual responses will be combined to calculate group means, require large group sizes; 10 animals per group are recommended. In large-animal studies, group sizes can usually be smaller because statistical variation can be minimized as each animal serves as its own control. Furthermore, animal losses from experimental manipulation are usually less in large-animal models.

Although the focus of the discussion for this assay has been detection of T-cell priming, the investigator should be aware that the assay has detected T-cell hyporesponsiveness to donor alloantigens in animals injected with MSCs [21]. In this case, T-cell proliferative responses from animals injected with allogeneic MSCs were significantly *lower* than the baseline response, suggesting that the animals were tolerized by the MSCs to donor alloantigens. Because tolerance is antigen specific, the response to third-party stimulator cells would need to be performed to claim that true tolerance was indeed induced in these animals.

The T-cell priming assay is a good indication of T-cell sensitization in vivo, but additional assays should be incorporated by the investigator to substantiate the conclusion. If possible, a histological evaluation of the implantation site should be done to determine whether the donor stem cells are still present and to assess the degree of inflammatory cell infiltration. In addition, evaluation of alloantibodies to donor cells is indicated in view of recent studies showing this response [21, 30].

Troubleshooting Table

Problem	Explanation	Potential Solutions
Low MLR response	Responder and stimulator cells are not sufficiently mismatched at MHC	Test different responder/stimulator combinations.
	Responder cells are compromised	Remove dead cells on the density gradient. Increase the number of responder cells per well. Use purified T cells as responder cells.
	Responder and stimulator cells are not in optimal culture configuration	Change responder-to-stimulator cell ratio.
	Culture conditions are not optimized	Try a different serum or percentage of serum in the culture medium. Change the duration of cell culture.
High background response in immunogenicity assay	Culture conditions are not optimized	Reduce the number of cells per well and/or culture duration. Try a different serum or percentage of serum in the culture medium.
Suppression by stem cells does not titrate out as cell number is decreased	Stem cells are contaminated with mycoplasma	Test cells for mycoplasma. Try a different lot of stem cells.
Outside wells on plate produce low responses, low medium volume in wells, or medium very yellow	Evaporation	Fill outer wells of plate with sterile phosphate-buffered saline. Shorten culture duration if possible.

11.7 Application Notes

To give a specific example of the multiple uses of the MLR assay, we have performed a study comparing syngeneic with allogeneic stem cells in mediating spinal fusion in a rat model (unpublished). Adipose-derived stem cells (ASCs) were produced from rats and characterized. They expressed a nonimmunogenic profile as shown by a lack of T-cell proliferation to allogeneic ASCs, as well as ASC-mediated suppression of the MLR. To determine whether these observations would translate in vivo, immune monitoring studies were carried out in rats transplanted with allogeneic ASCs as part of a scaffold-based spinal fusion study.

A total of 56 Fischer strain rats were randomly assigned to four different treatment cohorts after bilateral decortication of the L4 and L5 transverse processes (n = 14 per cohort). ASCs, derived from Fischer or ACI rats, were seeded on scaffolds and implanted in Fischer recipients according to the following treatments: (1) no treatment, (2) scaffold only, (3) syngeneic ASCs + scaffold, or (4) allogeneic ASCs + scaffold. Half of each group was sacrificed at 4 weeks after implantation and the remaining animals were sacrificed at 8 weeks. In addition to evaluating spinal fusion at both time points, T-cell proliferative responses to donor ACI strain spleen cells were assessed to determine whether ACI ASCs induced an immune response in recipient Fischer rats. Recipient Fischer lymph node cells were assessed for T-cell proliferation to ACI spleen cells by one-way MLR assays.

The results from this study are currently being evaluated. They should provide valuable information regarding whether allogeneic ASCs produced in our laboratory, combined with a scaffold and utilized for spinal fusion, induced an immune response in recipient rats. This information will be critical in deciding whether to perform further studies in large-animal models to test the universal donor strategy.

11.8 Summary Points

1. The MLR is a screening tool to estimate whether a stem cell population will be rejected after transplantation to an allogeneic immunocompetent recipient.
2. Initial experiments can utilize the MLR assay to assess the immunological properties (immunogenicity, suppression) of stem cells produced in the investigator's laboratory.
3. The MLR can be used to assess T-cell responses in animals treated with allogeneic stem cells.
4. Appropriate baseline controls must be performed in each MLR assay; these are the responses with which the stem cell responses are compared.
5. The MLR assay should be used in association with other readouts of immune rejection in preclinical studies (histological sections, alloantibody studies, stem cell survival).

Acknowledgments

I thank the numerous collaborators with whom I have worked throughout the years who have contributed the framework in which to perform, develop, and refine the MLR assay. Special thanks are given to Jeff Gimble for his valuable insight as well as to my wife, Marla, who tried in vain to teach me statistical analysis and who ate dinners alone too many times while I was performing MLR assays in the lab.

References

[1] Di Nicola, M., et al., "Human Bone Marrow Stromal Cells Suppress T-Lymphocyte Proliferation Induced by Cellular or Nonspecific Mitogenic Stimuli," *Blood*, Vol. 99, 2002, pp. 3838–3843.
[2] Bartholomew, A., et al., "Mesenchymal Stem Cells Suppress Lymphocyte Proliferation in Vitro and Prolong Skin Graft Survival in Vivo," *Exp. Hematol.*, Vol. 30, 2002, pp. 42–48.
[3] Tse, W. T., et al., "Suppression of Allogeneic T-Cell Proliferation by Human Marrow Stromal Cells: Implications in Transplantation," *Transplantation*, Vol. 75, 2003, pp. 389–397.
[4] Klyushnenkova, E., et al., "T Cell Responses to Allogeneic Human Mesenchymal Stem Cells: Immunogenicity, Tolerance, and Suppression," *J. Biomed. Sci.*, Vol. 12, 2005, pp. 47–57.
This is a good reference for using the MLR assay to obtain immunogenicity, suppression, and tolerance data about MSCs.
[5] Puissant, B., et al., "Immunomodulatory Effect of Human Adipose Tissue-Derived Adult Stem Cells: Comparison with Bone Marrow Mesenchymal Stem Cells," *Br. J. Haematol.*, Vol. 129, 2005, pp. 118–129.
[6] McIntosh, K., et al., "The Immunogenicity of Human Adipose Derived Cells: Temporal Changes in Vitro," *Stem Cells*, Vol. 24, 2006, pp. 1246–1253.
[7] Chang, C. J., et al., "Placenta-Derived Multipotent Cells Exhibit Immunosuppressive Properties That Are Enhanced in the Presence of Interferon-Gamma," *Stem Cells*, Vol. 24, 2006, pp. 2466–2477.
[8] Weiss, M. L., et al., "Immune Properties of Human Umbilical Cord Wharton's Jelly-Derived Cells," *Stem Cells*, Vol. 26, 2008, pp. 2865–2874.

[9] Wolbank, S., et al., "Dose-Dependent Immunomodulatory Effect of Human Stem Cells from Amniotic Membrane: A Comparison with Human Mesenchymal Stem Cells from Adipose Tissue," *Tissue Eng.*, Vol. 13, 2007, pp. 173–183.

[10] Koch, C.A., P. Geraldes, and J. L. Platt, "Immunosuppression by Embryonic Stem Cells," *Stem Cells*, Vol. 26, 2008, pp. 89–98.

[11] Hori, J., et al., "Neural Progenitor Cells Lack Immunogenicity and Resist Destruction as Allografts," *Stem Cells*, Vol. 21, 2003, pp. 405–416.

[12] Meisel, R., et al., "Human Bone Marrow Stromal Cells Inhibit Allogeneic T-Cell Responses by Indoleamine 2,3-Dioxygenase-Mediated Tryptophan Degradation," *Blood*, Vol. 103, 2004, pp. 4619–4621.

[13] Aggarwal, S., and M. F. Pittenger, "Human Mesenchymal Stem Cells Modulate Allogeneic Immune Cell Responses," *Blood*, Vol. 105, 2005, pp. 1815–1822.

[14] Nasef, A., et al., "Immunosuppressive Effects of Mesenchymal Stem Cells: Involvement of HLA-G," *Transplantation*, Vol. 84, 2007, pp. 231–237.

[15] Chabannes, D., et al., "A Role for Heme Oxygenase-1 in the Immunosuppressive Effect of Adult Rat and Human Mesenchymal Stem Cells," *Blood*, Vol. 110, 2007, pp. 3691–3694.

[16] Sato, K., et al., "Nitric Oxide Plays a Critical Role in Suppression of T-Cell Proliferation by Mesenchymal Stem Cells," *Blood*, Vol. 109, 2007, pp. 228–234.

[17] Yañez, R., et al., "Adipose Tissue-Derived Mesenchymal Stem Cells Have in Vivo Immunosuppressive Properties Applicable for the Control of the Graft-Versus-Host Disease," *Stem Cells*, Vol. 24, 2006, pp. 2582–2591.

[18] Fang, B., et al., "Favorable Response to Human Adipose Tissue-Derived Mesenchymal Stem Cells in Steroid-Refractory Acute Graft-Versus-Host Disease," *Transplant. Proc.*, Vol. 39, 2007, pp. 3358–3362.

[19] Le Blanc, K., and O. Ringdén, "Immunomodulation by Mesenchymal Stem Cells and Clinical Experience," *J. Intern. Med.*, Vol. 262, 2007, pp. 509–525.

[20] Liechty, K. W., et al., "Human Mesenchymal Stem Cells Engraft and Demonstrate Site-Specific Differentiation after in Utero Transplantation in Sheep," *Nat. Med.*, Vol. 6, 2000, pp. 1282–1286.

[21] Beggs, K. J., et al., "Immunologic Consequences of Multiple, High-Dose Administration of Allogeneic Mesenchymal Stem Cells to Baboons," *Cell Transplant.*, Vol. 15, 2006, pp. 711–721.
This is a good reference that describes the use of the T-cell priming assay in a large-animal model.

[22] Dai, W., et al., "Allogeneic Mesenchymal Stem Cell Transplantation in Postinfarcted Rat Myocardium: Short- and Long-Term Effects," *Circulation*, Vol. 112, 2005, pp. 214–223.

[23] Sudres, M., et al., "Bone Marrow Mesenchymal Stem Cells Suppress Lymphocyte Proliferation in Vitro but Fail to Prevent Graft-Versus-Host Disease in Mice," *J. Immunol.*, Vol. 176, 2006, pp. 7761–7767.

[24] Inoue, S., et al., "Immunomodulatory Effects of Mesenchymal Stem Cells in a Rat Organ Transplant Model," *Transplantation*, Vol. 81, 2006, pp. 1589–1595.

[25] Min, C.-K., et al., "IL-10-Transduced Bone Marrow Mesenchymal Stem Cells Can Attenuate the Severity of Acute Graft-Versus-Host Disease after Experimental Allogeneic Stem Cell Transplantation," *Bone Marrow Transplant.*, Vol. 39, 2007, pp. 637–645.

[26] Nauta, A. J., et al., "Donor-Derived Mesenchymal Stem Cells Are Immunogenic in an Allogeneic Host and Stimulate Donor Graft Rejection in a Nonmyeloblative Setting," *Blood*, Vol. 108, 2006, pp. 2114–2120.

[27] Eliopoulos, N., et al., "Allogeneic Marrow Stromal Cells Are Immune Rejected by MHC Class I- and Class II-Mismatched Recipient Mice," *Blood*, Vol. 106, 2005, pp. 4057–4065.

[28] Spees, J. L., et al., "Internalized Antigens Must Be Removed to Prepare Hypoimmunogenic Mesenchymal Stem Cells for Cell and Gene Therapy," *Mol. Ther.*, Vol. 9, 2004, pp. 747–756.

[29] Li, Y., et al., "Allogeneic Bone Marrow Stromal Cells Promote Glial–Axonal Remodeling without Immunologic Sensitization after Stroke in Rats," *Exp. Neurol.*, Vol. 198, 2006, pp. 313–325.
This is a good reference that describes the use of the T-cell priming assay in a small-animal model.

[30] Poncelet, A. J., et al., "Although Pig Allogeneic Mesenchymal Stem Cells Are Not Immunogenic in Vitro, Intracardiac Injection Elicits an Immune Response in Vivo," *Transplantation*, Vol. 83, 2007, pp. 783–790.
This is another good reference that describes the use of the T-cell priming assay in a large-animal model. It describes the use of third-party cells in standardizing the assay as well.

[31] Hing, K. A., L. F. Wilson, and T. Buckland, "Comparative Performance of Three Ceramic Bone Graft Substitutes," *Spine J.*, Vol. 7, 2007, pp. 475–490.

[32] Beggs, K. J., et al., "Evidence for Selective Suppression of Alloreactivity by Mesenchymal Stem Cells," *Blood*, Vol. 98, 2001, p. 648a.

[33] Krampera, M., et al., "Role for Interferon-Gamma in the Immunomodulatory Activity of Human Bone Marrow Mesenchymal Stem Cells," *Stem Cells*, Vol. 24, 2006, pp. 386–398.

CHAPTER

12

A Novel Method for the Preservation of Embryonic Stem Cells Using a Quartz Capillary Freezing System

Heidi Y. Elmoazzen and Mehmet Toner

Center for Engineering in Medicine
Department of Surgery, Massachusetts General Hospital
Harvard Medical School, Shiners Hospital for Children
Boston, MA 02114

Abstract

To have widespread application of embryonic stem cells, effective long-term storage of these cells is essential. There are currently two approaches to achieving cryopreservation of cells: the conventional slow-freezing approach, which uses low cooling rates; and the vitrification approach, which uses rapid cooling rates. With slow freezing, the cryoprotectant concentrations used are low and nontoxic to the cells. However, the challenge is that slow freezing is associated with injury resulting from ice formation. Vitrification involves the solidification of a supercooled liquid while maintaining the absence of ice, such that a glass is formed. However, to achieve vitrification, rapid cooling rates and very high toxic concentrations of cocktails of cryoprotectants are required. The ideal cryopreservation protocol, then, would be one that combines the benefits of conventional slow freezing (reduced toxicity secondary to low cryoprotectant levels) with the benefits of vitrification (absence of intracellular ice crystal formation). A method of cellular cryopreservation using quartz capillary freezing has shown that the process of vitrification can be optimized by maximizing the rate at which the sample is cooled, which allows for the use of lower cryoprotectant concentrations. The quartz capillary freezing technique can be used to preserve embryonic stem cells.

| Key Terms | Cryopreservation
slow freezing
vitrification
mouse embryonic stem cells
human embryonic stem cells
quartz capillaries |

12.1 Introduction

Embryonic stem (ES) cells are undifferentiated cells derived from the pluripotent cells of the inner cell mast of the blastocyst. ES cells are characterized functionally by two main features: their ability to propagate indefinitely and the capacity for differentiation into cells from all three embryonic germ layers. These unique characteristics of ES cells and their ability, theoretically, to produce an unlimited supply of differentiated cells, holds tremendous promise in regenerative medicine, clinical medicine, developmental biology, toxicity screening in vitro, as well as tissue engineering. However, to have widespread application of ES cells, effective long-term storage and transportation of these cells are essential. Cryopreservation is often the most viable option for the long-term storage of cells and tissues, and the ability to "stop time" in cryogenic storage for indefinite periods of time offers huge practical benefits. Often, preservation takes place at dry ice temperatures (–80°C) or in liquid nitrogen (–196°C). At temperatures this low, cells can often be stored for many years in a biologically stable state, because chemical reactions are limited. There are currently two main approaches to achieve cryopreservation of mammalian cells and tissues: traditional slow-freezing protocols and vitrification.

12.1.1 Slow-freezing protocols

During slow freezing, the cells are cooled to temperatures below their equilibrium freezing point and ice is seeded in the extracellular media. As ice forms in the extracellular solution, there is a progressive increase in the external solute concentration. As a result, the cell dehydrates, and the formation of intracellular ice is avoided. However, there are some disadvantages to using this approach. Cellular injury is thought to be the result of exposing the cells to highly concentrated intracellular and extracellular solutions and/or mechanical interactions between the cells and ice [1]. Other disadvantages to slow freezing are the result of limitations in practicality. Slow-freezing methods require the cooling rate as well as the seeding temperature to be accurately controlled, which may be responsible for the variable results obtained when using the slow-freezing technique.

12.1.2 Vitrification protocols

As a result of many of the problems resulting from ice formation inside cells during freezing, current approaches toward preservation attempt to eliminate ice formation by vitrification [2]. Vitrification involves the solidification of a supercooled liquid by adjusting the composition and cooling rate such that the crystal phase is avoided and there is an absence of both intracellular and extracellular ice, and a glassy state is formed (amorphous solidification). If cooling occurs rapidly enough, this glassy state can be induced in most liquids. Even pure water can be vitrified; however, cooling rates on the order of 10^8°C/minute are required [3]. The addition of cryoprotectants such as dimethyl sulfoxide, ethylene glycol, and propane-1,2-diol (PrOH) greatly decreases these prohibitively high cooling rates. In general, for concentrations of cryoprotective agents (CPAs) more than 60% weight/weight, homogeneous nucleation is avoided, allowing the solution to vitrify at a slow cooling rate. Because the concentrations of cryoprotectants needed to achieve vitrification are so high, one of the primary challenges in vitrifying cells and tissues is cryoprotectant toxicity. To reduce the exposure to toxic cryoprotectants and to prevent extreme dehydration, the cells are exposed to the cryoprotectants for short periods of times and usually are added stepwise. As a result, in order for vitrification to be a successful process, the cryoprotectant needed to vitrify must be decreased to a nontoxic level and the cooling rate must be increased to accommodate this reduction and allow vitrification to occur. The higher the cooling rate, the lower the concentration needed to vitrify.

12.1.3 Increasing cooling rates for vitrification

A number of innovations have been used to increase the cooling rate for vitrification by reducing the final volume. A minimal volume of cryoprotectant containing the cells is exposed directly to liquid nitrogen. Several devices have been developed to increase the cooling rates. The easiest and most common approach lies in placing the cells in a container such as a thin open straw in which cells are placed in a narrow plastic tube and quenched into liquid nitrogen [4]. This method has since been modified to the Cryotop [5] for oocyte cryopreservation. Similarly, electron microscopy grids have been used [6] that have since been modified to the Cryoloop [7]. The cooling rates for these devices are in the range of 2,000 to 30,000°C/minute, and generally concentrations of more than 4M are required.

12.1.4 Quartz capillary system

It is of great interest to develop a novel approach to achieve vitrification of mammalian cells using a low nontoxic concentration of cryoprotectants, which combines the advantages of the existing slow-freezing and vitrification approaches while avoiding their shortcomings [8]. Theoretically, this can be done by ultrafast cooling (>100,000°C/minute) of mammalian cells to a vitrified/glassy state at cryogenic temperatures. This is possible because the higher the cooling rate, the lower the required cryoprotectant concentration for vitrification [9], and even pure water can be vitrified when the cooling rate is high [10, 11]. Recently, a new technique for mammalian cell cryopreservation that takes advantage of the unique properties of quartz crystal capillaries has been developed [12]. The small dimensions of the quartz capillary (QC) (The Charles Supper Company) compared with other cooling devices (Table 12.1) and the extremely high thermal conductivity of quartz compared with other materials, including traditionally used plastics (Table 12.2), allows for significantly higher cooling rates compared with conventional plastic straws and vials. As such, we have shown this freezing technique to be significantly more efficient than conventional vitrification techniques. The thin-walled QC is transparent and has an inner diameter of 0.18 mm and a wall thickness of 0.010 mm, which is much smaller than other devices (Figure 12.1).

12.1.5 Apparent vitrification of CPA-laden solutions

One convenient way for determining nonvitrification is the appearance of opacity (or visible ice formation) when cooling solutions below their freezing point. If there is no observable opacity, it is called *apparent vitrification*. Although opacity could be easily identified using the traditional plastic straw and the open pulled straw (OPS) by the naked eye, it is very difficult to do so using the quartz microcapillary because of its small

Table 12.1 Dimensions of Various Vitrification Devices

Materials	Outer Diameter (mm)	Inner Diameter (mm)	Wall Thickness (mm)
Traditional straw	2	1.7	0.15
Open pulled straw	0.95	0.8	0.075
Grid (0.5-μL microdrop)	1.24	N/A	N/A
Quartz capillary	0.2	0.18	0.01

N/A, not applicable.

Table 12.2 Thermal Properties of Various Materials

Materials	Density (kg/m^3)	Specific Heat (J/kg/K)	Thermal Conductivity
Solution	1,022	3,800	0.54
Plastics	**1,200**	**1,500**	**0.2**
Glass	2,200	850	0.8
Quartz	**2,649**	**710**	**8**
Stainless steel	7,817	460	16.3
Sapphire	3,970	419	27.2
Gold	19,300	129	320
Copper	8,920	385	385
Silver	10,490	232	406
Diamond	3,500	502	1,000

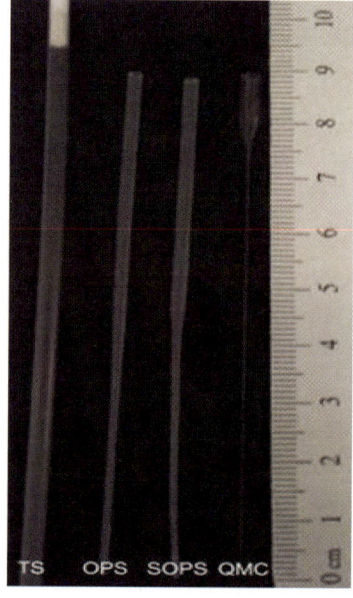

Figure 12.1 A comparison of cooling devices, including the traditional straw (TS), the open pulled straw (OPS), the superfine open pulled straw (SOPS), and the quartz capillary (QC).

dimension. He et al. [12] developed an experimental setup to visualize the opacity in the QC during cooling by directing two focused lights generated from two fiberoptic lamps on the capillary held against a dark background (Figure 12.2). Various total CPA concentrations from 12% to 30% by volume with 2% increments were studied. Further opacity studies were performed using the QC for solutions with various concentrations of sucrose or trehalose (0.2–1M) and PrOH in cell medium. The threshold CPA concen-

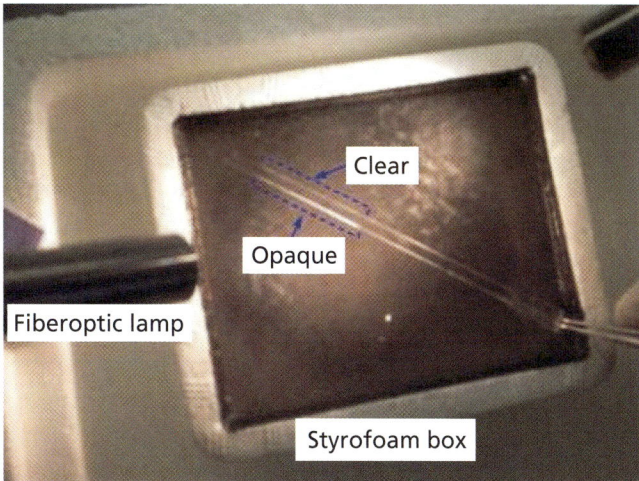

Figure 12.2 Experimental setup used to determine the threshold cryoprotectant concentration required for complete avoidance of visible opacity during ultrafast cooling solutions in the QC. Shown are two QCs loaded with solutions of different concentrations of 1,2-propanediol after plunging into liquid nitrogen. The top one, with 2M 1,2-propanediol, is clear (vitrified); the bottom one, with 1M 1,2-propanediol, is opaque (not vitrified).

tration required for apparent vitrification was as low as 1.9M when using the combination of QC and 1,2-propanediol. Further experiments were also performed using stem cell medium with 0.2–1.0M trehalose plus 1.5M (11% volume), 2M (15% volume), and 2.5M (19% volume) PrOH. No opacity was observed after plunging the QC loaded with these solutions into liquid nitrogen. Based on the results of He et al. [12], solutions of 2M PrOH and 0.5M trehalose were used for the vitrification studies.

12.1.6 Slush nitrogen

In addition to optimizing the sample container, alterations in the cryogenic liquid can also increase the desired cooling rates. One approach is to use slush nitrogen to reduce the insulating vapor layer that forms on the surface of the sample when it is plunged from room temperature into liquid nitrogen [13–15]. With these necessary improvements in mind, Risco et al. [16] explored the capability of QCs plunged into a two-phase slush nitrogen and compared it with the thermal performance of the conventional OPS. The solution within the sample containers consisted of 1.5M PrOH and 0.3M sucrose in 1× phosphate-buffered saline (PBS). Significantly higher cooling and rewarming rates were achieved through the use of the QCs. The cooling rates when quenching the OPS or the QCs into liquid nitrogen were approximately 5,700 and 30,000°C/minute, respectively. When plunged into slush nitrogen, the cooling rate for the OPS and the QCs increased significantly to 40,000 and 250,000°C/minute, respectively [16]. When the technique of OPS in liquid nitrogen is compared with that of QC in slush nitrogen, the difference is evident. The use of QC in slush nitrogen increases the cooling rate by one order of magnitude over other approaches developed to reach high cooling rates for cell vitrification. When thawed in a 37°C water bath, the warming rates for the QCs were significantly higher when plunged from slush nitrogen compared with the OPS and compared with thawing from liquid nitrogen. Warming rates of approximately 100,000°C/minute were obtained. The advantages of rewarming QC from slush nitrogen are obvious, taking into account the importance of achieving high warming rates to avoid devitrification and recrystallization.

12.2 Experimental Design

He et al. [12] recently demonstrated the use of the QC system with mouse ES cells and showed successful recovery of stem cells after cryopreservation. In their study, QCs with an outer diameter of 0.2 mm and a wall thickness of 0.01 mm were used to achieve ultrafast vitrification at a low and nontoxic level of cryoprotectants (2M PrOH and 0.5M extracellular trehalose). The efficacy of QC-assisted vitrification for maintaining murine ES cell viability, attachment, proliferation, and pluripotency was demonstrated. Risco et al. [16] demonstrated the benefits of using slush nitrogen over liquid nitrogen with the QC system. The following describes how these experiments were conducted.

12.3 Materials

12.3.1 Required equipment

- Sterile biosafety cabinet
- Centrifuge
- Incubator
- Vacuum pump
- Microscope

12.3.2 Supplies

- Pipets
- Pipet aid
- Styrofoam container
- QCs, 0.2 mm (Charles Supper Company)
- Liquid nitrogen
- Tissue culture flasks, 75 cm^2
- Ice
- Ice bucket
- Syringe

12.3.3 Cells and reagents

- R1 murine ES cell line, which expresses green fluorescent protein (GFP) under control of an Oct4 promoter
- Fetal bovine serum
- 1,2 Propanediol (Sigma)
- Trehalose (Pfanstienl Laboratories)

- Knockout Dulbecco's modified Eagle's medium (DMEM) supplemented with 15% knockout serum replacement (Invitrogen) containing 1,000 U/mL LIF (Chemicon)
- 1× PBS
- Trypsin

12.4 Methods

12.4.1 Murine ES cell culture

For the purpose of evaluating the maintenance of ES cell pluripotency, a GFP reporter cell system is used. The R1 murine ES cell line, which expresses GFP under control of the Oct4 promoter, was kindly provided by Andras Nagy (University of Toronto) [17]. The ES cell maintenance media consists of knockout DMEM supplemented with 15% knockout serum replacement (Invitrogen) containing 1,000 U/mL leukemia inhibitory factor (LIF) (Chemicon). Feeder layer-free ES cells are continually passaged in 0.1% gelatin-coated 75-cm^2 flasks in 5% CO_2 humidified air at 37°C.

12.4.2 Preparing slush nitrogen

To make slush nitrogen, a vacuum chamber and pump are used. A Styrofoam container holding 750 mL liquid nitrogen is placed inside the chamber. The vacuum pressure in the chamber is then reduced to 6,500 Pa. The nitrogen is left at this pressure for 15 minutes and is then removed. As a result, two-phase slush nitrogen is obtained. Liquid nitrogen has a temperature of –196°C. The slush nitrogen has a temperature of roughly –205 to –210°C. The main benefit of quenching with the slush over liquid nitrogen, however, does not come from this temperature difference, but from a reduction of vaporization when submitted to relatively high temperatures. This reduction of vaporization exposes the sample to a more direct contact with the cryogenic media, and in this way increases the cooling rate. To maximize this effect, the slush should be used within a couple minutes of removal from the vacuum chamber.

12.4.3 Cryopreservation of murine ES cells by vitrification

On the day of experiment, lightly trypsinize the attached murine ES cells for 3 to 5 minutes and then collect. Pellet the cells at 100×g for 5 minutes and resuspended in cold stem cell medium (on ice) for further use. Spin down the cells at 100×g for 3 to 5 minutes and resuspended in 1 mL solution made of ES cell maintenance medium with 1.5M 1,2-propanediol for 10 minutes. Then, spin down the cells at 100×g for 3 to 5 minutes and resuspend in a solution made of ES cell maintenance medium with 2M 1,2-propanediol and 0.5M trehalose at $10 \cdot 10^6$ cells/mL for another 10 minutes before cooling. The pH of all solutions is carefully adjusted to 7.2 to 7.4. The cell suspension is loaded into a quartz microcapillary tube by capillary action with a solution length of 4 cm in the capillary. The cell suspension in the quartz microcapillary is cooled by plunging the QC as fast as possible into slush nitrogen and is left in the slush nitrogen for 3 to 5 minutes. Warm the cryopreserved cell suspension by plunging the QC as fast as possible into 1× PBS with 0.2M trehalose at room temperature. Expel the cell suspension in the quartz microcapillary into 1 mL warm (37°C) ES cell maintenance medium with 0.2M trehalose and incubate for 10 to 15 minutes at 37°C. Transfer the 1 mL ES cell suspension into 9 mL warm fresh stem cell maintenance medium and incubate for another 10 to 15 minutes. Spin down the cells and resuspend in 1.5 mL fresh ES cell maintenance medium at room temperature, and culture in a 35-mm Petri dish coated with 25 µg/mL fibronectin (Chemicon) for further study.

12.5 Anticipated Results

12.5.1 Cell attachment and proliferation after vitrification

Immediate cell viability after cryopreservation can be assessed using a standard live/dead assay kit of fluorescent probes—calcein AM and ethidium homodimer (Invitrogen)—to check the cell membrane integrity. After warming the QC, expel a small droplet (2–3 µL) of the cell suspension into a Petri dish with warm ES cell maintenance medium with trehalose (0.2M) and the fluorescent probes (9 µM calcein AM and 9 µM ethidium homodimer) [12]. Incubate for 5 to 10 minutes at 37°C for dye uptake. The cell-containing droplet is then covered with a coverslip and the cell membrane integrity is evaluated using an inverted microscope (10× objective). Cells that exclude ethidium homodimer (red) and retain the fluorescent calcein (green) are counted as viable. The total number of cells under each field is determined using the corresponding phase field. At least 15 randomly selected fields of view were used for each sample on each day. The immediate cell viability is calculated as the ratio of the number of viable cells to the number of total cells per field (10×). The immediate cell viability using a vitrification solution of PrOH with 0.5M trehalose should be around 80%.

To check the cell viability after vitrification cryopreservation, the cell attachment and proliferation or growth after vitrification is determined by counting the number of cells per field under a 10× objective in a 35-mm Petri dish. At least 15 randomly selected fields of view are used for each sample. The attachment efficiency is calculated as the ratio of the total number of cells per field of a cryopreserved sample to that of the control nonfrozen sample at day 1. To assess the proliferation or growth rate of the attached cells, the total number of cells per field of view (10×) for both the control and cryopreserved samples in the 35-mm Petri dish is further countered every day for 3 days. The proliferation or growth rates of the ES cells after vitrification should be very similar to the proliferation of the control cells. There should be a robust increase in the number of cells in the field of view over a 3-day period and there should be a population doubling time of approximately 21 hours [12].

12.5.2 Pluripotent properties of ES cells after vitrification

To determine whether the ES cells retained their pluripotent properties after cryopreservation, three different types of assays that are characteristic to murine ES cells are performed [12]: the expression of transcription factor Oct4, the expression of membrane surface glycoprotein SSEA-1, and the elevated expression of the enzyme alkaline phosphatase. For immunofluorescence staining of SSEA-1, ES cells are fixed using 4% paraformaldehyde, permeabilized with 0.4% triton X-100, and blocked against nonspecific binding with

12.5 Anticipated Results

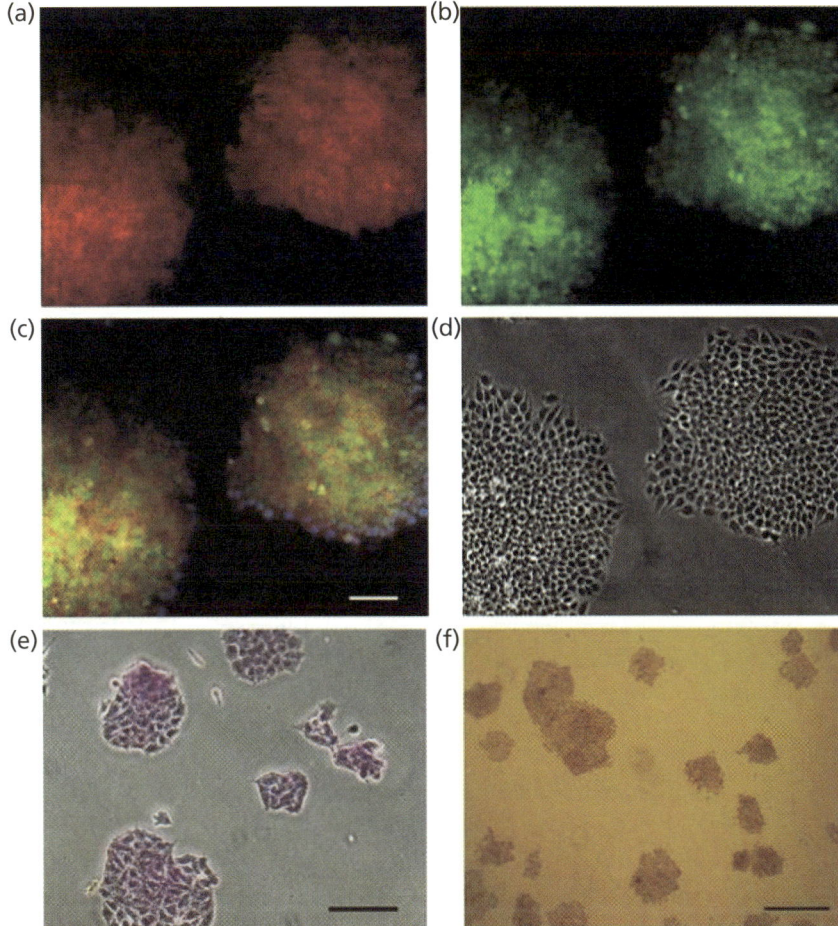

Figure 12.3 Immunofluorescence and histochemical analysis for maintenance of undifferentiated properties of the pluripotent ES cells after vitrification. (a, b) Fluorescence micrographs display high levels of staining for the surface glycoprotein SSEA-1 (a) and Oct4 transcriptional activity as denoted by GFP expression (b). (c) The merged view of the red and green channels indicates extensive coexpression of the two markers and 4′, 6-diamidina-2-phenylindole (DAPI) nuclei staining (blue). (d) Phase contrast image shows cells with a high nuclei-to-cytoplasm ratio and compact colony formation typical of pluripotent ES cells. (e, f) Histochemical staining shows strong expression for alkaline phosphatase at 10× magnification (e), which was seen to be well distributed within each colony as observed at a lower 4× magnification (f). Scale bars, 100 µm (A–D), 200 µm (E), and 500 µm (f).

2% bovine serum albumin. Monoclonal antibody against SSEA-1 (clone MC-480) was purchased from Chemicon. Antibody localization of SSEA-1 is performed using a Texas Red conjugated goat antimouse F(ab′)2 fragment antibody (Rockland). The histochemical staining of alkaline phosphatase is done by incubating naphthol AS-BI phosphate and Fast Red violet solutions (Chemicon) with 4% paraformaldehyde-fixed ES cells for 15 minutes. The undifferentiated properties of the pluripotent ES cells can be verified by the high levels of staining for the membrane surface glycoprotein SSEA-1 [Figure 12.3 (a)] and expression of the green fluorescent transcription factor Oct4 [Figure 12.3 (b)]. The merged view of the red (SSEA-1) and green (Oct4) channels indicates extensive coexpression of the two markers and DAPI nuclei staining [blue, Figure 12.3(c)]. Phase contrast imaging [Figure 12.3 (d)] shows cells with high nuclei-to-cytoplasm ratios and compact colony formation typical of pluripotent ES cells. Histochemical staining shows strong expression for alkaline phosphatase at high magnification [Figure 12.3 (e)], which was seen to be well distributed within each colony as observed at a lower magnification [Figure 12.3 (f)]. Collectively, the robust expression of the different markers that are characteristic to murine ES cells, along with proper ES cell morphology, suggests that the murine ES cells retained their undifferentiated properties as pluripotent cells after cryopreservation by vitrification.

12.6 Discussion and Commentary

A QC vitrification technique has been developed that uses ultrafast cooling rates that lead to vitrification at low, nontoxic intracellular concentrations of cryoprotectants (2M). Traditional vitrification approaches require high cryoprotectant concentrations (usually more than 4M), which is often toxic to cells and requires multiple loading steps [18–20]. It has been demonstrated that mammalian cells can be successfully cryopreserved by vitrification at a concentration that is nontoxic and close to concentrations used for traditional slow-freezing protocols (1–2M) [21, 22]. When using the QC technique with slush nitrogen, cooling rates of 250,000°C/minute are obtained. The QC approach has been used with mouse ES cells and showed successful recovery of stem cells after cryopreservation using the QC [12].

Troubleshooting Table

Problem	Explanation	Potential Solutions
The vitrification solution does not appear to vitrify	The plunging rate of the QC in nitrogen is not fast enough	The QCs should not be plunged straight into liquid nitrogen. The straw should be held above the liquid nitrogen with its length parallel to the surface, and then the tip of the straw should be plunged by rotating the straw downward around the operator's wrist so that the tip is plunged at a speed greater than 1 m/second.
No vacuum pump is available to make slush nitrogen	Vacuum pumps are not common lab equipment	Liquid nitrogen can be used instead of slush nitrogen. However, a technique of plunging, in which the straw is held above the liquid nitrogen with its length parallel to the surface and then the tip of the straw is plunged by rotating the straw downward around the operator's wrist so that the tip is plunged at a speed greater than 1 m/second.
QCs keep breaking	The QCs are very fragile	With more practice, the quartz becomes much easier to handle.
The QCs are currently an open system, so there are potential issues of contamination	There is no effective method for sealing the capillaries yet	We are developing effective approaches to sealing the capillaries at both ends, such as using Critoseal, a clay sealant used for sealing hematocrit tubes and various waxes. The sealant needs to withstand cryogenic temperatures.

12.7 Application Notes

Although there are published methods for the cryopreservation of both mouse and human ES cells using traditional cryopreservation approaches, there is no currently available technique that combines the benefits of both preservation techniques in one procedure. There are currently two approaches to achieving cryopreservation of ES cells: the conventional slow-freezing approach [23–26], which uses low cooling rates; and the vitrification approach [25–28], which uses rapid cooling rates. With slow freezing, the cryoprotectant concentrations used are low and nontoxic to the cells. A novel method of cellular cryopreservation using QC freezing has shown that the process of vitrification can be optimized by maximizing the rate at which the sample is cooled, which allows for the use of lower cryoprotectant concentrations similar to the range of cryoprotectants used in slow-freezing protocols while avoiding ice formation. The QC freezing technique can be used to preserve murine ES cells. We anticipate that the methodology, with some modifications, could also be used to preserve human ES cells, and preliminary results have been promising.

12.8 Summary Points

1. A novel ultrafast vitrification approach for cryopreservation of sensitive mammalian cells using a small QC has been developed.
2. The cryoprotectants used were 2M 1,2-propanediol and 0.5M extracellular trehalose. The intracellular concentration (2M) of cryoprotectants is in the range of that used for slowing freezing.
3. Biological assays show that trehalose and 1,2-propanediol protect murine ES cells from cryoinjury during cryopreservation by ultrafast cooling (vitrification). More than 70% of ES cells attach well, proliferate normally, and retain the undifferentiated properties of pluripotent cells after vitrification using the combination of 2M 1,2-propanediol and 0.5M trehalose.
4. These results indicate that vitrification by ultrafast cooling using a very low concentration of intracellular cryoprotectants (e.g., 2M 1,2-propanediol) is a viable and effective approach for the cryopreservation of murine ES cells and potentially other important mammalian cells.
5. QCs in slush nitrogen can be used to obtain cooling rates of 250,000°C/minute.
6. The combination of 200-μm QCs, slush nitrogen, and low cryoprotectant concentrations has the potential to improve cryopreservation of various cell types, including human ES cells.

Acknowledgments

We thank the National Institutes of Health for funding this research (NIH EB 02340).

References

[1] Mazur, P., S. P. Leibo, and E. H. Chu, "A Two-Factor Hypothesis of Freezing Injury: Evidence from Chinese Hamster Tissue-Culture Cells," *Exp. Cell Res.*, Vol. 71, 1972, pp. 345–355.
[2] Fahy, G. M., et al., "Vitrification as an Approach to Cryopreservation," *Cryobiology*, Vol. 21, 1984, pp. 407–426.
[3] Johari, G. P., A. Hallbrucker, and E. Mayer, "The Glass Liquid Transition of Hyperquenched Water," *Nature*, Vol. 330, 1987, pp. 552–553.
[4] Vajta, G., et al., "Open Pulled Straw (OPS) Vitrification: A New Way to Reduce Cryoinjuries of Bovine Ova and Embryos," *Mol. Reprod. Dev.*, Vol 51, 1998, pp. 53–58.
[5] Kuwayama, M., et al., "Highly Efficient Vitrification Method for Cryopreservation of Human Oocytes," *Reprod. Biomed. Online*, Vol. 11, 2005, pp. 300–308.

[6] Martino, A., N. Songsasen, and S. P. Leibo, "Development into Blastocysts of Bovine Oocytes Cryopreserved by Ultra-rapid Cooling," *Biol. Reprod.*, Vol. 54, 1996, pp. 1059–1069.
[7] Lane, M., et al., "Containerless Vitrification of Mammalian Oocytes and Embryos," *Nat. Biotechnol.*, Vol. 17, 1999, pp. 1234–1236.
[8] Han, X., et al., "Investigations on the Heat Transport Capability of a Cryogenic Oscillating Heat Pipe and Its Application in Achieving Ultra-fast Cooling Rates for Cell Vitrification Cryopreservation," *Cryobiology*, Vol. 56, 2008, pp. 195–203.
[9] Berejnov, V., et al., "Effects of Cryoprotectant Concentration and Cooling Rate on Vitrification of Aqueous Solutions," *J. Appl. Crystallogr.*, Vol. 39, 2006, pp. 244–251.
[10] Bhat, S. N., A. Sharma, and S. V. Bhat, "Vitrification and Glass Transition of Water: Insights from Spin Probe ESR," *Phys. Rev. Lett.*, Vol. 95, 2005, pp. 235702.
[11] Bruggeller, P., and E. Mayer, "Complete Vitrification in Pure Liquid Water and Dilute Aqueous Solutions," *Nature*, Vol. 288, 1980, pp. 569–571.
[12] He, X., et al., "Vitrification by Ultra-fast Cooling at a Low Concentration of Cryoprotectants in a Quartz Micro-capillary: A Study Using Murine Embryonic Stem Cells," *Cryobiology*, Vol. 56, 2008, pp. 223–232.
[13] Luyet, B., "On Various Phase Transitions Occurring in Aqueous Solution at Low Temperatures," *Ann. N. Y. Acad. Sci.*, Vol. 85, 1960, pp. 549–569.
[14] Mazur, P., et al., "Contributions of Cooling and Warming Rate and Developmental Stage to the Survival of *Drosophila* Embryos Cooled to −205 Degrees C," *Cryobiology*, Vol. 30, 1993, pp. 45–73.
[15] Sjoestrand, F. S., and L. G. Elfvin, "The Granular Structure of Mitochondrial Membranes and of Cytomembranes as Demonstrated in Frozen-Dried Tissue," *J. Ultrastruct. Res.*, Vol. 10, 1964, pp. 263–292.
[16] Risco, R., et al., "Thermal Performance of Quartz Capillaries for Vitrification," *Cryobiology*, Vol. 55, 2007, pp. 222–229.
[17] Nagy, A., et al., "Derivation of Completely Cell Culture-Derived Mice from Early-Passage Embryonic Stem Cells," *Proc. Natl. Acad. Sci. U. S. A.*, Vol. 90, 1993, pp. 8424–8428.
[18] Fahy, G. M., et al., "Improved Vitrification Solutions Based on the Predictability of Vitrification Solution Toxicity," *Cryobiology*, Vol. 48, 2004, pp. 22–35.
[19] Fahy, G. M., et al., "Cryopreservation of Organs by Vitrification: Perspectives and Recent Advances," *Cryobiology*, Vol. 48, 2004, pp. 157–178.
[20] Rall, W. F., and G. M. Fahy, "Ice-Free Cryopreservation of Mouse Embryos at −196 Degrees C by Vitrification," *Nature*, Vol. 313, 1985, pp. 573–575.
[21] Karlsson, J. O., and M. Toner, "Long-Term Storage of Tissues by Cryopreservation: Critical Issues," *Biomaterials*, Vol. 17, 1996, pp. 243–256.
[22] Mazur, P., "Freezing of Living Cells: Mechanisms and Implications," *Am. J. Physiol.*, Vol. 247, 1984, pp. C125–C142.
[23] Kashuba Benson, C. M., J. D. Benson, and J. K. Critser, "An Improved Cryopreservation Method for a Mouse Embryonic Stem Cell Line," *Cryobiology*, Vol. 56, 2008, pp. 120–130.
[24] Valbuena, D., et al., "Efficient Method for Slow Cryopreservation of Human Embryonic Stem Cells in Xeno-Free Conditions," *Reprod. Biomed. Online*, Vol. 17, 2008, pp. 127–135.
[25] Zhou, C. Q., et al., "Cryopreservation of Human Embryonic Stem Cells by Vitrification," *Chin. Med. J. (Engl.)*, Vol. 117, 2004, pp. 1050–1055.
[26] Miszta-Lane, H., et al., "Effect of Slow Freezing Versus Vitrification on the Recovery of Mouse Embryonic Stem Cells," *Cell Preserv. Technol.*, Vol. 5, 2007, pp.16–24.
[27] Li, T., et al., "Bulk Vitrification of Human Embryonic Stem Cells," *Hum. Reprod.*, Vol. 23, 2008, pp. 358–364.
[28] Reubinoff, B. E., et al., "Effective Cryopreservation of Human Embryonic Stem Cells by the Open Pulled Straw Vitrification Method," *Hum. Reprod.*, Vol. 16, 2001, pp. 2187–2194.

CHAPTER 13

In Vivo MR Tracking of hESC-Derived Oligodendrocyte Precursors in Mouse Brain

Heechul Kim,[1] Candace Kerr,[2] and Jeff W. M. Bulte[3]

[1]Russell H. Morgan Department of Radiology and Radiological Science, Division of MR Research Cellular Imaging Section, Vascular Biology Program, Institute for Cell Engineering
The Johns Hopkins University School of Medicine
Baltimore, MD 21205

[2]Stem Cell Biology Program
Department of Gynecology and Obstetrics
The Johns Hopkins University School of Medicine
Baltimore, MD 21205

[3]Russell H. Morgan Department of Radiology and Radiological Science, Division of MR Research Cellular Imaging Section, Vascular Biology Program, Institute for Cell Engineering
Department of Gynecology and Obstetrics
Department of Chemical and Biomolecular Engineering
Department of Biomedical Engineering
Johns Hopkins University School of Medicine
Baltimore, MD 21205

Abstract

Human embryonic stem cells are pluripotent stem cells and a potentially infinite source for transplant therapy against human disease. For successful transplant treatment, transplanted stem cells must be able to be tracked noninvasively in the body. Magnetic resonance imaging is a clinically applicable technology for tracking transplanted cells in vivo. To accomplish this, cells need to be magnetically prelabeled in vitro, usually with dextran-coated superparamagnetic iron oxides and transfection agents. We describe here current methodologies for magnetic labeling of human embryonic stem cell-derived oligodendrocyte precursors and their tracking with magnetic resonance imaging after transplantation in the mouse brain.

Key Terms

Central nervous system
human embryonic stem cells
transplantation
cell therapy
magnetic resonance imaging
cell tracking
superparamagnetic iron oxide

13.1 Introduction

Cell therapy using human embryonic stem (hES) cells has significant potential for the treatment of many diseases. hES cells are pluripotent and can differentiate into a variety of cell types, including neurons, glial cells, cardiomyocytes, hepatocytes, hematopoietic precursors, osteoblasts, keratinocytes, and endothelial cells.

The central nervous system is the most complex system in the body, but its ability to accomplish an effective replacement of resident cells that are lost by aging or disease falls far short of the regenerative capacity observed in most other organ systems. Thus, stem cell therapy would likely be most advantageous in the treatment of neurological disease. Although there are few clinical trials of hES cells applied to human neurological disease, experimental therapeutic cell transplantation has been studied in human disease models, including Parkinson's disease, spinal cord injury, brain ischemia, and multiple sclerosis.

To develop clinical cell therapy protocols further for the treatment of neurological diseases, it is critically important to determine, noninvasively, whether transplanted cells migrate to targeted lesions and how long these cells survive during the treatment period. Noninvasive in vivo imaging offers the opportunity to determine the biodistribution and migration of cells after transplantation into the central nervous system. The ideal imaging modality is capable of three-dimensional, single-cell imaging; has a high (soft) issue imaging resolution; has a high sensitivity and specificity; is nontoxic; does not suffer from label dilution; and does not transfer label to adjacent host cells.

Commercially available technologies, including X-ray computed tomography, magnetic resonance imaging (MRI), optical imaging, ultrasound, single photon emission computed tomography (SPECT), and positron emission tomography (PET) have been used for in vivo imaging in experimental animal models. SPECT and PET utilize radiolabeled and positron-emitting molecules to report on the expression level of a target, including the activity of cells. The advantage of SPECT and PET is the high sensitivity level for detecting subtle biological changes using limited quantities of the imaging agent, but both these methods require radioactivity. MRI is a very attractive noninvasive imaging modality because it does not rely on ionizing radiation and offers a spatial resolution of tens of microns, providing clear advantages, such as high resolution and sensitivity, over other imaging methodologies. MRI has therefore been a preferred in vivo modality to track cells after transplantation into the central nervous system.

13.2 Experimental Design

In order for transplanted cells to be detected on the MR images, they must be magnetically labeled to aid in discrimination from the surrounding native tissue. Magnetic labeling of cells also requires a contrast agent. The currently preferred contrast agents for magnetic labeling are superparamagnetic iron oxides (SPIO), because they are biocompatible and exert strong effects on T2 relaxation. However, SPIO by itself cannot be taken up by nonphagocytic stem cells; this limitation is addressed with a variety of labeling techniques. Most often, stem cells are labeled with the clinically approved, dextran-coated SPIO Feridex (Berlex Laboratories). In this chapter, we briefly describe the methodology for the preparation of magnetic labeling of cells using Feridex, followed by MRI tracking of hES cell-derived oligodendrocyte precursors after transplantation into rodent mouse brain.

13.3 Materials

- Mice or rats
- Undifferentiated hES cells (e.g., HES1 line; WiCell Research Institute)
- Mitomycin-c-treated primary mouse embryo fibroblasts (Chemicon)
- hES cell medium: 80% Dulbecco's modified Eagle's medium (DMEM)/F12 (Invitrogen), 20% knockout serum (Invitrogen), 1% penicillin–streptomycin (Sigma), 1% L-glutamine (Specialty Media), 1% nonessential amino acids (Specialty Media), 0.007 μL/mL β-mercaptoethanol (Sigma), supplemented with 4 μg/mL human recombinant fibroblast growth factor 2 (FGF2; R&D Systems)
- Differentiation medium: 50% DMEM/F12, 50% neural basal media (Invitrogen), 1% B27 supplementation (Invitrogen), 0.5% N2 supplementation (Invitrogen), 1% insulin (Sigma), 500 μg/mL bovine serum albumin (Sigma), 250 ng/mL gentamicin (Invitrogen), and 0.007 μL/mL β-mercaptoethanol
- Human recombinant noggin, epidermal growth factor (EGF), FGF4, and platelet-derived growth factor (PDGF) (all from R&D Systems)
- Ca/Mg-free phosphate-buffered saline (PBS)
- Ultralow attachment dishes (Corning)
- Matrigel (BD)
- Collagenase type IV
- 0.05% Trypsin/ethylenediaminetetraacetic acid (EDTA) solution (Invitrogen)
- Feridex (Berlex)
- Transfection agent, such as poly-L-lysine (PLL; molecular weight, 350–400 kDa; Sigma), Lipofect (Gibco), Superfect (Qiagen), FuGENE (Roche), and protamine sulfate (American Pharmaceuticals Partner)
- Anesthetics: ketamine (80–100 mg/kg) + xylazine (5–10 mg/kg)
- Betadine
- Puralube ointment
- Heating pad
- Stereotactic brain apparatus (Stoelting)
- Surgical tools: needle holder, scissors, forceps, scalpel blade, scalpel handle, 4-0G silk suture
- Syringe, 1 mL
- Hamilton syringe, 10 μl, with needle (26G)
- Isoflurane anesthesia machine (Surgivet)
- Respiratory module for small animal (SA instruments)
- MR scanner (e.g., 9.4T Bruker horizontal bore magnet)
- MR surface coil

13.4 Methods

13.4.1 Maintenance and differentiation of hES cells

For further details about hES cell cultures, please see previous studies.
1. Culture undifferentiated hES cells on an inactivated mouse embryo fibroblast feeder layer on a 0.1% gelatin-coated plate.
2. Change medium daily for 5 days.
3. Split hES cells using 0.05% trypsin/EDTA.
4. Maintain hES cell cultures.
5. For differentiation, collect hES cells from their culture dish using 1 µg/mL collagenase type IV for 5 minutes in a 37°C incubator, then scrape mechanically.
6. Transfer detached hES cell colonies (embryoid bodies) into ultralow attachment dishes and incubate with differentiation medium, supplemented with human recombinant FGF2 (20 µg/mL), FGF4 (20 µg/mL), and noggin (200 µg/mL).
7. After 14 days, transfer formed embryoid bodies to matrigel-coated dishes and incubate with differentiation medium supplemented with human recombinant FGF2 (20 µg/mL) and FGF4 (20 µg/mL).
8. After 5 days, change media to differentiation medium supplemented with human recombinant FGF2 (20 ng/mL) and EGF (20 µg/mL).
9. After 5 days, change media to differentiation medium supplemented with human recombinant FGF2 (20 µg/mL) and PDGF (20 µg/mL).
10. After 15 days, cells are ready for magnetic labeling.

13.4.2 Preparation of magnetically labeled cells

An example is given for the use of PLL as transfection agent.
1. Add Feridex from stock (11.2 mg Fe/mL) to prepare a medium solution containing 50 µg Fe/mL. Mix well before proceeding to step 2.
2. Add PLL from stock (1.5 mg/mL, in sterile water) to the medium solution with Feridex to a final concentration of 1.5 µg/mL. Mix well.
3. Incubate the PLL–Feridex medium for 60 minutes at room temperature using a rotating shaker. This allows the formation of PLL–Feridex complexes through electrostatic interactions.
4. Discard old media from the culture dish, and then replace with 50% differentiation media and 50 % of the media containing PLL–Feridex complexes.
5. Incubate cells for 2 days in a 37°C incubator. Shorter incubation times will result in a lesser uptake of iron.

13.4.3 Confirmation of magnetically labeled cells: Histochemical staining

Prior to transplantation, confirmation that cells are magnetically efficiently labeled is mandatory. Perl's reaction or Prussian Blue staining is a simpler and faster procedure compared with immunohistochemistry using an antidextran (Feridex coat) antibody.
1. Prepare a neutral fast red (NFR) solution by dissolving 100 mg NFR in 100 mL deionized water.

2. Add 5g aluminum sulfate and bring to a boil while stirring. Cool and filter the NFR solution and add a grain of thymol as a preservative. The NFR solution will remain stable for several weeks.
3. Fix plate or slide with cells with 4% paraformaldehyde for 10 minutes.
4. Wash cells three times using PBS.
5. Incubate slides for 30 minutes with 2% potassium ferrocyanide in 6% HCl.
6. Wash cells and counterstain with NFR for about 5 minutes (depending on freshness of NFR).
7. Wash cells three times using PBS.
8. Observe cells using light microscope.
9. A more sensitive staining for iron can be achieved using diaminobenzidine (DAB) enhancement of the Prussian Blue product. To this end, cells are incubated with unactivated 140 µg/mL DAB solution (in deionized water) for 15 minutes in the dark.
10. Without washing, cells are then incubated with 140 µg/mL DAB solution activated with 0.03% H_2O_2, for 15 minutes in the dark.
11. Wash slides and counterstain with either NFR or hematoxylin. For optimal sensitivity of detection, noncounterstained slides are preferred.
12. Embed slides and apply coverslip.

An example of hES cells labeled with PLL–Feridex and stained with DAB-enhanced Prussian Blue staining is shown in Figure 13.1.

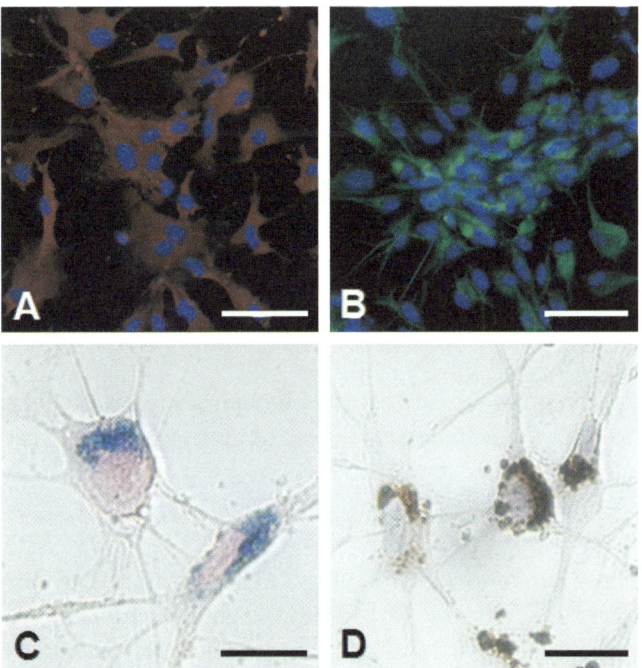

Figure 13.1 (a, b) Immunofluorescent staining for oligodendrocyte lineage markers [anti-Oligo1, red (a); anti-2′,3′-cyclic nucleotide 3′-phosphodiesterase (anti-CNPase), green (b)] demonstrates proper differentiation of hES cells into oligodendrocyte precursors. Oligodendrocyte precursors are then incubated with PLL–Feridex complexes (25 µg Fe/mL) for 48 hours. (c, d) Nonenhanced (c) and DAB-enhanced (d) Prussian Blue staining reveals an efficient intracellular uptake of superparamagnetic iron particles (brown). Scale bars, 60 µm (a, b) and 20 µm (c, d).

13.4.4 Transplantation procedure

To prevent immunorejection of human cells, mice can be given 10 mg/kg cyclosporine or rapamycin/FK506 by intraperitoneal injection 1 day prior to transplantation, and subsequently each day until the end of the study.

1. Prepare labeled hES derived oligodendrocyte precursors for transplantation as follows: After magnetic labeling, wash cells twice with PBS and then harvest cells using 0.05% trypsin/EDTA. Spin trypsinized cells for 5 minutes at 200g and then wash using PBS. Count cell number using a hemocytometer and assess viability of Feridex-labeled cells using trypan blue staining. Maintain the tube containing cells on ice until transplantation.
2. Anesthetize the mouse intraperitoneally with ketamine/xylazine (for dose, see Section 13.3).
3. When the mouse shows no toe pinch reflex, shave the fur from the skull using electrical clippers.
4. Place the mouse into a stereotaxic device (e.g., Stoelting).
5. Apply eye ointment solution (e.g., Puralube) to prevent the eyes from drying out.
6. Securely immobilize the mouse head using the nose, tooth, and ear bars.
7. Apply disinfectant solution, such as Betadine, on the area of the skull to be exposed using sterile cotton swabs to ensure sterility.
8. Longitudinally incise skin to expose the skull.
9. Find the bregma in the mouse skull and confirm the correct coordinate in the right lateral ventricle (anteroposterior, 0 mm bregma; lateral, 1 mm).
10. Drill at the correct coordinate in the skull and make a small burr hole in the skull.
11. Inject a Hamilton syringe (26G) forward to the small hole and lower the filled needle into the correct coordinate (vertical, –3 mm from skull).
12. Transplant cells ($5 \cdot 10^5$ in 5 μL sterile PBS) into the right lateral ventricle. At this point, perform the injection slowly over 10 minutes to avoid injuring the tissue by a rapid increase in pressure.
13. After injection, slowly remove the Hamilton syringe from the mouse and then suture the wound closed.
14. Apply Betadine disinfectant solution to the wound.
15. Place the mouse on a warming pad for recovery and then return the mouse to its cage.
16. Apply an analgesic, such as topical bupivacaine (Buprenex, 30 mg/mL) or Ketofen (2–5 mg/kg subcutaneously) every 12 hours for 2 days.

13.4.5 MRI procedure

After transplantation, magnetically labeled cells are tracked using a high-field animal MR imager (e.g., a Bruker 9.4T horizontal bore spectrometer) equipped with a volume surface coil (Figure 13.2). The following procedure describes how T2-weighted MR images can be obtained, optimized for tracking SPIO-labeled cells in vivo in the brain:

1. Anesthetize the mouse using isoflurane gas at 2% and 0.5-L/minute airflow for about 2 minutes. Administer an eye ointment solution to prevent the eyes from drying out.

13.4 Methods

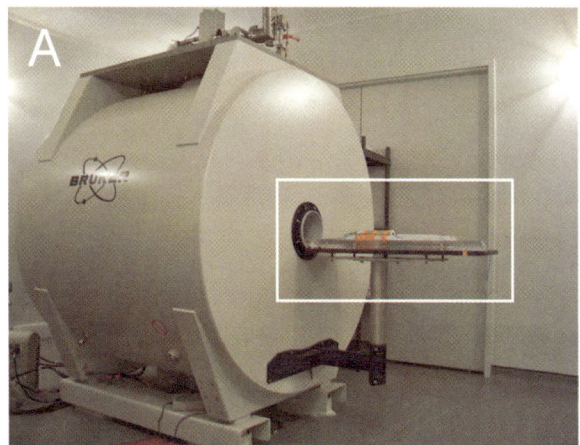
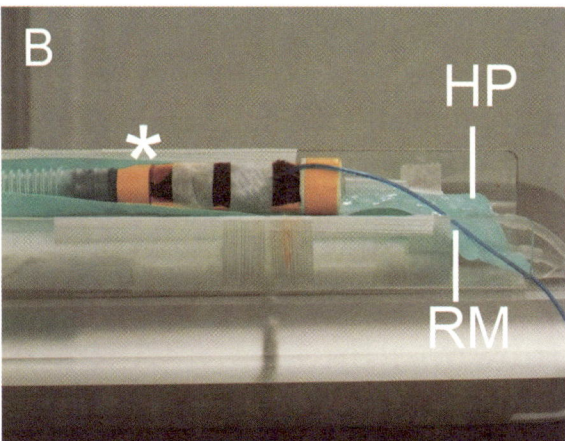
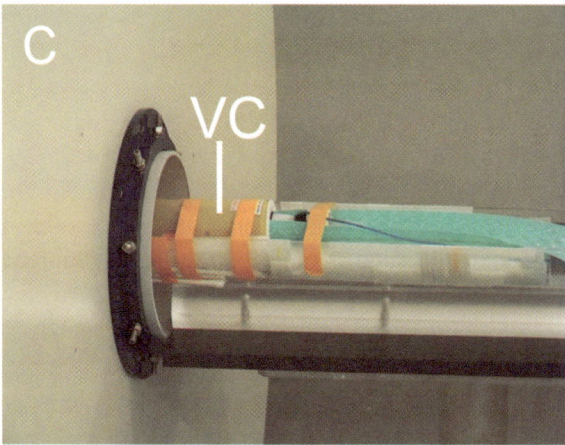

Figure 13.2 (a) High-field MRI setup exemplified for a Bruker 9.4T horizontal bore scanner. (b) The mouse is positioned in a nose cone (asterisk) connected to a vaporizer delivering 1% to 2% isoflurane. The animal cradle also contains a heating pad (HP) and a respiratory monitor (RM). (c) The assembly is then placed into the volume coil (VC) and moved into the center of the MR imager.

2. Place the mouse into a specially designed, custom-constructed acrylic container that is connected to isoflurane gas at 1% to 2% and 0.5-L/minute airflow to maintain anesthesia.
3. Attach respiratory monitor to detect the breathing rate of the mouse. Maintain breath rate at 30 to 80 breaths/minute by adjusting the flow of isoflurane.
4. Immobilize the head with surgical tape.
5. Move and adjust the animal container and the surface coil. The mouse head should be located at the center of the surface coil. Immobilize the surface coil to the head with surgical tape.
6. Scan the mouse head using the a "localizer" sequence with the following parameters: pulse sequence, rapid acquisition with relaxation enhancement (RARE); repetition time (TR), 2000 msec; echo time (TE), 12.5 msec; RARE factor, 8; field of view (FOV), 4×4 cm; resolution, 312×312 μm; number of averages, 1; total scan time, 32 seconds. This localizer scan is to determine and confirm that the animal is positioned correctly and the spatial coordinates are set for further scanning.
7. Adjust the imaging plane and then use a fast low-angle shot sequence with the following parameters: TR, 400 msec; TE, 6 msec; FOV, 1.4×1.4 cm; resolution, 70×70 mm; number of averages, 1; total scan time, 1 minute 20 seconds. This step is required for a detailed adjustment of the scanning field for the eventual T2-weighted three-dimensional RARE sequence imaging.
8. Adjust the imaging plane for the next T2-weighted three-dimensional RARE sequence with the following parameters: TR, 1,400 msec; TE, 11.31 msec; RARE factor, 4; FOV, $1.4 \times 1.4 \times 1.2$ cm; resolution, $109 \times 109 \times 375$ mm; number of averages, 1; total scan time, 23 minutes 53 seconds.
9. After finishing the MRI, place the mouse on a warming pad for recovery and return the mouse to its cage. A representative MR image using the three-dimensional RARE sequence is shown in Figure 13.3.

13.4.6 Data analysis

There are several methods to analyze in vivo cell migration patterns and to compare images obtained at various time points for each individual mouse. Anatomic structures, such as the anterior commissure, the corpus callosum, and the ventricular system, serve as the primary landmarks for orientation using an atlas of the brain. For cellular imaging analysis after intracerebroventricular transplantation, the maximal distance of the migration of transplanted cells is calculated according to the number of MR slices counted from the most proximal site of hypointense MR signal at the ventricular edge to the most distant site of hypointense signal. Downward migration in the internal capsule, fornix, or stria medullaris, and lateral migration in the corpus callosum are visualized in coronal images and measured as the number of axial or sagittal slices spanning the hypointense signal.

13.5 Anticipated Results

For each MRI cell-tracking experiment, it is mandatory that PLL–Feridex-incubated cells are confirmed to have been efficiently labeled. Successful labeling is manifested by a

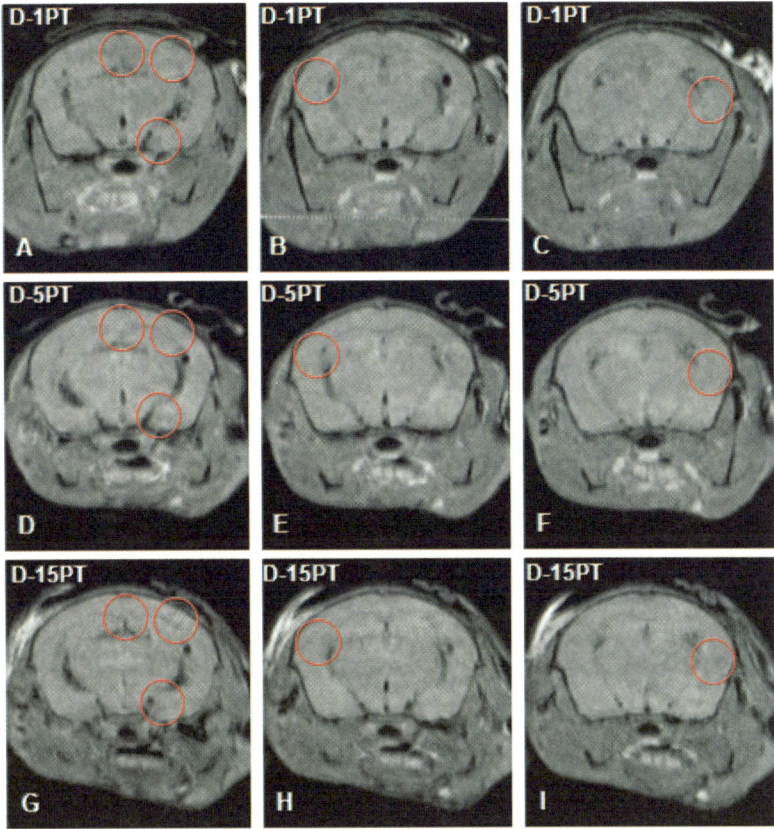

Figure 13.3 Representative MR images of experimental autoimmune encephalomyelitis (EAE) mouse brain receiving an intracerebroventricular transplant of $5 \cdot 10^5$ Feridex-labeled hES cell-derived oligodendrocyte precursors. (a–c) On day 1 posttransplantation (PT), hypointense MRI signals can be observed mainly in the ventricle, with few cells present in the cerebral cortex (red circles). (d–i) On day 5 PT (d–f) and day 15 PT (g–i), the hypointense MRI signal gradually decreases within the ventricle and more cells can be found in the cerebral cortex (red circles), suggesting cell migration from the ventricles into the cerebral cortex.

Prussian Blue-positive product that enhances with DAB staining (Figure 13.1). After transplantation, magnetically labeled transplanted cells will induce a hypointense signal (black) on the MR images, primarily located in the ventricular system, resulting from the induction of microscopic field homogeneities and the resulting dephasing of protons. Over time, cells partially differentiated into the glial lineage (e.g., hES cell-derived oligodendrocyte precursors) will migrate into the brain while primarily following white matter tracts (e.g., the corpus callosum, fimbria). Other studies have found that inflammatory brain lesions, such as those found in EAE, induces recruitment and faster migration, although few published data are available.

13.6 Discussion and Commentary

We anticipate in vivo tracking of transplanted hES cells to become an important technique for the application of cell therapy to human (neurodegenerative) disease. Because of its excellent soft-tissue contrast, whole-body imaging ability, and high resolution,

MRI is ideally suited to detect transplanted cells in vivo. To this end, transplanted cells must be magnetically labeled before transplantation. Several techniques exist (e.g., receptor-mediated endocytosis, the use of transfection agents, or electroporation). A new direction may be the use of fluorinated nanoparticles for ^{19}F tracer imaging of neural stem cells, which can be combined with conventional ^1H MRI. There are, however, some limitations with the use of MRI to track transplanted stem cells after labeling with nanoparticles. Certain stem cells are characterized by a high proliferation and differentiation ability. Labeled stem cells may also divide asymmetrically, even further diluting cytoplasm of stem cells. In this scenario, cells can only be tracked for shorter time periods. Furthermore, regardless of labeling, stem cells may die after transplantation and the label-containing cell debris may be taken up by scavenging host cells such as macrophages, making proper interpretation of which cell is which difficult. This suggests that iron particles in the stem cells could be taken up by activated macrophages, but this is also undetectable by MRI.

Ideally, one would want to use MRI reporter genes, which has been the Holy Grail for MRI cell tracking for some time. Reporter genes are not also indefinitely reproduced in rapidly or asymmetrically dividing daughter cells, enabling long-term cell tracking, but they can also report on stem cell survival and differentiation. There are some experimental approaches toward creating a suitable MRI reporter gene, but none so far has proved to provide a robust, widely applicable cell-tracking system. Thus, MRI cell tracking using SPIO nanoparticles is the best available approach we have, which is supported by the three recent clinical studies that have used this approach.

Troubleshooting Table

Problem	Explanation	Potential Solutions
Formation of precipitate when Feridex and PLL are mixed	Aggregation and formation of large complexes of Feridex and PLL	Add Feridex to the medium first and mix well before adding PLL. Adjust ratio of Feridex to PLL. PLL with wrong molecular weight is being used.
Reflux of injection fluid during transplantation into ventricle	Inappropriate injection speed/pressure or using wrong stereotactic coordinates for injection	Check correct coordinates of lateral ventricle, which differs in neonates and adults. After injection, very slowly remove syringe backward for at least 1 minute.
MR images are not covering the entire brain or display (wraparound artifacts)	Incorrect alignment adjustment, centering of animal, or setting of FOV	Check localizer image for properly chosen coordinates from the center field, and check used MRI parameters, or "reshim" and start over.
Blurry MR images	Animal is waking up, moving its head, displacing the MR signal	Check whether fixation of head is still in place and if the animal is no longer being anesthetized (e.g., isoflurane bottle running low or empty).

13.7 Application Notes

Two applications are highlighted here that underline the unique advantage and strength of MRI cell tracking. The first one is MRI cell tracking in an animal model of EAE. Migration of Feridex-labeled neurospheres transplanted intracerebroventricularly was monitored for 30 days after transplantation. The migration distance from the ventricular wall was measured as described in Section 13.4.6. Only MRI has the resolution to measure precisely the actual distance in millimeters of migration per day. A large variability in the speed of migration was observed, which was found to correlate with the clinical disease score. Also, based on histology for inflammatory markers, it was hypothesized that inflammation induces targeted and enhanced migration of cells from the ventricle into the brain parenchyma.

A second application is a clinical one, albeit not with stem cells. ^{111}Indium oxine-and Feridex-labeled dendritic cells, primed with melanoma antigens, were used as cancer vaccines to boost the immune system of stage III melanoma patients. To this end, cells were injected in draining lymph nodes under ultrasound guidance. Although the main aim of the study was to determine cell migration to nearby lymph nodes, a surprising finding was that cell injections to lymph nodes under ultrasound guidance missed the target in half the patients. Only with MRI, and not radionuclide imaging, could it be shown that cells were accidentally injected into either the surrounding muscles or perinodal fat rather than the draining lymph node. These results demonstrate the importance of MR labeling, not only in assessing cell biodistribution and migration after injection, but also the potential to guide targeting of the injections in real time using MR-compatible devices. For applications of hES cells in neurodegenerative diseases such as Parkinson's disease, spinal cord injury, amyotrophic lateral sclerosis, and multiple sclerosis, noninvasive evaluation of the accuracy of targeted intraparenchymal cell injections will be of critical importance and, thus, MRI cell tracking may become an important clinical tool for the future to bring stem cell-based therapy into clinical use.

13.8 Summary Points

1. MRI is a well-established, noninvasive technique to detect transplanted cells in vivo.
2. SPIO is a magnetic nanoparticle contrast agent for MRI, and labeling of cells with this material is required to distinguish labeled cells from the surrounding tissue. Feridex, a dextran-coated SPIO, is commercially available and clinically approved, and several protocols exist to label cells effectively.
3. As long as the transplanted cells proliferate slowly and remain viable, MRI cell tracking enables serial monitoring of the spatial and temporal dynamics of the fate of transplanted cells unmatched by any other noninvasive imaging technique.

Acknowledgments

We gratefully acknowledge the support of the Maryland Stem Cell Research Fund (TEDCO ESC07-06-29-01), the National Multiple Sclerosis Society (RG3630), and the National Institutes of Health (RO1 NS045062).

References

[1] Rice, C. M., C. A. Halfpenny, and N. J. Scolding, "Stem Cells for the Treatment of Neurological Disease," *Transfus. Med.*, Vol. 13, 2003, pp. 351–361.
[2] Carpenter, M. K., et al., "Enrichment of Neurons and Neural Precursors from Human Embryonic Stem Cells," *Exp. Neurol.*, Vol. 172, 2001, pp. 383–397.

[3] Liang, P., et al., "Neuronal and Glial Differentiation following Culture of the Human Embryonic Cortical Stem Cells," *Hum. Cell*, Vol. 16, 2003, pp. 151–156.
[4] Mummery, C., et al., "Cardiomyocyte Differentiation of Mouse and Human Embryonic Stem Cells," *J. Anat.*, Vol. 200, 2002, pp. 233–242.
[5] Baharvand, H., et al., "Differentiation of Human Embryonic Stem Cells into Hepatocytes in 2D and 3D Culture Systems in Vitro," *Int. J. Dev. Biol.*, Vol. 50, 2006, pp. 645–652.
[6] Kaufman, D. S., et al., "Hematopoietic Colony-Forming Cells Derived from Human Embryonic Stem Cells," *Proc. Natl. Acad. Sci. U. S. A.*, Vol. 98, 2001, pp. 10716–10721.
[7] Bielby, R. C., et al., "In Vitro Differentiation and in Vivo Mineralization of Osteogenic Cells Derived from Human Embryonic Stem Cells," *Tissue Eng.*, Vol. 10, 2004, pp. 1518–1525.
[8] Green, H., K. Easley, and S. Iuchi, "Marker Succession during the Development of Keratinocytes from Cultured Human Embryonic Stem Cells," *Proc. Natl. Acad. Sci. U. S. A.*, Vol. 100, 2003, pp. 15625–15630.
[9] Levenberg, S., et al., "Endothelial Cells Derived from Human Embryonic Stem Cells," *Proc. Natl. Acad. Sci. U. S. A.*, Vol. 99, 2002, pp. 4391–4396.
[10] Ben-Hur, T., et al., "Transplantation of Human Embryonic Stem Cell-Derived Neural Progenitors Improves Behavioral Deficit in Parkinsonian Rats," *Stem Cells*, Vol. 22, 2004, pp. 1246–1255.
[11] Keirstead, H. S., et al., "Human Embryonic Stem Cell-Derived Oligodendrocyte Progenitor Cell Transplants Remyelinate and Restore Locomotion after Spinal Cord Injury," *J. Neurosci.*, Vol. 25, 2005, pp. 4694–4705.
[12] Kim, D. Y., et al., "Effect of Human Embryonic Stem Cell-Derived Neuronal Precursor Cell Transplantation into the Cerebral Infarct Model of Rat with Exercise," *Neurosci. Res.*, Vol. 58, 2007, pp. 164–175.
[13] Aharonowiz, M., et al., "Neuroprotective Effect of Transplanted Human Embryonic Stem Cell-Derived Neural Precursors in an Animal Model of Multiple Sclerosis," *PLoS ONE*, Vol. 3, 2008, p. e3145.
[14] Ben-Hur, T., et al., "Serial in Vivo MR Tracking of Magnetically Labeled Neural Spheres Transplanted in Chronic EAE Mice," *Magn. Reson. Med.*, Vol. 57, 2007, pp. 164–171.
[15] Judenhofer, M. S., et al., "Simultaneous PET-MRI: A New Approach for Functional and Morphological Imaging," *Nat. Med.*, Vol. 14, 2008, pp. 459–465.
[16] Burdette, J. E., "In Vivo Imaging of Molecular Targets and Their Function in Endocrinology," *J. Mol. Endocrinol.*, Vol. 40, 2008, pp. 253–261.
[17] Modo, M., M. Hoehn, and J. W. Bulte, "Cellular MR Imaging," *Mol. Imaging*, Vol. 4, 2005, pp. 143–164.
[18] Bulte, J. W., and D. L. Kraitchman, "Monitoring Cell Therapy Using Iron Oxide MR Contrast Agents," *Curr. Pharm. Biotechnol.*, Vol. 5, 2004, pp. 567–584.
[19] Reubinoff, B. E., et al., "Neural Progenitors from Human Embryonic Stem Cells," *Nat. Biotechnol.*, Vol. 19, 2001, pp. 1134–1140.
[20] Reubinoff, B. E., et al., "Embryonic Stem Cell Lines from Human Blastocysts: Somatic Differentiation in Vitro," *Nat. Biotechnol.*, Vol. 18, 2000, pp. 399–404.
[21] Arbab, A. S., et al., "Efficient Magnetic Cell Labeling with Protamine Sulfate Complexed to Ferumoxides for Cellular MRI," *Blood*, Vol. 104, 2004, pp. 1217–1223.
[22] Bulte, J. W., et al., "Preparation of Magnetically Labeled Cells for Cell Tracking by Magnetic Resonance Imaging," *Methods Enzymol.*, Vol. 386, 2004, pp. 275–299.
[23] Walczak, P. et al., "Instant MR Labeling of Stem Cells Using Magnetoelectroporation," *Magn. Reson. Med.*, Vol. 54, 2005, pp. 769–774.
[24] Paxinos, G., and K. B. J. Franklin, *The Mouse Brain: In Stereotactic Coordinates*, San Diego: Academic Press, 2001.
[25] Bulte, J. W., et al., "Neurotransplantation of Magnetically Labeled Oligodendrocyte Progenitors: Magnetic Resonance Tracking of Cell Migration and Myelination," *Proc. Natl. Acad. Sci. U. S. A.*, Vol. 96, 1999, pp. 15256–15261.
[26] Bulte, J. W., et al., "Magnetodendrimers Allow Endosomal Magnetic Labeling and in Vivo Tracking of Stem Cells," *Nat. Biotechnol.*, Vol. 19, 2001, pp. 1141–1147.
[27] Frank, J. A., et al., "Clinically Applicable Labeling of Mammalian and Stem Cells by Combining Superparamagnetic Iron Oxides and Transfection Agents," *Radiology*, Vol. 228, 2003, pp. 480–487.
[28] Walczak, P., et al., "Magnetoelectroporation: Improved Labeling of Neural Stem Cells and Leukocytes for Cellular Magnetic Resonance Imaging Using a Single FDA-Approved Agent," *Nanomedicine*, Vol. 2, 2006, pp. 89–94.
[29] Gilad, A. A., et al., "MR Tracking of Transplanted Cells with 'Positive Contrast' Using Manganese Oxide Nanoparticles," *Magn. Reson. Med.*, Vol. 60, 2008, pp. 1–7.
[30] Ruiz-Cabello, J., et al., " In Vivo 'Hot Spot' MR Imaging of Neural Stem Cells Using Fluorinated Nanoparticles," *Magn. Reson. Med.*, Vol. 60, 2008, pp. 1506–1511.
[31] Walczak, P., et al., "Applicability and Limitations of MR Tracking of Neural Stem Cells with Asymmetric Cell Division and Rapid Turnover: The Case of the Shiverer Dysmyelinated Mouse Brain," *Magn. Reson. Med.*, Vol. 58, 2007, pp. 261–269.

[32] Pawelczyk, E., et al., "In Vitro Model of Bromodeoxyuridine or Iron Oxide Nanoparticle Uptake by Activated Macrophages from Labeled Stem Cells: Implications for Cellular Therapy," *Stem Cells*, Vol. 26, 2008, pp. 1366–1375.

[33] Genove, G., et al., "A New Transgene Reporter for in Vivo Magnetic Resonance Imaging," *Nat. Med.*, Vol. 11, 2005, pp. 450–454.

[34] Cohen, B., et al., "Ferritin as an Endogenous MRI Reporter for Noninvasive Imaging of Gene Expression in C6 Glioma Tumors," *Neoplasia*, Vol. 7, 2005, pp. 109–117.

[35] Gilad, A. A., et al., "Artificial Reporter Gene Providing MRI Contrast Based on Proton Exchange," *Nat. Biotechnol.*, Vol. 25, 2007, pp. 217–219.

[36] Gilad, A. A., et al., "Developing MR Reporter Genes: Promises and Pitfalls," *NMR Biomed.*, Vol. 20, 2007, pp. 275–290.

[37] de Vries, I. J., et al., "Magnetic Resonance Tracking of Dendritic Cells in Melanoma Patients for Monitoring of Cellular Therapy," *Nat. Biotechnol.*, Vol. 23, 2005, pp. 1407–1413.

[38] Toso, C., et al., "Clinical Magnetic Resonance Imaging of Pancreatic Islet Grafts after Iron Nanoparticle Labeling," *Am. J. Transplant.*, Vol. 8, 2008, pp. 701–706.

[39] Zhu, J., L. Zhou, and F. Xing Wu, "Tracking Neural Stem Cells in Patients with Brain Trauma," *N. Engl. J. Med.*, Vol. 355, 2006, pp. 2376–2378.

About the Editors

Biju Parekkadan, Ph.D. is an instructor in surgery and bioengineering in the Department of Surgery at Massachusetts General Hospital and Harvard Medical School in Boston, MA. He received his Ph.D. in chemical and medical engineering from the Harvard-MIT Division of Health Sciences and Technology in 2008. Dr. Parekkadan research interests lie in the development of mesenchymal stem cell immunotherapy for clinical use.

Martin L. Yarmush, M.D., Ph.D. is the Helen Andrus Benedict professor of surgery and bioengineering in the Harvard-MIT Division of Health Science and Technology and the director of the Center for Engineering in Medicine at Massachusetts General Hospital in Boston, MA. He received in Ph.D. in biophysical chemistry at The Rockefeller University and his M.D. from Yale University School of Medicine. Dr. Yarmush is internationally renowned for his work in tissue engineering and regenerative medicine.

List of Contributors

Gregor B. Adams
Eli and Edythe Broad Center for Regenerative Medicine and Stem Cell Research
Keck School of Medicine
University of Southern California
1450 Biggy Street (NRT 4507)
Los Angeles, CA 90033

Tomokazo Amano
Center for Regenerative Biology and Department of Animal Science
University of Connecticut
Storrs, CT 06269

G. Delbert Antwiler
CaridianBCT
Lakewood, CO 80215

Sangeeta N. Bhatia
Laboratory for Multiscale Regenerative Technologies
Division of Health Sciences and Technology/Electrical Engineering and Computer Science
Massachusetts Institute of Technology
77 Massachusetts Avenue, E19–502D
Cambridge, MA 02139
Division of Medicine, Brigham & Women's Hospital
Boston, MA 02115

Paolo Bianco
Stem Cell Laboratory
Biomedical Science Park San Raffaele
Dipartimento di Medicina Sperimentale
Sapienza University of Rome
Viale regina Elena 324
00161 Rome, Italy

Jeff W. M. Bulte
Russell H. Morgan Department of Radiology and Radiological Science, Division of MR Research
Cellular Imaging Section, Vascular Biology Program, Institute for Cell Engineering
Department of Gynecology and Obstetrics
Department of Chemical and Biomolecular Engineering
Department of Biomedical Engineering
Johns Hopkins University School of Medicine
217 Traylor Building
720 Rutland Avenue
Baltimore, MD 21205-2195

Ken W. Y Cho
Department of Developmental and Cell Biology
University of California Irvine
Irvine, CA, 92697

Bong Geun Chung
Department of Biomedical Engineering
University of California Irvine
Irvine, CA, 92697

Irina M. Conboy
Department of Bioengineering
University of California, Berkeley
174 Stanley Hall
Berkeley, CA 94720-1762

Michael J. Conboy
Department of Bioengineering
University of California, Berkeley
Berkeley, CA 94720

George Q. Daley
Division of Pediatric Hematology/Oncology, Children's Hospital Boston
Department of Biological Chemistry and Molecular Pharmacology, Harvard Medical School
Harvard Stem Cell Institute
Howard Hughes Medical Institute
One Blackfan Circle, Karp 7215
Boston, MA 02115

Heidi Y. Elmoazzen
Center for Engineering in Medicine
Department of Surgery, Massachusetts General Hospital
Harvard Medical School, Shiners Hospital for Children
51 Blossom Street
Boston, MA 02114

Christopher J. Flaim
Departments of Bioengineering and Medicine
University of California–San Diego
La Jolla, CA 92093

Noo Li Jeon
Department of Biomedical Engineering
University of California Irvine
3120 Natural Science II
Irvine, CA, 92697

Candace Kerr
Stem Cell Biology Program
Department of Gynecology and Obstetrics
The Johns Hopkins University School of Medicine
Baltimore, MD 21205

Heechul Kim
Russell H. Morgan Department of Radiology and Radiological Science, Division of MR Research
Cellular Imaging Section, Vascular Biology Program, Institute for Cell Engineering
The Johns Hopkins University School of Medicine
Baltimore, MD 21205

Hyung Joon Kim
Department of Biomedical Engineering
University of California Irvine
Irvine, CA, 92697

Paul H. Lerou
Division of Newborn Medicine
Brigham & Women's Hospital and Children's Hospital Boston
Harvard Medical School
Boston, MA 02115

Kevin R. McIntosh
Cognate BioServices, Inc.
1448 S. Rolling Road
Baltimore, MD 21227

Ian K. McNiece
Interdisciplinary Stem Cell Institute
University of Miami
Miami, FL 33136

Kim T. Nguyen
Interdisciplinary Stem Cell Institute
University of Miami
Miami, FL 33136

Hiroshi Ohta
Laboratory for Genomic Reprogramming, Center for Developmental Biology
RIKEN
2-2-3 Minatojima-minamimachi, Chuo-ku Kobe 650-0047, Japan

Louise E. Purton
Department of Medicine at St. Vincent's Hospital
St. Vincent's Institute, The University of Melbourne,
9 Princes Street, Fitzroy, Victoria, 3065, Australia

Benedetto Sacchetti
Stem Cell Laboratory
Biomedical Science Park San Raffaele
Dipartimento di Medicina Sperimentale
Sapienza University of Rome
Rome, Italy

David T Scadden
Center for Regenerative Medicine, Massachusetts General Hospital
Boston, MA 02114
Harvard Stem Cell Institute
Cambridge, MA 02138

Hwa-Sung Shin
Department of Biomedical Engineering
University of California Irvine
Irvine, CA, 92697

Sadie L. Smith
Department of Molecular, Cellular and Developmental Biology
Yale University
New Haven, CT 06520

Aixu Sun
Department of Developmental and Cell Biology
University of California Irvine
Irvine, CA, 92697

Li-Ying Sung
Institute of Biotechnology
National Taiwan University
Taipei 106, Taiwan ROC

Mehmet Toner
Center for Engineering in Medicine
Department of Surgery, Massachusetts General Hospital
Harvard Medical School, Shiners Hospital for Children
Boston, MA 02114

Gregory H. Underhill
Laboratory for Multiscale Regenerative Technologies
Division of Health Sciences and Technology/Electrical Engineering and Computer Science
Massachusetts Institute of Technology
Cambridge, MA 02139

Teruhiko Wakayama
Laboratory for Genomic Reprogramming, Center for Developmental Biology
RIKEN
2-2-3 Minatojima-minamimachi, Chuo-ku, Kobe 650-0047, Japan

Akiko Yabuuchi
Division of Pediatric Hematology/Oncology
Children's Hospital Boston
Harvard Medical School
Boston, MA 02115

Xiangzhong Yang
Center for Regenerative Biology and Department of Animal Science
University of Connecticut
1392 Storrs Road, Unit 4243
Storrs, CT 06269

Index

A

Acrylamide gel substrate fabrication, 66–67
Activation, in nuclear transfer, 11–12
Adipose-derived stem cells (ASC), 163
Aging studies
 experimental design for, 130
 materials, 131
 methods, 131–36
 parabiosis in, 125–39
Aliquot, 92
Allogeneic stem cells, 144
Allogeneic transplantation, 143
American Type Culture Collection (ATCC), 61, 162
Analysis of variance (ANOVA), 96, 99
Anastomosis, 126
Animal species, parabiosis and, 126
Apoptosis, 76
Artificial organ design, 138
Astrocytes, 84–85
Autologous cells, 147

B

Bert, Paul, 127
Biocompatibility, of hollow-fiber bioreactor, 53
Biohazardous waste, 153
Biomarkers, for identification of MSC, 58
Biomedical applications, of parabiosis, 127–28
Bioreactor
 defined, 50
 gas transfer mechanism for, 55
 hollow-fiber, 53–54
Bioreactor design and implementation, 49–62
 application notes, 61–62
 closed system, 52
 discussion and commentary, 60
 experimental methods, 51–56
 general system description, 51
 hollow-fiber bioreactor, 53–54
 materials, 51–56
 monitoring, 56
 oxygenator design, 55–56
 results for, 56–59
 troubleshooting table for, 61
 user interface, 56
Blastocyst injection, generation of embryonic stem cells by, 42
Blastocyte stage, 32
BMP-responsive element (BRE), 85
BMP signaling, ESC response to, 85–86
Bone formation, 118
Bone marrow (BM)
 cogenic, 101
 HSC and progenitor cells in, 90–91
 loading whole into CES, 58–59
 obtaining, 120
 osteoprogenitors, 110–11
 single-cell suspensions, 109–10
 therapeutic dose of MSC grown from, 61
 transplant, 49
 whole cells, 91–94
Bone marrow transplantation
 process for, 97
 troubleshooting table for, 97
Bone morphogenic protein 4 (BMP-4), 79, 85–86
Bouin's fixative, 99, 100
Bradley, Ray, 95

Index

C

Carrel, Alexis, 137
Cell doubling time, 59
Cell expansion system (CES), 50
   automated, 60
   cell load, 56
   defined, 51
   fluid circuit, 54–55
   growing, 56
   harvesting, 56
   IC/EC media exchange, 56
   loading whole bone marrow into, 58–59
   manual function, 56
   monitoring, 56
   prime, 56
   prototype, 51
   user interface, 56
Cell surface adhesion, 53
Cesarean section, 45
Chemotaxis, 76
Chimeras, 126
   generation, 16
   mouse, 40
Cloning, 1
Closed system, 52
   gas control in, 52
Clostridium histolyticum, 112
Cogenic bone marrow cells, 101
Colony-forming cell (CFC) assays, 90, 95
   troubleshooting table, 97
Colony-forming unit-fibroblast (CFU-F), 108
Colony-forming unit-spleen (CFU-S) assay, 90, 98–100
   data acquisition, 99–100
   discussion and commentary, 100
   equipment, 99
   interpretation, 99–100
   materials for, 98
   methods, 99
   reagents, 98
   results, 99–100
   troubleshooting table for, 100
Competitive repopulating units (CRU) assay, 90
   calculation of frequency, 102
Concanavalin A (Con A), 147, 151
Conjoined identical twins, 126
Culture drops, diagram of, 29
Cumulus cells, preparation of, 6
Current Protocols in Immunology, 152
Cytokines, 96
Cytometry, 145
Cytospins, 96

D

Differentiation
   hematopoietic markers, 90
   of hNSC into astrocytes, 84–85
   of stem cells, microfluidic culture platforms for, 75–87
   test for harvested cells, 58
Direct injection, in nuclear transfer, 7–10
Donor cells
   fibroblast cells, 7
   fresh cumulus cells, 6
   frozen hematopoietic cells, 7
   injection of, 8
   preparation of, 6–7
Dynabeads magnet, 91
   depletion using, 93

E

EC loop, 54
Embryo culture, 12–13
Embryonic stem cell derivation
   materials for, 13
   methods for, 14–19
   of ntES cells, 14–15
Embryonic stem cells (ESC), 40, 64, 76
   culture conditions and, 41–42
   derivation of, 1–21
   generation of mice from, 39–48
   mouse, 79
   response to BMP signaling, 85–86
   response under controlled gradient condition, 79–80
Embryo transfer, 12–13, 17
Engineering, parabiotic, 139
Enucleation
   methods for, 5–6
   pipettes, 4
   preparation of, 4
Eppendorf tube, 153
Equipment
   for colony-forming unit-spleen (CFU-S) assay, 99
   for limiting dilution assay, 101
   for lineage depletion, 91
   for methylcellulose-based in vitro colony-forming assay, 95
   for mouse nuclear transfer, 2

Erythroid colonies (BFU-E & CFU-E), 95, 96
ES cell characterization, 34
    alkaline phosphatase staining, 34
    immunohistochemistry, 34
    karotyping and fluorescence in situ hybridization, 34
Ethylenediaminetetraacetic acid (EDTA), 66
Experimental design
    for aging studies, 130
    for extracellular matrix microarrays, 65
    for generation of mice from embryonic stem cells, 42–45
    for microfluidic culture platforms, 76–80
    for mixed lymphocyte reaction assay, 146–51
    skeletal stem cells, 108–9
    stem cell niche in vivo, 119
Extracellular matrix (ECM), 64
    protein mixtures, 67
    proteins, 65, 67–68
Extracellular matrix microarrays, 63–73
    acrylamide gel substrate fabrication, 66–67
    application notes, 72
    cell culture on, 68
    data analysis, 69
    discussion and commentary, 70
    ES cell differentiation and, 71
    experimental design, 65
    fabrication of, 65, 67
    implementation, 65
    materials for, 65–66
    methods, 66–69
    preparation of substrates for, 66
    results, 69–70
    silanization treatment, 66
    staining, imaging, and data acquisition, 68–69
    troubleshooting table, 71–72

F

Fetal bovine serum (FBS), 145, 160
Fiber bundle packing density, 53
Fibroblast cells
    embryonic, 79
    preparation of, 7
    transfer of, example, 10
Ficoll-Hypaque cells, 93, 94
Ficoll-Hypaque column, loading, 92
Ficoll-Hypaque density gradient, 153, 154
Fischer strain rats, 163

Flow cytometry, test for harvested cells, 58
Fluorescein isothiocyanate (FITC), 77, 79
Fluorescent-assisted cell sorting (FACS), 90
Fluoromount-G, 68
Foster mothers, in animal preparation, 5
4n embryos
    generation by aggregation, 43
    generation by blastocyst injection, 42
    preparation of, 41
Fusion method, for nuclear transfer, 10–11

G

Gas permeability, 53
Generalized Linear Model, 18
Genetic defects, 144
Germline transmission test, 17
Good manufacturing practice (GMP), 50, 51
Granulocyte (CFU-G), 95
Granulocyte/erythroid/macrophage/megakaryocyte (CFU-GEMM), 95
Granulocyte/macrophage (CFU-GM), 95

H

Haploid oocyte, 24
Harvesting function, in CES, 56
Hematopoiesis, 89
Hematopoietic cells
    preparation of, 7
    viability of, 10
Hematopoietic microenvironment, 107–16
Hematopoietic stem cells (HSC), 108
    defined, 90
    niche, 117, 119
    targeting niche, 123
Heterochronic transplant studies, 128–29
Heterotopic ossicles, analysis of, 112
Heterozygosity, diagram of, 25
Holding pipettes, 4
Hollow-fiber bioreactor
    biocompatibility and stability, 53
    cell surface adhesion, 53
    fiber bundle packing density, 53
    gas permeability, 53
    hydraulic permeability, 53
    membrane sieving coefficient, 53
    parameters of fibers, 53
Hollow-fiber oxygenator, 52
    design of, 55
Host embryos, preparation of, 42–43
H-thymidine, 146, 152, 155

Index

Human leukocyte antigen (HLA), 144
Human neural stem cells (hNSC), 76, 81–82
   differentiation of into astrocytes, 84–85
   proliferation in gradient chamber, 83–84
   quantitative analysis of proliferation, 84
Human stem cells (HSC)
   colony-forming cells *versus*, 98
   quantification of, using limiting dilution assay, 100–104
Hybrid microfluidic platform, 77–79, 80
   fabrication of, 81
Hydraulic permeability, 53

I

Immunocytochemistry, 78, 83
Immunogenicity assay, 146–48
   basic features, 146
   data acquisition, 155–57
   discussion and commentary, 161
   graphic representation, 156
   interpretation, 155–57
   performance of, 154
   plate setup, 147, 148
   responder cells, 146
   results, 155–57
   simulator cells, 147
   small animals, 147–48
   statistical guidelines for, 155–57
Immunophenotypic enumeration, 120, 121
Immunostaining, 15, 68
Immunosuppression therapy, 136, 138
Induced pluripotent stem (iPS) cells, 47
Injection
   direct, 7–10
   of donor cells, 8
   failed, example of, 9
   important points about, 9–10
   of ntES cells, 16
   pipettes, 4
Inner cell mass (ICM), 24
Institutional Animal Care and Use Committee guidelines, 82
Intracytoplasmic sperm injection, 46
In vitro characterization, of ntES cells, 15–16
In vivo assays, radiation of mice for, 97
In vivo characterization, of ntES cells, 16–18
In vivo transplantation, of skeletal stem cells, 109, 111
Iscove's Modified Dulbecco's Medium, 153

J

Jagged-1, 70
Joining, physiology of, 126–27

K

Karotyping, 15, 34
Kg1a cells, 61
   growth of, 62

L

Leukemia inhibitory factor (LIF), 79, 86
Limiting dilution assay
   buffers and materials, 101
   data acquisition, 102–3
   discussion and commentary, 103–4
   equipment, 101
   interpretation, 102–3
   methods, 101–2
   quantification of HSC using, 100–104
   reagents, 101
   results, 102–3
   troubleshooting table for, 104
Lineage depletion
   experimental design of whole bone marrow cells, 90–91
   materials for, 91–94
   troubleshooting table for, 94

M

Major histocompatability (MHC), 144
Materials
   for aging studies, 131
   for bioreactor design and implementation, 51–56
   for colony-forming unit-spleen (CFU-S) assay, 98
   for extracellular matrix microarrays, 65–66
   for generation of mice from embryonic stem cells, 41–42
   for limiting dilution assay, 101
   for lineage depletion of whole bone marrow cells, 91–94
   for methylcellulose-based in vitro colony-forming assay, 95
   for microfluidic culture platforms, 80–83
   for nuclear transfer, 2–4
   for skeletal stem cell transplantation, 109
   for stem cell niche in vivo, 120
   for T-cell priming assay, 152

Media recipe, for mouse parthenogenetic embryonic stem cells, 27–28
Membrane sieving coefficient, 53
Mesenchymal stem cells (MSC), 49, 50, 56, 107, 158
  biomarkers for identification of, 58
  columns, 94
  defined, 108
  depletion using beads, 93
  harvested cells as, 57
  loading bone marrow into CES, 58–59
  loading preselected, 59
  sources, 57
  therapeutic dose of, 61
Metcalf, Don, 95
Methylcellulose-based in vitro colony-forming assay, 95–96
  data acquisition, 96
  discussion and commentary, 96
  equipment, 95
  interpretation, 96
  materials, 95
  methods, 95–96
  reagents, 95
  results, 96
Mice
  aging studies and, 132, 134
  euthanization of, 99
  neural stem cells, 82–83
  radiation of for in vivo assays, 97
  treatment with PTH, 120–21
Mice, generation from embryonic stem cells, 39–48
  application notes, 47
  comparison of birthrates from different methods, 46
  discussion and commentary, 45–46
  electrofusion of two-cell stage embryos, 43
  experimental design, 41
  4n embryos by aggregation, 43
  4n embryos by blastocyst injection, 44
  host embryo preparation, 42–43
  materials, 41–42
  methods, 42–45
  removal of zona pellucida, 43
  results, 45
  troubleshooting table, 46
Microfluidic culture platforms, 75–87
  application notes, 87

data acquisition, 83–86
differentiation of neural progenitor cells, 76–77
discussion and commentary, 86
experimental design, 76–80
gradient-generating devices, 77
hybrid, 77–79
immunocytochemistry, 83
interpretation, 83–86
results, 83–86
troubleshooting table for, 86
vacuum platform, 78
Microfluidic device, fabrication of, 80–81
Microfluidic vacuum platform, 78
Millipore water, 66
MiniMACS magnetic column, 110
Mitogenic controls, for T-cell priming assay, 151
Mixed lymphocyte reaction (MLR) assay, 143–64
  application notes, 163–64
  data acquisition, 155–60
  discussion and commentary, 160–63
  experimental design, 146–51
  as immunological tool, 145
  interpretation, 155–60
  materials, 152
  methods, 152–55
  plate culture, 155
  results, 155–60
  statistical guidelines for, 155–60
  troubleshooting table, 163
Morphology, test for harvested cells, 57
Mouse ESC (mESC), 79
Mouse hematopoietic stem cells, analysis of, 89–105
  experimental design of lineage depletion of whole bone marrow cells, 90–91
  limiting dilution assay and, 100–104
  materials for lineage depletion of whole bone marrow cells, 91–94
  methylcellulose-based in vitro colony-forming assay, 95–96
Mouse ntES cells, derivation of, 13
Mouse nuclear transfer
  discussion and commentary, 19
  equipment for, 2
  reagents for, 2–3
  time schedule for, 17–18

Mouse parthenogenetic embryonic stem cells, derivation of, 23–37
  chromosome dynamics in, 25
  data acquisition, 35
  discussion and commentary, 35–36
  equipment, 26–27
  interpretation, 35
  materials, 24–29
  media recipe for, 27–28
  methods for, 28–35
  reagents, 24–26
  results for, 35
  troubleshooting table for, 36
Mouse progenitor cells, analysis of, 89–105
  experimental design of lineage depletion of whole bone marrow cells, 90–91
  limiting dilution assay and, 100–104
  materials for lineage depletion of whole bone marrow cells, 91–94
  methylcellulose-based in vitro colony-forming assay, 95–96
Mouse strain, 26
Murine cells, 115
Murine fertilization, 25
Myelotoxic injury, 119

N

National Human Neural Stem Cell Resource, 81
Navier-Stokes convection and diffusion model, 79
Neural progenitor cells, differentiation of, 76–77
Neural stem cells (NSC), 76
  culture, 82
  culturing cells inside microfluidic chamber, 82–83
  human, 76, 81–82
  mouse, 82–83
Nonosteoconductive carriers, 115
Notch ligand, 70
ntES cells
  derivation of, 14–15, 17–18, 19
  ES mice derivation from, 47
  establishment of cell line, 14
  injection of, 16
  in vitro characterization of, 15–16
  in vivo characterization of, 16–18
Nuclear transfer, 1–21. *See also* Cloning
  activation, 11–12
  animal preparation, 5
  direct injection, 7–10
  discussion and commentary, 19
  embryo culture and transfer, 12–13
  of embryos from different donor cell types, 18
  equipment for mouse, 2
  fusion method, 10–11
  materials for, 2–4
  medium preparation, 4
  methods for, 4–13
  oocyte collection, 5
  preparation of pipettes, 4
  reagents for mouse, 2–3
  troubleshooting table, 19–21
  in vitro development of, 18

O

Occupational Safety and Health Administration (OSHA), 153
Oocyte donors, in animal preparation, 5
Oocyte enucleation, layout for droplets of, 5
Organ transplantation, 137
Oxygenator design, 55–56

P

Parabiosis
  in aging research, 125–39
  animal species and, 126
  biomedical applications of, 127–28
  defined, 125, 126
  discussion and commentary, 137–39
  heterochronic, 129
  history of, 127–28
  physiology of joining, 126–27
  postoperative care, 135
  protocol, 131–32
  separation and, 135–36
  steps in, 132
  troubleshooting diseases, 136–37
  in utero, 126
Parabiotic disease
  side effects associated with, 137
  troubleshooting, 136–37
Parabiotic engineering, 139
Parabiotic intoxication, 136–37
Parathyroid hormone (PTH), 118
  diagrammatic representation of, 119
  treatment, 120

treatment, for mice, 120–21
treatment after transplant, 121
Parthenogenesis, 23
defined, 24
Pellet cells, 153
Peripheral blood mononuclear cell (PBMC), 146, 150, 153
p(hap) embryos
derivation of, 32–34
generation of, 31–32
p(hap) ES cells. See Haploid oocyte
Phytohemagglutinin, 147
Pipettes
enucleation, 4
holding, 4
injection, 4
for nuclear transfer, 4
Plasma treatment, 81
Plate setup
for immunogenicity assay, 147, 148
for suppression assay, 149, 151
p(MI) embryos
derivation of, 32–34
generation of, 30
p(MII) embryos
derivation of, 32–34
generation of, 30–31
Poisson statistics, 101, 102
Primary mouse embryonic fibroblast (PMEF), 14
Printing buffer, preparation of, 67
Progeny, production of, 45
Proliferation
of hNSC, 84
of stem cells, microfluidic culture platforms for, 75–87
T-cell, 148

R

Radiation, of mice for in vivo assays, 97
Reagents
in CES fluid circuit, 54
for colony-forming unit-spleen (CFU-S) assay, 98
for limiting dilution assay, 101
for lineage depletion, 91
for methylcellulose-based in vitro colony-forming assay, 95
mice and, 42
for mouse nuclear transfer, 2–3
for mouse parthenogenetic embryonic stems cells, 24–26
Recipient mothers, in animal preparation, 5
Reconstructed oocytes
activation of, 11–12
chromatin remodeling dynamics in, 12
droplet layout for washing, 11
hand alignment of, 11
Regenerative medicine, 125–39
Responder cells
immunogenicity assay, 146
preparation of populations, 153–54
for T-cell priming assay, 150
RT-PCR
for ntES cells, 16
primers for, 16

S

Safety, in T-cell priming assay, 153
Sensitization, studies of, 162
Siamese twins. See Conjoined identical twins
Silanization treatment, 66
Skeletal stem cells, 107–16
application notes, 114–15
discussion and commentary, 113–14
experimental design, 108–9
heterotopic ossicles, analysis of, 112
materials for, 109
methods, 109–12
results, 112–13
troubleshooting table for, 114
in vivo transplantation of, 109, 111
Specificity controls, for T-cell priming assay, 150
SpotArray 24 (Perkin Elmer) system, 67
SpotBot 2 (Telechem) system, 67
Standard deviation, 158
Stem cell biology, hybrid microfluidic platform for, 77–79
Stem cell immunogenicity, 143–64
Stem cell niche, defined, 118
Stem cell niche in vivo, 117–23
application notes, 123
discussion and commentary, 122
experimental design, 119
materials, 120
methods, 120–21
results, 121–22
troubleshooting table, 122

Stem cells
  allogeneic, 144
  neural, 76
  skeletal, 107–16
  suppression, 143–64
  therapeutic potential of, 75
StemCell Technologies, 96, 103
Stem cell therapies, 50
Stimulator cells
  immunogenicity assay, 147
  irradiated, 156
  preparation of populations, 154
  radiated, 154
  for T-cell priming assay, 150
Streptavidin Dynabeads, 91
Stromal cell isolation, 109
Substrates, preparation of, 66–67
Supernatants, 94
Suppression, stem cells, 143–64
Suppression assay, 148–49
  basic features, 148
  data acquisition, 157–58
  data summary, 157
  discussion and commentary, 162
  graphic representation, 157
  interpretation, 157–58
  plate setup, 149
  results, 157–58
  statistical guidelines for, 157–58
Suppression titer, 162

T

T-cell hyporesponsiveness, 162
T-cell priming assay, 145, 149–51, 162
  basic features, 149–50
  data acquisition, 158–60
  data summary, 159
  discussion and commentary, 162–63
  graphic representation, 159
  human and large-animal studies, 153–54
  interpretation, 158–60
  materials, 152
  media preparation, 153
  methods, 152–55
  mitogenic controls, 151
  performance of, 155
  plate setup, 151
  preparation of responder cell populations, 153
  responder cells, 150
  results, 158–60
  safety and, 153
  small-animal studies, 153–54
  specificity controls, 150
  statistical guidelines for, 158–60
  stimulator cells, 150
T-cell proliferation, 148, 160, 162, 163
T-cell response, 144
T cells, 143, 149
  activation markers on, 145
Teratoma induction, 34–35
Tetraploid embryos, as hosts, 39–48
Tissue regeneration, 144
T lymphocytes, 143, 149
Transplantation, 108
  allogeneic, 143
  histology of, 113
  organ, 137
Trichostatin A (TSA) treatment, 12
Troubleshooting table
  for bioreactor design and implementation, 61
  for CFU assay, 97
  for CFU-S assay, 100
  for extracellular matrix microarrays, 71–72
  for generation of mice from embryonic stem cells, 46
  for limiting dilution assay, 104
  for lineage depletion, 94
  for microfluidic culture platforms, 86
  for mixed lymphocyte reaction assay, 163
  for mouse parthenogenetic embryonic stem cells, 36
  for nuclear transfer, 19–21
  for skeletal stem cells, 114
  for stem cell niche in vivo, 122
Trypsinization, 82
Two-tailed *t*-test, 155
Tyrode's solution, 43

U

Universal donor, 144

Z

Zona pellucida, 43

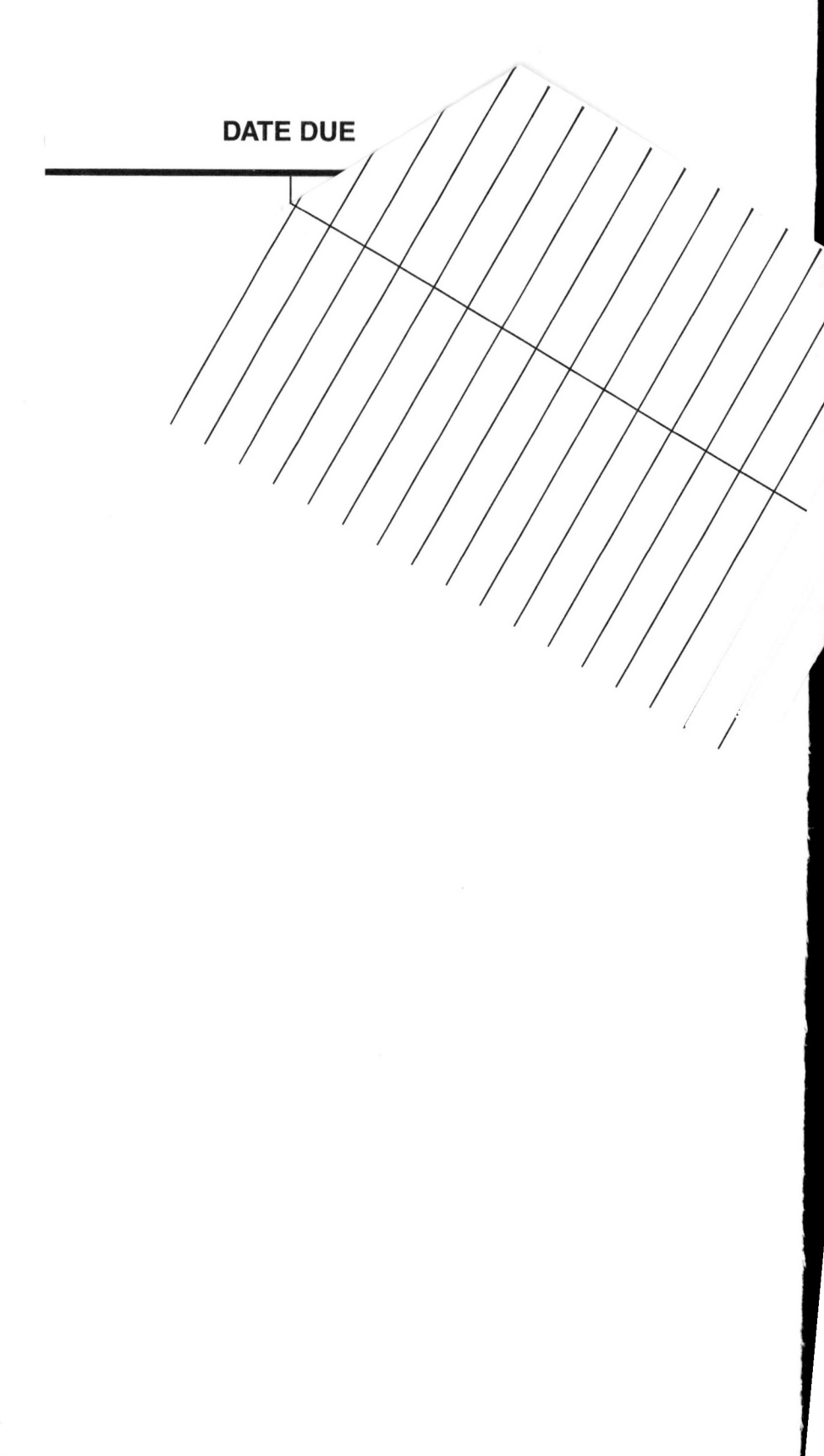